APPLIED CLINICAL INFORMATICS

FOR NURSES

Edited by

Susan Alexander, DNP, RN, ANP-BC, ADM-BC
Clinical Associate Professor
University of Alabama, Huntsville
Huntsville, Alabama

Karen H. Frith, PhD, RN, NEA-BC
Professor
University of Alabama, Huntsville
Huntsville, Alabama

Haley Hoy, PhD, ACNP
Assistant Professor
University of Alabama, Huntsville
Nurse Practitioner
Vanderbilt Medical Center
Nashville, Tennessee

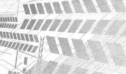

JONES & BARTLETT
LEARNING

World Headquarters
Jones & Bartlett Learning
5 Wall Street
Burlington, MA 01803
978-443-5000
info@jblearning.com
www.jblearning.com

Jones & Bartlett Learning books and products are available through most bookstores and online booksellers. To contact Jones & Bartlett Learning directly, call 800-832-0034, fax 978-443-8000, or visit our website, www.jblearning.com.

Production Credits

Executive Publisher: William Brottmiller
Senior Editor: Amanda Martin
Associate Managing Editor: Sara Bempkins
Production Editor: Amanda Clerkin
Senior Marketing Manager: Jennifer Stiles
Art Development Editor: Joanna Lundeen
VP, Manufacturing and Inventory Control: Therese Connell

Composition: Aptara®, Inc.
Cover Design: Kristin E. Parker
Director of Photo Research and Permissions: Amy Wrynn
Cover Image: © vs148/ShutterStock, Inc. (abstract geometric design); © wongwean/ShutterStock, Inc. (binary code)
Printing and Binding: Edwards Brothers Malloy
Cover Printing: Edwards Brothers Malloy

To order this product, use ISBN: 978-1-284-04996-1

Library of Congress Cataloging-in-Publication Data
Applied clinical informatics for nurses/[edited by] Susan Alexander, Karen H. Frith, Haley Hoy.
  p. ; cm.
  Includes bibliographical references and index.
  ISBN 978-1-284-02700-6
  I. Alexander, Susan, 1969- editor of compilation.   II. Frith, Karen H., editor of compilation.   III. Hoy, Haley M., editor of compilation.
  [DNLM: 1. Nursing Informatics. WY 26.5]
  RT50.5
  610.730285—dc23
                                                                          2014001383
6048
Printed in the United States of America
18 17 16   10 9 8 7 6 5 4 3

Contents

Preface

FOR WHOM IS THIS TEXT WRITTEN?

This is a contributed text designed for nurses who are interested in expanding their knowledge about technology and informatics as applied in the setting of health care. The chapters are written by a diverse group of contributors who have experience in both designing and using health informatics applications. The content is broad in scope, covering topics beginning with an overview of basic concepts in informatics and proceeding to a discussion of application of the concepts in selected healthcare delivery settings. Though advanced concepts are included in the text, they are discussed in a manner that is highly readable for nursing students. The text includes multiple examples and case studies that will aid students in immediately linking the content to the clinical environment.

WHY IS THIS TEXT IMPORTANT FOR THE STUDENT NURSE?

This text stems from the recognition of the need for improvements in nurses' skill sets in the use of health information technology. Nursing is a high-tech field, requiring a wide variety of competencies ranging from basic computer abilities to advanced skills with medical devices and lifesaving equipment. Nurses are the largest group of healthcare providers in the United States, with statistics from the U.S. Department of Labor, Bureau of Labor Statistics, indicating that there are more than 2.6 million nurses employed in the United States (in 2012). The ability of nurses to use health information technologies safely and efficiently to improve patient care cannot be ignored. It is essential that all nurses have minimum levels of competency to use health information technology in all aspects of patient care in both outpatient and inpatient settings.

Perhaps the most appropriate place to begin the integration of technology and informatics in patient care is for the pre-licensure nurse. If this group of nurses enters the workforce with the skill sets, clinical experience, and the expectation to integrate health information technologies into practice, many of the issues that confound healthcare organizations now may cease to exist. This is not an unusual phenomenon. Consider the example of universal precautions for blood and body fluids. The use of universal precautions began in response to the HIV and hepatitis B outbreaks in the 1980s. The integration of universal precautions in patient care caused great upheaval. Millions of dollars were spent in reeducating healthcare providers, redesigning hospital rooms and units, and in revising nursing curricula to teach the foundational practice of universal precautions. The nursing graduates of today have been taught the need for handwashing from the first day of class, and it is simply no longer an issue. Likewise, as informatics knowledge and skills become more embedded in nursing education and in practice settings, the more informatics will be accepted as an indispensable component of nursing practice and patient care.

WHAT MAKES THIS TEXT UNIQUE?

This text is written primarily for the pre-licensure nurse who has experience in the use of diverse hardware and software applications and who is now ready to apply those skills in the healthcare setting. A distinctive feature of this text is its flexibility. While it could be used in a focused informatics course, it could also be integrated into a nursing program that elects to teach designated informatics concepts at different points throughout the program. In addition, this text is distinctive because its content largely adheres to the competencies described in the American Association of Colleges of Nursing's *Essentials of Baccalaureate Education for Professional Nursing Practice* (2008).

The text is divided into three sections. Section I introduces concepts and issues relevant to the field of clinical informatics. A review of the culture of health care and the use of health information technology in the United States, with a summary of information science principles, sets the stage for a discussion of the nurse's role in healthcare informatics in the 21st century. In Chapter 3, Section I, the reader is presented with strategies to obtain, evaluate, and apply evidence for nursing practice with the use of informatics tools.

Sections II and III contain chapters with more isolated content, not necessarily building on one another. The content and resources in the chapters of Sections II and III could be used in multiple areas of the nursing curricula. The material contained in Sections II and III is a rather basic discussion of advanced concepts. It is purposely designed to stimulate the interest of the reader and to initiate discussion and interaction between students and teachers on the enormous possibilities for use of healthcare technologies, now and in the future.

Acknowledgments

There are many to whom we are grateful for their assistance in making the idea for this text become a reality. Our students, whose rich blend of backgrounds and talents make life endlessly interesting, helped us to understand the need for creating a textbook that could build on existing computer skills and enhance informatics competencies to improve patient care. Studying to become a nurse in the 21st century involves more than learning the basic skills of caring for patients at the bedside. Technology is interwoven into many of the nurses' tasks, and we applaud those nurses who realize the importance of competence with technology and informatics early in their careers. This is not an easy task, but effective use of health information technologies will lead to important advancements in patient care.

We would like to thank the staff at Jones & Bartlett Learning for their encouragement and guidance. The JBL production team is a pleasant and talented group. Special thanks also go to Amanda Martin, our optimistic and supportive Senior Editor, who shared our vision of crafting a book that would integrate informatics content into nursing curricula in a manner both clinically relevant and exciting for nursing students. Amanda has been unfailingly gracious over the past months, while managing to keep this project on course! Sara Bempkins, our Associate Managing Editor, has been patient and flexible in offering editorial assistance, yet somehow kept us all on track in meeting (most) of our deadlines.

We are grateful to the talented and diverse group of authors who contributed their expertise to the writing of this text. Though their positions range from computer scientists to physicians and, of course, nurses, each of our contributors understands the role that informatics will continue to play in achieving high-quality patient care. They also understand the need to challenge our nursing students to apply more advanced informatics concepts in varied healthcare settings.

Finally, we must acknowledge the unceasing support from our families. While they did not always understand our motives for taking on the project of creating a book, they remained positive and calming in ways that only families can do. Alan, Kendal, Ashley, and Trey—we love you all.

Susan Alexander
Karen H. Frith
Haley Hoy

Contributors

Ellise D. Adams, PhD, RN, CNM
Associate Professor
University of Alabama, Huntsville
Huntsville, Alabama

Susan Alexander, DNP, RN, ANP-BC, ADM-BC
Clinical Associate Professor
University of Alabama, Huntsville
Huntsville, Alabama

Faye E. Anderson, DNS, RN, NEA-BC
Associate Professor
University of Alabama, Huntsville
Huntsville, Alabama

Gennifer Baker, MSN, RN, CCNS
Director of Nursing Practice
Huntsville Hospital
Huntsville, Alabama

Janie T. Best, DNP, RN, ACNS-BC, CNL
Assistant Professor
Blair College of Health
Queens University of Charlotte
Charlotte, North Carolina

Jane M. Carrington, PhD, RN
Assistant Professor
Community & Systems Health Science Division
College of Nursing
University of Arizona
Tucson, Arizona

Elizabeth Clark, BA, BSN, RN
Huntsville Hospital
Huntsville, Alabama

Evan Corley, BS
University of Alabama, Huntsville
Huntsville, Alabama

Kelly M. East, MS, CGC
Genetic Counselor
HudsonAlpha Institute for Biotechnology
Huntsville, Alabama

Crayton Fargason Jr., MD, MBA
Professor
University of Alabama, Birmingham
Medical Director
Children's of Alabama
Birmingham, Alabama

Karen H. Frith, PhD, RN, NEA-BC
Professor
University of Alabama, Huntsville
Huntsville, Alabama

Haley Hoy, PhD, ACNP
Assistant Professor
University of Alabama, Huntsville
Nurse Practitioner
Vanderbilt Medical Center
Nashville, Tennessee

Emil Jovanov, PhD
Associate Professor
Department of Electrical and Computer Engineering
University of Alabama, Huntsville
Huntsville, Alabama

Steffi Kreuzfeld, MD
Research Associate
Deputy Director
Institute for Preventive Medicine
University of Rostock
Rostock, Germany

Neil E. Lamb, PhD
Director of Educational Outreach
HudsonAlpha Institute of Biotechnology
Huntsville, Alabama

Manil Maskey, MS
Research Scientist II
Information Technology and Systems Center
University of Alabama, Huntsville
Huntsville, Alabama

Aleksandar Milenkovic, PhD
Associate Professor
Department of Electrical and Computer Engineering
University of Alabama, Huntsville
Huntsville, Alabama

Mladen Milosevic, PhD
Research Assistant
Department of Electrical and Computer Engineering
University of Alabama, Huntsville
Huntsville, Alabama

Stephanie Norman-Lenz, BSN, RN
Nurse Informaticist
Children's of Alabama
Birmingham, Alabama

Rahul Ramachandran, PhD
Informatics and Data Management
National Aeronautics and Space Administration
George C. Marshall Space Flight Center
Huntsville, Alabama

Kimberly D. Shea, PhD, RN
Assistant Professor
Community & Systems Health Science Division
College of Nursing
University of Arizona
Tucson, Arizona

Regina Stoll, MD
Director
Institute of Preventive Medicine
University of Rostock
Rostock, Germany

Mariah Strickland, BSN, RN
Nurse Informaticist
Children's of Alabama
Birmingham, Alabama

Brenda Talley, PhD, RN, NEA-BC
Associate Professor
College of Nursing
University of Alabama, Huntsville
Huntsville, Alabama

Diana Hankey-Underwood, MS, WHNP-BC
Nurse Practitioner
Center for Aging
Huntsville, Alabama

Xiaohua Sarah Wu, MSN, RN, FNP-BC
University of Rochester Medical Center
Strong Memorial Hospital
Rochester, New York

Reviewers

Kim Siarkowski Amer, PhD, RN
Associate Professor
School of Nursing
DePaul University
Chicago, Illinois

Judith Bailey, RN, MS
Cedar Crest College
Allentown, Pennsylvania
Lehigh Valley Health Network
Allentown, Pennsylvania

Margaret Benham-Hutchins, PhD, RN
Texas Woman's University
College of Nursing
Denton, Texas

Ann M. Bowling, PhD, RN, CPNP-PC, CNE
Wright State University
Miami Valley College of Nursing and Health
Dayton, Ohio

Deborah Cheater, MS, RN, CNE
Nursing Instructor
Carl Albert State College
Poteau, Oklahoma

Mary Anne Blum Condon, PhD
Chair and Professor
Averett University
Danville, Virginia

David J. Crowther, PhD, RN, CNS
Associate Professor
Angelo State University
San Angelo, Texas

Kathleen Dunemn, PhD, APRN, CNM
Associate Professor
University of Northern Colorado
Greeley, Colorado

Tresa Kaur Dusaj, PhD(c), RN-BC, CNE, CHSE
Monmouth University
Long Branch, New Jersey

Beth Elias, PhD, MS
Assistant Professor
University of Alabama, Birmingham
School of Nursing
Birmingham, Alabama

Sally K. Fauchald, PhD, RN
The College of St. Scholastica
Department of Graduate Nursing
Duluth, Minnesota

Rebecca Hill, DNP, MSN, FNP-C
Assistant Professor
Massachusetts College of Pharmacy and Health Sciences
Boston, Massachusetts

Janice M. Jones, PhD, RN, CNS
Clinical Professor
University at Buffalo School of Nursing
Buffalo, New York

Lynn M. Klima, MSN, RN
Faculty
School of Nursing
Siena Heights University
Adrian, Michigan

Barbara A. Miller, PhD, RN, ACNS-BC
Assistant Professor
Darton State College
Albany, Georgia

Catherine S. Moe, MS, RN, CNE
Assistant Professor
Lakeview College of Nursing
Danville, Illinois

Angela Mountain, RN, MS, CMSRN
Assistant Professor
Texas A&M Health Sciences Center

Colleen Neal, MS, RN
Assistant Professor
Texas A&M Health Science College of Nursing

Anita K. Reed, MSN, RN
Department Chair Adult and Community Health Practice
Saint Joseph's College
St. Elizabeth School of Nursing
Lafayette, Indiana

Tina Reinckens, RN, MA
Coppin State University
Baltimore, Maryland

Marisa L Wilson, DNSc, MHSc, RN-BC
University of Maryland School of Nursing
Baltimore, Maryland

Annette M. Weiss, PhD, RN, CNE
Assistant Professor and RN to BSN Program Director
Misericordia University
Dallas, Pennsylvania

About the Editors

Susan Alexander, DNP, RN, ANP-BC, ADM-BC, is a Clinical Associate Professor of Nursing at the University of Alabama in Huntsville. She has more than 20 years of experience in nursing, with experience in a variety of both inpatient and outpatient settings, having earned her Doctor of Nursing Practice degree in 2009. In addition to her faculty responsibilities, she is certified by the American Nurses Credentialing Center as an Adult Health Nurse Practitioner and in Advanced Diabetes Management. She is a member of a research team that is studying the use of mobile applications to facilitate networking, transfer of information, and ease of patient care among healthcare providers in the field of organ donation and transplantation. Dr. Alexander serves as a reviewer for the Health Resources and Services Administration, *Online Journal of Issues in Nursing*, McMaster Online Rating of Evidence, and Multimedia Educational Resources for Learning and Online Teaching (MERLOT) Health Sciences. She has authored articles on topics including implementation of software applications for health professionals and the use of online teaching strategies and mobile applications for healthcare providers in transplant. In addition, she is a contributor to *Distance Education in Nursing, Third Edition* (2013, Springer). Dr. Alexander was the recipient of a 2013 American Association of Nurse Practitioners State Award for Excellence.

Karen H. Frith, PhD, RN, NEA-BC, is a Professor of Nursing at the University of Alabama in Huntsville. She has been a nurse educator since 1992 and has an active program of research in health services focusing on nurse staffing and patient outcomes. She cofounded a startup company that has developed decision support software for nurse leaders to improve patient and organizational outcomes. She is a member of the American Organization of Nurse Executives (AONE) and served for 2 years on the national Patient Safety Committee for AONE. She is a member of Healthcare Information and Management Systems Society (HIMSS), Sigma Theta Tau International

Honor Society of Nursing, and the Southern Nursing Research Society. She serves as reviewer (of grants and articles) for Sigma Theta Tau; Health Resources and Services Administration, *Journal of Nursing Administration*, *Online Journal of Issues in Nursing*, *Computers, Informatics, Nursing, Journal of Health & Medical Informatics*, and *Nurse Educator*, among others. She has authored more than 30 articles in peer-reviewed journals, authored the book, *Distance Education in Nursing, Third Edition*, contributed chapters to three other books, and presents nationally. Her previous clinical positions experience is in cardiovascular surgical intensive care, coronary intensive care, and orthopedics. She is board certified by the American Nurses Credentialing Center as Nurse Executive, Advanced (NEA-BC).

Haley Hoy, PhD, ACNP, is an acute care nurse practitioner and Interim Associate Dean at the University of Alabama in Huntsville. She has been a nurse practitioner for more than 15 years and is a leader in technology and transplant nursing. Her current research interests include the role of technology and web- and mobile-based applications for the transplant community, in addition to nurse and community attitudes toward organ donation. She has research grants from the North American Transplant Coordinators Organization (NATCO) and from the University of Alabama in Huntsville (Faculty Distinguished Research grant recipient). She is an active member of the American Association of Nurse Practitioners, the North American Transplant Coordinators Organization, and the Medical Automation Organization. She was the recipient of the 2011 American Association of Nurse Practitioners State Award for Excellence and the Advanced Transplant Provider Award. She is board certified by the American Nurses Credentialing Center and continues to practice as a nurse practitioner at Vanderbilt Medical Center in the Department of Lung Transplantation.

Concepts and Issues in Clinical Informatics

CHAPTER 1

Overview of Informatics in Health Care

Susan Alexander, DNP, RN, ANP-BC, ADM-BC

CHAPTER LEARNING OBJECTIVES

1. Review the history of the development of clinical informatics in the United States.
2. Define and discuss key concepts relating to clinical informatics and information science.
3. Describe the present culture of health care in the United States.
4. Describe the role of clinical informatics in contemporary health care in the United States.

KEY TERMS

Clinical informatics
Data (datum)
Fragmentation
Healthcare providers (HCPs)

Information
Knowledge
Nursing informatics
Wisdom

CHAPTER OVERVIEW

The purposes of this chapter are to provide an overview of health information technology (IT) used in contemporary nursing practice and briefly describe the history of clinical informatics. Clinical informatics can provide possible solutions to existing problems in the U.S. healthcare system including fragmentation, access to care, and care of special populations. Nurses who understand clinical informatics will likely improve healthcare delivery and patient safety.

INFORMATICS IN NURSING PRACTICE

The role of the 21st century nurse is complex, requiring interaction with multiple medical devices and health IT. Nurses at all levels of educational preparation and in all healthcare settings use technology every day in practice. In addition to becoming expert users, it is increasingly likely that nurses, because of their rich experience in patient care, will be called upon to participate in the design of new clinical systems for delivering high-quality and efficient care. The case study that follows illustrates how technology is integral to all parts of healthcare delivery for **healthcare providers (HCPs)**, patients, and healthcare settings (see **Box 1-1**).

Box 1-1   Case Study

Cody arrives for her scheduled 12-hour hospital shift as a circulating surgical registered nurse (RN). After she swipes her name badge at the double doors, the doors slowly swing open for her to proceed to the same-day surgery unit. Another swipe of her badge through the time clock yields a "beep," and Cody knows her day has officially begun. At the desk, Cody greets her coworkers and glances at the large monitor hanging on the wall in the nurses' station where the day's schedule of patients, procedures, their providers, and other notes are posted. "It's going to be another busy day," she thinks to herself. Cody finds the patient, Mr. Jones, who she is scheduled to move from preop to the operating room (OR) suite, noting that he is to undergo a robotic prostatectomy. She picks up a clipboard and touches the screen. The patient's name begins to blink, letting other staff know that the patient will soon be in the OR suite.

At the patient's bedside, Cody introduces herself to the patient and the family and notes the planned surgery. She uses a bar-code scanner on the patient's bracelet, and she notes the completed consent documents on her electronic clipboard. Releasing the brakes on the patient's gurney, Cody and Mr. Jones bid farewell to his family members, and they move slowly down the hall to the OR. As Mr. Jones' gurney moves into the OR, a transponder that is embedded in the gurney is detected by a scanner immediately inside the OR door. This information is both imported directly into the electronic health record (EHR) and used to update the monitor in the nurses' station. In the OR, she assists with transferring the patient to the OR table and positions him comfortably. The anesthetist places a mask over the patient's face and, after full anesthesia is achieved, the surgery begins.

Less than 4 hours later, the surgery is complete, and Cody assists in moving Mr. Jones back to the gurney for transfer to the post-anesthesia care unit (PACU). As the gurney moves through the door of the suite, the scanner again detects the transponder, updating the EHR and notifying the PACU that the patient is on his way. In the PACU, Mr. Jones' vital signs, oxygen saturation, and heart rhythm will be monitored until he awakens. Once he is stable, Mr. Jones can be moved to his room on the medical-surgical unit.

After an uncomplicated postoperative recovery period, Mr. Jones is ready to be discharged. As Mr. Jones' surgeon and nurse practitioner perform morning rounds, they prepare Mr. Jones for discharge. The nurse on the medical-surgical unit confirms that Mr. Jones' discharge medications are reconciled with his prescriptions for pain medications and electronically transmitted from the EHR to the pharmacy. As the unit nurse completes her discharge teaching for Mr. Jones and his family, further instructions are printed. A follow-up appointment request is faxed to the surgeon's office from the EHR.

HISTORY OF CLINICAL INFORMATICS DEVELOPMENT_____

In the 21st century, it is difficult to imagine providing patient care in any setting without the use of computer technology. It is surprising that the word "computer" can be traced to 1646 (Merriam-Webster, 2013). The word "computer" literally means "one who computes." In the 19th century, the word "computer" was used to describe the activities of humans who labored to create tables of numerical values used in science, mathematics, and engineering. Despite painstaking work, the tables contained a high rate of errors, a phenomenon recognized by Charles Babbage, an English mathematician and scholar. In 1821, Babbage began construction of the first mechanical computer, known as the "Analytical Engine" (The Great Idea Finder, 1997–2007), designed to compute the values of polynomial functions, which eventually earned him the title of "Father of Computing" (http://www.charlesbabbage.net/). Babbage's colleague, Augusta Ada Lovelace (Countess Lovelace), a mathematician, is attributed with the first efforts at programming a computer when she authored the first algorithm intended to be processed by a computer (San Diego Computer Science Center, 1997). Though the Analytical Engine did not have the capability for practical daily use, it possessed many features found in modern computers, such as the ability to read data from punch cards, store data, and perform arithmetic operations (The Great Idea Finder, 1997–2007). The Analytical Engine was the conceptual and technical basis for the highly developed technology in use today.

Over time, the value of computers and technology in the collection and manipulation of data became readily apparent. Through its work in establishing and maintaining ongoing population records, the U.S. Census Bureau recognized the ability of digital computers to process large amounts of information. The Universal Automatic Computer (UNIVAC) was designed especially for the needs of the Census Bureau (see **Figure 1-1**). The first version of UNIVAC (UNIVAC I) was used to conduct a portion of the population census in 1950 and then the entire economic census in 1954 (U.S. Census Bureau, n.d.). UNIVAC is widely viewed as the first successful civilian computer, ushering in the dawn of the computer age in information processing.

While a full history of the development of computers into the hand-held models we use today is not within the scope of this text, a brief review of significant changes in the use of computers and technology in health care is warranted. Robert Ledley, a dentist who also studied physics, is credited with invention of the first full-body computed tomography (CT) scanner. Dr. Ledley had a deep interest in how the fields of pattern recognition and image analysis could be applied to patient care through the use of computers and founded the National Biomedical Research Foundation in 1960, a nonprofit organization dedicated to the promotion of computing methods among biomedical scientists. He was also a founding fellow of the American College of Medical Informatics. Dr. Ledley foresaw the role of technology in issues of patient

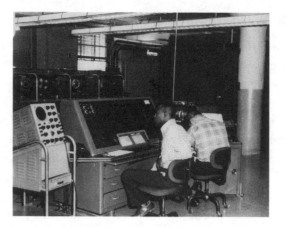

FIGURE 1-1 Photo of UNIVAC 1105 used in the 1960 census, at Census Bureau.
Source: http://www.census.gov/history/www/innovations/technology/univac_i.html

care such as recordkeeping, imaging, and diagnosis in settings ranging from private office practices to acute care facilities. Today, the use of technologically driven devices such as electrocardiogram machines, ventilators, and intravenous pumps necessitates a degree of technical skill in every clinician.

The increasing incorporation of technology into health care quickly resulted in an accumulation of data as HCPs realized that not only could computers be used at the point of patient care, but they also could collect and store data useful for later patient care. Specialty fields, developed by people with interest in data manipulation and its application, arose from this need to maintain and apply analysis of data to patient care. The field of clinical informatics is an example. Data storage and maintenance are also of interest to the federal government, because huge databases containing billions of data points on patients are available for researchers to answer clinical questions.

A review of the history of clinical informatics would not be complete without a discussion of nursing's contribution to the field and to the development of nursing informatics (NI) as a science in the public and private sectors. In the late 1950s, Harriet Werley became the first nurse researcher at the Walter Reed Army Research Institute and was asked to join a small group of people who were consulting about the possibilities of using computers in health care. Werley was instrumental in promoting research on what would later emerge as the field of NI (Ozbolt & Saba, 2008). The American Medical Informatics Association (AMIA) recognizes many important nurse leaders as NI pioneers. While this text cannot highlight all, it is important to understand the contributions that have shaped the discipline of NI.

Dr. Patricia Abbott, who might be best known for her work in helping to develop NI as a specialty field, was a member of the team of authors who crafted the initial American Nurses Association Scope and Standards of Practice for Nursing Informatics (AMIA, n.d.). Dr. Abbott also worked with the American Nurses Credentialing Center to develop the first certification exam in NI. Dr. Virginia Saba, another pioneer of NI, actively participated in initiating academic technology programs and healthcare IT systems (AMIA, n.d.). Dr. Saba has coordinated distance learning projects for nurses and served on national healthcare standards committees. Dr. Kathleen McCormick has been a clinical trial researcher and NI scientist within the National Institutes of Health Clinical Center and the National Institute on Aging, and she is an elected member of the National Academy of Sciences, Institute of Medicine (AMIA, n.d.).

Activities of NI pioneers are not limited to the field of nursing. Dr. Marion Ball has provided service to the public sector as a member of the Institute of Medicine and on the Board of Regents of the National Library of Medicine (AMIA, n.d.). She has worked with multiple national and international committees, including serving as president of the International Medical Informatics Association and as a board member of the AMIA. Dr. Ball was also invited to serve as an international advisor to the Board of the China Hospital Information Management Association. Roy L. Simpson, vice president, NI, Cerner Corporation, worked with colleagues to develop the Nursing Minimum Data Set and to develop online nursing administration and NI master's programs (AMIA, n.d.).

NI pioneers are also active in the areas of educating and fostering the NI workforce of tomorrow. Dr. Linda Thede is professor emeritus at the College of Nursing at Kent State University, where she has developed and taught NI programs (AMIA, n.d.). Dr. Susan K. Newbold, a healthcare informatics consultant based in Franklin, TN, worked to found CARING, an NI group that was established in 1982. She also participates in teaching NI to nursing students at multiple curricular levels (AMIA, n.d.). Dr. Susan J. Grobe developed the Nursing Education Module Authoring System, which consists of a set of software programs that faculty can use to create modules on the nursing process. Dr. Grobe was one of the first of two nurse fellows elected to the American College of Medical Informatics (AMIA, n.d.).

CLINICAL INFORMATICS AND NURSING INFORMATICS DEFINED

Clinical informatics is a broad term that encompasses all medical and health specialties, including nursing, and addresses the ways information systems are used in the day-to-day operations of patient care. The domains of clinical informatics include

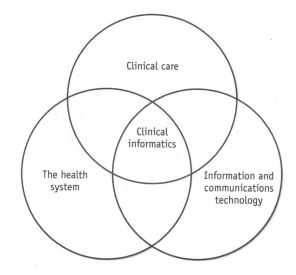

FIGURE 1-2 Domains of clinical informatics.

Source: Reproduced from AMIA Board White Paper: Core Content for the Subspecialty of Clinical Informatics by Reed M Gardner, J Marc Overhage et al. for the AMIA Board of Directors, Journal of the American Medical Informatics Association 16(2), copyright © 2009 with permission from BMJ Publishing Group Ltd.

health systems, clinical care, and information and communication technologies (see **Figure 1-2**). The purpose of clinical informatics is to improve patient care by using methods and technologies from established disciplines such as computer science and information science.

Nursing informatics is a specialty in the discipline of nursing, and it is classified as a special interest group in professional organizations whose focus is clinical informatics. NI is defined by the International Medical Informatics Association's Nursing Informatics Special Interest Group (2009) as the "science and practice [that] integrates nursing, its information and knowledge, with management of information and communication technologies to promote the health of people, families, and communities worldwide." Because of the emphasis on promoting health, the study of NI is a natural fit for nurses who are dedicated to quality care for patients. As described in subsequent chapters, the understanding of NI concepts is not a "nice to know" set of knowledge, skills, and values; rather, it is a requirement for effective nursing practice (Thede, 2012).

The role of clinical informatics is becoming increasingly important and can be seen in almost every aspect of patient care, from the bedside to the patient's bill. Use of powerful clinical informatics tools can be used to support processes of care, such as promoting the flow of information between those who are involved in the delivery of care across HCPs in large delivery systems. At the macro-system level, clinical informatics tools can be used to assess specific outcomes of care for groups, such as the efficacy of annual influenza vaccinations or fall prevention programs.

CLINICAL INFORMATICS CONCEPTS

Informatics is a science, with its beginnings in how **data** are processed and communicated between systems. What are data? Data are values or measurements, bits of information that can be collected and transformed, allowing one to answer a question or to create an end product, such as an image. Data are created with every patient contact. Nurses and other HCPs use their education and experience to assemble data in a clinical context to create **information**, which gives insight about patient care. Information can then be used to plan care for patient aggregates, increase the efficiency of organizations, improve quality of care, prevent medical errors, increase efficiency of care, and potentially reduce unnecessary costs. **Knowledge** creation concerns the ways that nurses and HCPs use the data and information they create to better understand and manage their practice. The proper use of knowledge to solve real-world problems and aid continuous improvement is what is known as **wisdom** (McGonigle & Mastrian, 2012).

Many different systems support the movement from data to information, information to knowledge, or knowledge to wisdom. Systems that support the transfer from data to information are known as information systems. Systems that support the transition from information to knowledge are decision-support systems, and those that apply knowledge through wisdom are known as expert systems (McGonigle & Mastrian, 2012). At each level, these systems contain computer, communications, and human elements.

Principles of informatics can apply to many different fields, from economics to health care. However, in clinical informatics, people with a background in health care use informatics tools, such as health information databases, medical imaging software, or point-of-care technologies to capture information and present it to other members of healthcare teams. The implementation of clinical informatics tools has the potential to create vast improvements in patient care by improving efficiency and reducing errors, which is a top priority for the United States.

HEALTH CARE IN THE UNITED STATES AND THE NEED FOR HEALTH INFORMATION MANAGEMENT

The United States spends more per capita on health care than any other country in the world. Health expenditures in the United States neared $2.6 trillion in 2010—more than 10 times the $256 billion spent in 1980, and costs are increasing annually

(Centers for Medicaid and Medicare Services [CMS], 2012). Despite the spending, a poll of public opinion on the present culture of health care in the United States would garner a variety of responses. While there are those who would express satisfaction, it is far more likely that more people would be unhappy about some aspect of the healthcare environment. This growing dissatisfaction has attracted attention. A recent report from the Institute of Medicine (IOM, 2011) draws attention to the poor health of U.S. citizens. Though the United States has the highest rate of per capita spending on health care, comparing our population of citizens under the age of 75 to those of peer countries finds that ours have higher rates of chronic diseases and disabilities (IOM, 2011). In a country with as many assets as the United States, particularly in the field of health care, how can this be the case? More importantly, what tools and strategies exist that can potentially change this situation?

Burden of Fragmentation

Missing medical information can be a detriment to care in many settings, but perhaps more so in areas of high acuity, in which HCPs may be forced to make rapid decisions that may be challenging to patient safety. A retrospective review of 3.6 million patient visits to acute care sites in Massachusetts from 2002–2007 revealed that 56.5% of the patients were multisite users or had used more than one acute care site within the 5-year period (Bourgeois, Olson, & Mandl, 2010). **Fragmentation** of care ultimately places patients at greater risk for poor outcomes, particularly if those patients have multiple or chronic conditions. Patients with chronic diseases such as type 2 diabetes mellitus (T2DM) are at risk for multiple complications that often necessitate management by subspecialists, such as ophthalmologists, nephrologists, podiatrists, and cardiologists. Initiating such referrals and follow-ups for patients with T2DM, while consistent with evidence-based guidelines, can be an arduous task for an HCP. Patients who do not receive needed referrals for treatment of complications may be forced to seek care in settings that are more expensive and less appropriate for chronic management, such as an emergency department (ED). Liu, Einstadter, and Cebul (2010) studied the effects of care fragmentation on a group of 683 adult patients with diabetes and chronic kidney disease. The primary outcome variable was the number of ED visits made during a 2-year period. Findings from the study revealed that patients who had fewer visits to primary HCPs had higher numbers of ED visits.

For optimal protection against transmissible diseases such as measles, mumps, and pertussis, childhood immunizations must be given at specified intervals and ages. Tracking the administration of childhood immunizations for each child, which may total 24 timed vaccinations during the first 18 months of life, is another area at risk for fragmentation and subsequent elevation in risk of acquiring childhood diseases (Centers for Disease Control and Prevention [CDC], 2013). The effects of fragmented health care have also been studied in immunization rates of children aged 19 to 35 months residing in four geographical areas (northern Manhattan, San Diego, Detroit, and rural Colorado), which have received federal designation as health professional shortage areas (Yusuf et al., 2002). HCPs must have reliable information in order to offer necessary immunizations; otherwise children may miss opportunities for vaccinations if providers decide to delay based on inaccurate or incomplete records from parents or other HCPs. Incomplete information from recent HCPs was associated with both overimmunization and underimmunization in this study (Yusuf et al., 2002). The utilization of community-wide immunization registries, containing information from all immunization providers in a community, was suggested as a solution to the dilemma of clinical questions regarding vaccinations (Yusuf et al., 2002).

Inaccurate or incomplete transfer of information, another example of the fragmentation that permeates health care today, can put vulnerable patients at risk of adverse events, hospital readmission, and even death in the transition from inpatient to home care (Davis, Devoe, Kansagara, Nicolaidis, & Englander, 2012). HCPs have identified the need for improved communication between healthcare systems, particularly for those patients who have conditions that have been identified as high risk for hospital readmission. In a qualitative study of 75 healthcare professionals, representing physicians, nurses, pharmacists, and other allied health professionals, poor cross-site communication was noted as a major gap in helping patients to transition from hospital to home (Davis et al., 2012). These gaps were amplified by the lack of interoperability between EHR systems of the facility and outpatient practice, and this was especially troubling to primary care providers who cited:

> A patient's there in front of me [after discharge], they've had a life changing event, and I'm sitting there without the information. You feel like an idiot . . . . I would think, "What kind of system do you guys have here? I almost died, and you don't even have the information." . . . That's embarrassing and I don't think it engenders a lot of confidence for your patients. (Davis et al., 2012, p. 1653)

The Promises of Clinical Informatics Systems

The adoption of clinical informatics systems has the potential to improve many of the issues troubling health care today in the United States, yet the full potential of clinical informatics tools remains to be realized. Improving efficiency of care for specific disease states, care settings, and populations is an area in which clinical informatics tools can make a positive impact. For example, a survey of 40 hospital infection preventionists suggests that expansion of the capabilities of the hospital EHR, in order to provide clinical decision prompts on patients who need closer inspection, would be of benefit in detecting and providing timely care for patients with hospital-associated infections. Improved awareness of regional health initiatives and public health reporting capabilities would increase communication and earlier detection (McKinney, 2013).

Improved Efficiency

Defragmentation, a strategy long used in fields such as engineering, computer science, and manufacturing, is a means of managing limited resources while improving the performance of a system. A myriad of applications for health IT and informatics incorporating defragmentation can be used to improve efficiency, even in the office environment, where millions of patients schedule appointments with HCPs every day. Conventional appointment scheduling, in which a block of time is scheduled to accommodate the needs of a patient, is a tradeoff between the need to maximize the productivity of an HCP while minimizing the wait time for a patient. A ranked list of most preferred to least preferred appointment time slots for providers was created for schedulers, designed to offer guidance on how to best schedule patient appointments to prevent provider schedule fragmentation (Lian, Distefano, Shields, Heinichen, Giampietri, & Wang, 2010). A computer model was developed to measure efficiency using two metrics: "acceptance rate (the number between the number of accepted appointments and the total number of appointment requests), and the utilization rate (the health care provider's actual service time divided by the total work time" (Lian et al., 2010, p. 128). The advanced appointment scheduling process was tested in four different specialty and primary care clinics. The aggregation of open time slots for HCPs that resulted from the implementation of the process was utilized in various ways, including the addition of new patient appointments in the open blocks of time.

Improving the Health Care of Older Adults

Older adults bear a higher burden of illness and frailty, and may transition frequently between healthcare systems, leading to higher costs and risk. More than 125 million Americans had at least one chronic disease in 2000, and this number is expected to grow to 157 million by the year 2020 (Wu & Green, 2000). A disproportionately large number of older adults are dealing with chronic illnesses. Potentially avoidable hospitalizations in older adult clients result in poor outcomes, which are unnecessary and create excessive expenditures. By improving communication across systems, clinical informatics may assist HCPs in meeting the challenges of caring for older adults. For example, the Regenstrief Medical Record System (RMRS), housed at the University of Indiana and serving the Indianapolis area, contains records from more than 1.3 million patients. As early as 1974, the RMRS began to deliver automatic reminders in the form of paper reports, creating reminders for preventive services such as fecal occult blood testing, mammography, and vaccinations—topics pertinent to the care of older adults. In a 2-year randomized trial involving 130 providers and more than 12,000 patients, investigators found that older adult patients of physicians who received reminders for influenza vaccinations were twice as likely to receive the vaccination as patients of physicians who did not receive electronically generated reminders (Weiner et al., 2003).

Challenges in Clinical Informatics

A key concept in clinical informatics is the purpose of the IT—to improve health of people, aggregates, communities, and populations. However, several barriers must be overcome if technology can really improve the U.S. healthcare system. The first and biggest barrier is the lack of system interoperability, which restricts the flow of data from one information system to others (Thede, 2012). There are many reasons for the interoperability problem, including the purchase of "best of breed" systems for specialty practices, the use of legacy systems that cost too much to upgrade, and integration processes that are too difficult to implement. Poor usability of health IT is the second barrier (Thede, 2012). When nurses and other HCPs are burdened with technology rather than helped by it, the health IT has been improperly designed for the user experience and for the workflow. A related and important third barrier is the failure to design health IT for human factors to prevent errors (Thede, 2012). The interaction of humans with technology is studied in other fields and applied in the design of technology and processes. In clinical informatics, attention to human factors is emerging and will become more prominent as a strategy to improve patient safety.

SUMMARY

HCPs recognized the impact of informatics to improve outcomes for patients more than 100 years ago. New applications for informatics-based tools continue to emerge, offering nurses and other HCPs ways to decrease fragmentation of care in their own settings. As informatics tools continue to be adapted for the field of health care, nurses will play an integral role in analysis, planning, and implementing ways health IT can be used to improve patient care.

> **www** ᐅ For a full suite of assignments and additional learning activities, use the access code located in the front of your book and visit www.jblearning.com. If you do not have an access code, you can obtain one at the site.

REFERENCES

American Medical Informatics Association. (n.d.). *Video Library 1: Nursing informatics pioneers.* Retrieved from http://www.amia.org/programs/working-groups/nursing-informatics/history-project/video-library-1

Bourgeois, F. C., Olson, K. L., & Mandl, K. D. (2010). Patients treated at multiple acute health care facilities: Quantifying information fragmentation. *Annals of Internal Medicine, 170*(22), 1989–1995.

Centers for Disease Control and Prevention. (2013). *2013 recommended immunizations for children from birth through 6 years old.* Retrieved from http://www.cdc.gov/vaccines/parents/downloads/parent-ver-sch-0-6yrs.pdf

Centers for Medicare and Medicaid Services, Office of the Actuary, National Health Statistics Group. (2012). *National health expenditures.* https://www.cms.gov/NationalHealthExpendData/downloads/tables.pdf. Retrieved from https://www.cms.gov/Research-Statistics-Data-and-Systems/Statistics-Trends-and-Reports/NationalHealthExpendData/downloads/tables.pdf

Davis, M. M., Devoe, M., Kansagara, D., Nicolaidis, C., & Englander, H. (2012). "Did I do as best as the system would let me?" Healthcare professionals' views on hospital to home care transitions. (2012). *Journal of General Internal Medicine, 27*(12), 1649–1656.

Institute of Medicine. (2011). *Health IT and patient safety: Building safer systems for better care.* Washington, DC: Committee on Patient Safety and Health Information Technology, Board on Health Care Services.

International Medical Informatics Association, Nursing Informatics Special Interest Group. (2009). *Definition.* Retrieved from http://imia-medinfo.org/ni/node/28

Lian, J., Distefano, K., Shields, S. D., Heinichen, C., Giampietri, M., & Wang, L. (2010). Clinical appointment process: Improvement through schedule defragmentation. *IEEE Engineering in Medicine and Biology Magazine, 29*(2), 127–134. doi: 10.1109/MEMB.2009.935718

Liu, C. W., Einstadter, D., & Cebul, R. D. (2010). Care fragmentation and emergency department use among complex patients with diabetes. *American Journal of Managed Care, 16*(6), 413–420.

McGonigle, D., & Mastrian, K. G. (2012). *Nursing informatics and the foundation of knowledge* (2nd ed.). Burlington, MA: Jones & Bartlett Learning.

McKinney, M. (2013). *Study: EHRs underutilized by preventionists.* Retrieved from http://www.modernhealthcare.com/article/20130225/NEWS/302259955

Merriam-Webster. (2013). *Computer.* Retrieved from http://www.merriam-webster.com/dictionary/computer

Ozbolt, J. G., & Saba, V. K. (2008). A brief history of nursing informatics in the United States. *Nursing Outlook, 56,* 199–205.

San Diego Computer Science Center. (1997). *Ada Byron, Countess of Lovelace.* Retrieved from http://www.sdsc.edu/ScienceWomen/lovelace.html

The Great Idea Finder. (1997–2007). *Ada Lovelace.* Retrieved from http://www.ideafinder.com/history/inventors/lovelace.htm

Thede, L. (2012). Informatics: Where is it? *OJIN: The Online Journal of Issues in Nursing, 17*(1). Retrieved from http://www.nursingworld.org/MainMenuCategories/ANAMarketplace/ANAPeriodicals/OJIN/Columns/Informatics/Informatics-Where-Is-It.html

U.S. Census Bureau. (n.d.). *UNIVAC I.* Retrieved from http://www.census.gov/history/www/innovations/technology/univac_i.html

Weiner, M., Callahan, C. M., Tierney, W. M., Overhage, M., Mamlin, B., Dexter, P. R., & McDonald, C. J. (2003). Using information technology to improve the health care of older adults. *Annals of Internal Medicine, 139,* 430–436.

Wu, S., & Green, A. (2000). *Projection of chronic illness prevalence and cost inflation.* Santa Monica, CA: RAND Corporation.

Yusuf, H., Adams, M., Rodewald, L., Pengjun, L., Rosenthal, J., Legum, S., & Santoli, J. (2002). Fragmentation of immunization history among providers and parents of children in selected underserved areas. *American Journal of Preventive Medicine, 23*(2), 106–112.

CHAPTER 2

Information Needs for the Healthcare Professional of the 21st Century

Haley Hoy, PhD, ACNP
Susan Alexander, DNP, RN, ANP-BC, ADM-BC
Evan Corley, BS
Gennifer Baker, MSN, RN, CCNS

CHAPTER LEARNING OBJECTIVES

1. Describe informatics competencies essential for the graduate nurse.
2. Understand the process of knowledge generation and management.
3. Review the importance of informatics in nursing workflow.
4. Describe a common change model, the Plan-Do-Study-Act model, and explain how it can be used in a healthcare setting.
5. Review ongoing educational needs for the nurse in the field of informatics.

KEY TERMS

Clinical decision-support systems (CDSS)
Continuing education
Data
Information
Information literacy
Information management

Information systems
Knowledge
Knowledge creation
Nursing informatics
Plan-Do-Study-Act (PDSA)

CHAPTER OVERVIEW

The world of technology in health care has undergone a profound shift over the past several decades. Technology that was once limited to use in a hospital-based critical care unit may now be seen in the homecare setting, or even delivered via a mobile application on a smartphone or tablet. In addition to proficiency in patient care skills

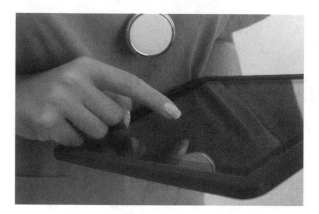

FIGURE 2-1 Today's nurses must possess competence in patient care, communication, and data management.
Source: © iStockphoto.com/hocus-focus

that have long been associated with the profession of nursing, such as injections and dressing changes, today's nurse must possess a degree of competence in patient care, communication, and data management technologies. Assisting the newly graduated nurse to acquire this varied skill set has also changed the face of prelicensure nursing education. This chapter reviews expectations for informatics content within nursing curricula and discusses selected examples of how informatics technologies can influence the daily workflow for nurses. Specific ways in which informatics is commonly used in healthcare settings to improve patient care, such as the Plan-Do-Study-Act model of quality improvement (QI), are presented. Finally, the chapter describes the integral role that information technology (IT) may play in a nurse's continuing education.

PROGRAM CURRICULAR CHANGES

Recent generations of nurses, born with their hands on computer keyboards and mobile devices, may seem to readily integrate IT into their nursing practice. Exposure to common software applications such as Microsoft Word or PowerPoint, which some nurses may have encountered initially only in the practice setting, is now offered in many elementary schools. This phenomenon has radically altered the expectations for content that needs to be included in curricula for the baccalaureate-prepared nurse (**Table 2-1**). The American Association of Colleges of Nursing (AACN, 2008), in *The Essentials of Baccalaureate Education for Professional Nursing Practice*, summarizes the need for informatics content in curricula: "Knowledge and

Table 2-1   AACN Essentials of Baccalaureate Education for Professional Nursing Practice. Essential IV: Information Management and Application of Patient-Care Technology
Demonstrate skills in using patient-care technologies, information systems, and communication devices that support safe nursing practice.
Use telecommunication technologies to assist in effective communication in a variety of health-care settings.
Apply safeguards and decision-making support tools embedded in patient-care technologies and information systems to support a safe practice environment for patients and healthcare workers.
Understand the use of clinical information systems to document interventions related to achieving nurse-sensitive outcomes.
Use standardized terminology in a care environment that reflects nursing's unique contribution to patient outcomes.
Evaluate data from all relevant sources, including technology, to inform the delivery of care.
Recognize the role of information technology in improving patient-care outcomes and creating a safe care environment.
Uphold ethical standards related to data security, regulatory requirements, confidentiality, and patients' right to privacy.
Apply patient-care technologies as appropriate to address the needs of a diverse patient population.
Recognize that redesign of workflow and care processes should precede implementation of care technology to facilitate nursing practice.
Participate in evaluation of information systems in practice settings through policy and procedure development.

Source: American Association of Colleges of Nursing. (2008). *The essentials of baccalaureate education for professional nursing practice.* Retrieved from http://www.aacn.nche.edu/education-resources/baccessentials08.pdf

skills in information management and patient care technologies are critical in the delivery of quality patient care" (p. 4).

Nursing education programs are working to implement health informatics education into present curricula, but this can be a difficult process. Time constraints and a shortage of nursing faculty with health informatics expertise have been cited as barriers to full integration of health informatics content in programs of study in the United States and abroad (Bartholomew, 2011). In a study of 186 students enrolled in healthcare professions in the United Kingdom, 61% reported that they desired more training in the use of clinical **information systems** (Bartholomew, 2011). It is essential that students understand that working with health information technologies (health IT) tools is a meaningful component of the professional nurse's skill set. Exposure to an academic electronic health record (EHR), and repeat opportunities to develop competency in use of the EHR, have been cited as important throughout the curricula. These exposures may be important approaches in assisting nursing students to meet the evolving health IT expectations in healthcare settings (Gardner & Jones, 2012).

INFORMATICS COMPETENCIES AND THE TIGER INITIATIVE

There are many different specific functions in the nursing informatics discipline, each with its own necessary competencies and responsibilities. The Technology Informatics Guiding Education Reform (TIGER) Initiative, formed in 2004, is a sustainable relationship between the Alliance for Nursing Informatics (ANI) and many other nursing organizations such as the American Nurses Association (ANA), the American Organization of Nurse Executives (AONE), and the AACN. The purpose of the TIGER initiative is to "identify information/knowledge management best practices and effective technology capabilities for nurses" (TIGER Initiative, 2007–2013). It was developed in response to the national goal of expanding the EHR to all citizens and in recognition of the nurse's role in meeting that goal. At its summit meeting, held in October and November 2006, a 3-year action plan was developed, detailing strategies to better prepare nurses to practice in an informatics-rich environment. Nine collaborative teams were created to address the action plan in specified areas, and each team developed a report describing the background and strategies for future work in its area. TIGER's activities have continued, including the creation of a comprehensive document designed to define the informatics competencies practicing nurses would need (Technology Informatics Guiding Educational Reform, 2009). Recommendations from the initiative are grouped into three levels: basic computer competency, information literacy, and information management.

Basic Computer Competency

The TIGER Informatics Competencies Collaborative (TICC) recommendations for basic computer competency are based on modules from the European Computer Driving License Qualifications (ECDL, 2013), which were developed in Europe to help provide standards for competency and routes to develop competency. The major computing functions covered in the ECDL include working with different hardware and operating systems, developing a file management system, working with printers and other output devices, protecting computers against malicious software, using word processing and spreadsheet software programs, finding information on the Internet, and collaborating via Internet-based and mobile technologies including social media, cloud computing, and shared calendars.

The full ECDL course requires more than 30 hours of study and is relatively expensive, so the TICC highlights four specific modules for nurses: Basic Computing Concepts, Using the Computer and Managing Files, Word Processing, and Web Browsing and Communication. This recommendation is based on relative importance, and the TICC recommends that all nurses have the complete competencies for the ECDL or a similar certification. Resources other than the ECDL include Computer Skills Placement (http://www.csplacement.com), a computer competency learning and skill assessment course, and the Healthcare Information Management System Society (HIMSS, http://www.himss.org), which offers the Health Informatics Training System (HITS) program and certification (TIGER, 2009).

Information Literacy Competency

TICC defines **information literacy** as "the ability to identify information needed for a specific purpose, locate pertinent information, evaluate the information, and apply it correctly" (TIGER, 2009). The process can be expanded into the five basic steps shown in **Box 2-1**.

Box 2-1   Five Steps to Information Literacy

1. Determine the nature and extent of the information needed.
2. Access needed information effectively and efficiently.
3. Evaluate information and its sources critically and incorporate information into knowledge base and value system.
4. Individually, or as a member of a group, use the information effectively to accomplish a specific purpose.
5. Evaluate the outcomes of the use of information.

Assessments of Information Literacy

The American Library Association (ALA) Information Literacy Competency Standards for Higher Education

http://www.ala.org/acrl/standards/informationliteracycompetency

Information Literacy in Technology (iLIT)

http://www.ilitassessment.com/

Information Management Competency

Information management is defined as the process of collecting data, processing, and presenting and communicating the data as information or knowledge (TIGER, 2009). This process is the initial step in the data-information-knowledge-wisdom continuum. Systems that perform this function are known as information systems, and the most important for nurses are those that pertain to EHRs, (EHRs; also called electronic medical records (TIGER, 2009). The current EHR standard is the EHR System Functional Model provided by the American National Standards Institute (ANSI; TIGER, 2009).

The ECDL provides the ECDL-Health syllabus that focuses on the core information management competencies needed in healthcare environments. The ECDL syllabus includes four categories: Concepts, due care, user skills, and policies and procedures. For pre-licensure nurses, the recommended skill set includes understanding the purpose and types of health information systems (HIS), adhering to confidentially, access, and security protocols, using an HIS effectively and safely, understanding how to navigate an HIS, and using decision support, clinical guidelines, and other features of an HIS to provide safe patient care. Based on this framework, the TICC has issued competency statements that pertain to each competency, which can be found on the TIGER Initiative website.

KNOWLEDGE MANAGEMENT AND TRANSFORMATION _____

The creation of knowledge is the first step in using IT efficiently and effectively. One thing healthcare practices do very well is create **data**. Detailed records are kept of patient histories, diagnoses, treatments, and the effects of treatments. With the help of IT, the data can be used to create a wealth of knowledge to improve the quality and efficiency of care. IT is the foundation of EHRs and **clinical decision-support systems (CDSS)**, technologies that continue to change the way health care is provided.

The **knowledge creation** process begins by structuring raw data into understandable, meaningful **information**. The next step is to turn that information into knowledge that can be used to support decision making. Graves and Corcoran provided a classic definition of **knowledge** as "information that has been synthesized so that relationships are identified and formalized" (1989, p. 230). For example, information is a series of a patient's vital signs. Knowledge comes with the formalization of rules to guide the interpretation of those vital signs. The utility of any knowledge is directly dependent on its perceived accuracy and validity. In the past, validity was based on the opinions of a few well-respected experts. However, with the advent of computing and the information age, validity is largely becoming based on the size and representativeness of the dataset upon which the knowledge is based. As healthcare providers (HCPs) continue transitioning to EHRs and other health IT languages, the breadth of available data will continue to increase, as will the need to interpret and synthesize data to create new knowledge and refine knowledge already in circulation.

The creation of knowledge from raw data is the foundation of informatics. It is a continuous process that requires the tools provided by IT and the expertise and interpretive skills of the practitioner. The efficacy of knowledge is directly related to the breadth of the data from which it is derived. As time progresses and the adoption of technologies such as the EHR continues, this process will become more important and more efficacious, and the skills required for knowledge creation will become more and more integral to the nursing process.

NURSES, INFORMATICS, AND NURSING WORKFLOW

Health IT has a profound effect on the way that nurses provide care for patients, regardless of the location of that care. In many cases the effects may be negative, by reducing the efficiency of nursing care processes, also called nursing workflow. Because workflow issues are so important, an entire chapter is devoted to the topic later in the book. However, a short description is warranted here to emphasize the role that nurses have when using health IT.

Quantitative research methods are often used to evaluate the implementation of informatics tools in nursing workflow, because these methods can describe details such as cost, time, and other factors that are often associated with health IT use in organizations. However, a more comprehensive understanding of the scope of health IT implementation in nursing workflow requires an assessment of the attitudes and perceptions of the nurses who will work directly with the technology. This type of information may be better captured with the use of qualitative research methods. In complex bedside procedures, such as the administration of intensive insulin therapy (IIT) in the patient with diabetes who is experiencing a hyperglycemic crisis, the use of a computer-assisted clinical decision-support system may be helpful. In a qualitative ethnographic study of 49 instances of nurses who used such a system embedded in a provider order-entry system to administer IIT to patients, researchers found that nurses felt that the documentation associated with use of the system presented a hindrance to patient care, but valued its ability to recommend insulin dosages based on their data input (Campion, Waitman, Lorenzi, May, & Gadd, 2011).

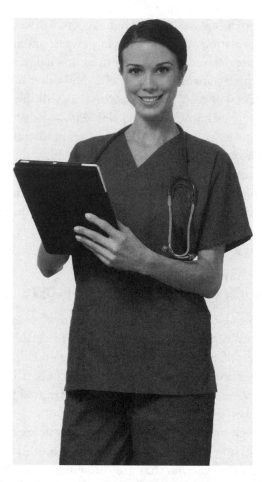

FIGURE 2-2   Describing the impact of health IT implementation upon nursing workflow necessitates assessment of nurses' attitudes and perceptions about the use of technology in patient care settings.
Source: © iStockphoto.com/EricHood

Health information exchanges (HIEs) are high-level systems that are designed to promote the rapid sharing of data across facilities. Although technological factors may certainly be essential in the success of an HIE, understanding how the HIE impacts users is also important. Unertl, Johnson, and Lorenzi (2012) conducted a 9-month qualitative ethnographic study, gathering data from six emergency departments and eight ambulatory clinics in the Southeastern United States. They found that HIEs were incorporated into workflow in user-specific roles; for example, nurses reported frequent access of HIEs to confirm patients' reports of care at other facilities within the exchange (Unertl, Johnson, & Lorenzi, 2012). Additional positive impacts of HIEs upon workflow were noted by participants in other ways, such as how they assist in medical decision making by supplying essential information when laypersons were unable to do so and facilitate referrals and transfers to other facilities.

In addition to providing practitioners with a more thorough dataset on which to base their clinical decisions, IT can be used to look at and improve the operating processes of organizations. These types of organizational improvements are often based on models of incremental change and analysis such as the Plan-Do-Study-Act (PDSA) model.

The **Plan-Do-Study-Act (PDSA)** model is a cyclical process that is made up of alternating phases of enacting changes and then assessing the effects of those changes (**Figure 2-3**). It is one of the models incorporated by the Institute for Healthcare Improvement (2012) as a framework in guides that organizations can adopt to promote system-wide changes. The first step of a PDSA cycle is to determine what

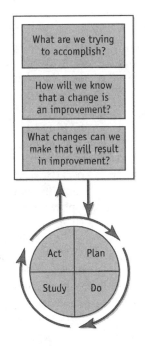

FIGURE 2-3   PDSA Model used in health care.

Source: http://www.ihi.org/knowledge/Pages/HowtoImprove/default.aspx. Reprinted by permission of Institute for Healthcare Improvement.

Box 2-2   Case Study: The Plan-Do-Study-Act Model

To illustrate how the PDSA Model works, consider the example of a particular group of residents. In this group, 34 residents took part in the Clinical Preventive Services Practice Improvement Model (CPS PIM) from July 2006 to June 2007. During their first block, each resident conducted five patient chart reviews, asked five patients to complete the CPS PIM patient survey, and met with clinic leaders to complete the CPS PIM systems survey (Oyler & Vinci, 2008). Once the data were amassed, they were broken down into groups. Data points included patient demographics, outcome measures (e.g., body mass index [BMI]), processes of care measures (e.g., whether height was recorded, whether a breast cancer screening was performed), and systems enhancements (e.g., whether records contained up-to-date medicine lists, if smoking cessation counseling was provided) (Oyler & Vinci, 2008). With the data broken down and categorized, the residents were able to easily see places where improvements could be made. In this case, the residents noticed that only 4% of patients met the goal for a BMI of less than 25, only 30% of patients' charts documented tobacco cessation counseling, and 20% of patients reported difficulty obtaining medication refills (Oyler & Vinci, 2008).

With key issues identified, the residents began to develop QI goals, which included: (1) increase the percentage of charts that had height recorded as a step to increase BMI screening, (2) increase the percentage of patients receiving smoking cessation counseling, and (3) improve the refill process. Once the goals were articulated, the residents were charged with developing and enacting a plan to achieve them and then reporting the results of their actions. To address the BMI issue, the residents worked with nurses to make height a part of their triage process, posted BMI charts throughout the clinic, and educated other residents on the importance of calculating and documenting BMI (Oyler & Vinci, 2008). These changes increased the documentation of height from 11% to 88%, and the documentation of BMI from 4% to 79%. To address the tobacco counseling problem, the residents again worked with the nursing staff, encouraging them to document smoking status and to provide patients who were currently smoking with a "readiness to quit" pamphlet. These changes improved documentation of smoking status from 41% to 67%. To address the problems with prescription refills, residents worked to educate other residents on how the prescription refill process works, placing a particular emphasis on the need to update the medication lists that the medication refill center uses whenever medication changes are made in the plan (Oyler & Vinci, 2008).

There are several important things to note from this example. From the very beginning, with the data-gathering phase, the goal was to get information on how the clinic operates from all viewpoints: from inside through looking at the charts, from the patient's view through the patient survey, and through the clinic management's view through the systems survey. This breadth of perspective is important because it shows that the different aspects of care are interrelated and interdependent. Along with a holistic view of the clinic, there must also be open and constructive communication between the different members of the team; the doctors and the nurses must be on the same page with each other, and also with the patients and the administrators. The problems to be addressed and the goals to be achieved should be well defined and specific so that they can be measured, and the plan of action must be understood and integrated by all the members of the team. The PDSA model is designed to be a continuous, cyclical process. As changes are implemented, they should be studied and analyzed and new changes should be planned and implemented on a consistent basis.

changes need to be made. Perhaps an HCP is not meeting benchmarks and needs to adjust his or her process to try to improve performance. Once the HCP knows what changes need to be made, he or she needs to determine how to measure the effectiveness of the changes. This could be achieved with any number of various metrics, depending on the specific situation. Once the HCP has a firm "Plan", the next step is to put it into action, or the "Do" phase. In this phase the changes are enacted and the HCP works for a set period of time with them in place. At the end of that time, the team comes together to study the results of the changes made in the "Do" phase. If the changes are found to be effective in addressing the issues defined in the "Plan" section, then the changes will be implemented permanently. If they are not, then the process begins again with a new planning stage.

The PDSA model shines because of its simplicity, but determining how to introduce it and utilize it in a clinical environment can be difficult. For this reason, the American Board of Internal Medicine (ABIM) created the CPS PIM (Oyler & Vinci, 2008). Given to internal medicine residents during their second postgraduate year, the CPS PIM is a quality assessment and improvement curriculum (QAIC) that is made up of two 1-month rotations. In the first month, the residents perform PIM chart reviews and patient and system surveys. During the second month, the data gathered are analyzed, and the residents use the PDSA cycle to enact changes that address areas where there is potential for QI (Oyler & Vinci, 2008).

QUALITY IMPROVEMENT TECHNIQUES AND NURSING INFORMATICS

Any system designed to assess and improve quality of care must begin with a thorough breakdown and understanding of the aims of the organization. The Institute of Medicine highlights six main aims of HCPs: effectiveness, safety, efficiency, patient-centeredness, timeliness, and equitability (Hughes, 2008). The QI system then must develop measures of quality that reflect these aims. Because of the complex and unpredictable nature of health care, measuring quality can be difficult; it is particularly hard to attribute the outcomes of treatment to any one particular cause. Another factor is whether an error or adverse event is likely to occur or is a rare, exceptional event (Hughes, 2008). Several groups have attempted to address this issue by researching, vetting, and endorsing measures of quality that have proven valid and reliable within a healthcare setting. The Agency for Healthcare Research and Quality (AHRQ) is the primary of these, and a breakdown of these measures can be found on its National Quality Measures Clearinghouse website (http://www.qualitymeasures.ahrq.gov/).

Using clinical guidelines, HCPs can begin to assess quality through benchmarking. With internal benchmarking, HCPs compare their current performance to their past performance. This is helpful in identifying best practices within an organization. In external benchmarking, performance is compared with those from other HCPs to see where it stands with respect to the community as a whole. Sources for comparative data for external benchmarking include the AHRQ's annual *National Healthcare Quality Report* and *National Healthcare Disparities Report*. There are also other more nursing-specific sources, such as the ANA's National Database of Nursing Quality Indicators (Hughes, 2008).

Quantitative measures of quality are useful, but they do not provide the entire picture. In order to use them to their fullest potential, a thorough understanding of the structures and processes that make up the workflow of the organization and an open and collaborative team approach to QI are vital. This is where continuous quality improvement (CQI) systems come in. With CQI systems, the belief is that there is always room for improvement in every aspect of the process. They are holistic systems that focus on every aspect of an organization and strive to make improvement the primary purpose of the organization. This includes defining processes, honing organizational management, working in teams, gathering and assessing data, and translating those assessments into changes in the function of the practice (Hughes, 2008). The continuous nature of these types of systems means constantly re-evaluating and assessing the changes made in the past. These systems are some of the most team-oriented, requiring a large commitment from the organization's leadership and its constituents, but can produce amazing results if implemented by a willing and committed staff. A detailed list of QI strategies and tools can be found at the AHRQ's website (http://www.innovations.ahrq.gov/innovations_qualitytools.aspx).

ONGOING EDUCATION AND NURSING INFORMATICS _____

Continuing education is required for all nurses to stay current in practice, meet their state-mandated continuing education units (CEUs), and fulfill requirements for certification/recertification in specialty practice. For example, 30 states in the United States require CEUs for renewal of the registered nurse (RN) license. Some states have special requirements for CEUs including education on human immunodeficiency virus/acquired immune deficiency syndrome, professional practice, pain management, bioterrorism, domestic violence, and reporting to public health authorities (ANA, 2011). For nurses with national certification in specialized nursing areas or in advanced practice roles, CEU requirements are more extensive and vary by the certification.

Table 2-2 Resources	
Resource	**Internet Address**
Agency for Healthcare Research and Quality: Quality Measures Website	http://www.qualitymeasures.ahrq.gov
Agency for Healthcare Research and Quality: Patient Safety Website	http://www.patientsafety.gov.
American Library Association Information Literacy Competency Standards for Higher Education	http://www.ala.org/ala/mgrps/divs/acrl/standards/informationliteracycompetency.cfm
American Nurses Association States Which Require Continuing Education for RN Licensure	http://nursingworld.org/MainMenuCategories/Policy-Advocacy/State/Legislative-Agenda-Reports/NursingEducation/CE-Licensure-Chart.pdf
ECDL Foundation	http://www.ecdl.org/programmes/ecdl_icdl
TIGER Initiative	http://www.tigersummit.com/About_Us.html

As clinical evidence rapidly evolves, an efficient means to gain access to education is available through the use of IT, particularly online programs offering CEUs (see **Table 2-2**). Many professional nursing organizations, for-profit companies, and universities offer quality educational material online (see the companion website to this text for resources). Nurses who wish to take CEUs by using online resources need to make sure that the CEUs will meet the requirements of state licensure or certification.

Online CEU offerings can take different forms: text documents with examination questions returned to CEU provider by email, fax, or U.S. mail; asynchronous webinars with embedded examination questions that upload to CEU providers; synchronous webinars with question-and-answer sessions; and interactive tutorials with embedded questions that upload to a CEU provider. The ANA hosts Twitter chats occasionally found at #ANAChat; nurses who Tweet can participate in the discussion and earn free CEUs. Podcasts are also methods by which nurses can obtain CEUs.

Even complete certificate programs are available online from organizations such as the Institute for Healthcare Improvement's *Open School*. Completion of a series of asynchronous tutorials in patient safety and QI provide, at the time of this writing,

26 hours of continuing education with a certificate of completion for nurses and other HCPs. Certainly, universities offer certificate programs online such as post-master's certificates in nursing education, **nursing informatics**, and geriatrics.

Other methods of professional development may not provide CEUs, but they can help clinicians stay abreast of developments in their areas of interest. For example,

---

Box 2-3   Case Study: Establishment and Utilization of the IT/Nursing Workflow Group

When change is inevitable for an organization, such as in a product, process, or pathway, it is in the best interests of the organization to include in the process of change those who would be defined as end users. The end user is someone who actually touches or uses whatever is being addressed. Involvement of end users assists in streamlining changes and creates an environment of appreciation and ownership that yields a greater volume of interest and increased morale.

Shannon's hospital is planning to upgrade the EHR admission assessment and charting workflow for nurses, and he is charged with getting direct care nurses involved in the process. Collaborative communication with a senior IT applications analyst resulted in a formal meeting for direct care nurses, held in a location away from the nursing units. Shannon schedules monthly meetings, allotting 4 to 5 hours for each, in order to provide an opportunity for the direct care nurses to voice concerns with the current charting and help make decisions regarding desired upgrades.

Several months before the scheduled upgrade, Shannon requested the nursing directors to ask each nursing manager to recruit a staff nurse to participate in the monthly meeting. Desired participants were described as direct care nurses who would be willing to speak up in a group of their peers and give honest input. Each would need to be proficient with EHR charting.

Each month the senior applications analyst worked with Shannon to establish an agenda for the meeting to coincide with the upgrade timeline. It was imperative that this group remained on task in order to meet the overall goal for the organization. Participation flourished in the beginning as workflow was redefined.

During the meetings prior to the upgrade, Shannon and the direct care nurses validated that there were several ways in which to chart multiple data elements. Identification of these multiple elements became a high priority, along with streamlining charting by nursing within the EHR. Duplication and cumbersome charting in the EHR were identified as nursing dissatisfiers, and as such became of high importance to nursing and hospital administration. The direct care nurses were glad to see that their concerns were heard and that they were trusted to work toward problem resolution.

Over the period of 9 months, Shannon was able to lead the direct care nursing workflow group in offering invaluable input into how nursing staff charts in the EHR. They minimized and streamlined charting pathways and gave input on the training materials for the upgrade roll out. Over time, staff nurse participation decreased and those who persisted brought vital worth to the project. These individuals also stepped up to assist in facilitating the education of their peers throughout the organization. This well-organized group created an improved charting path that was embraced by other bedside nurses throughout the hospital.

web-conferencing or voice over Internet with Skype or other methods can connect nurses to specialists in their areas of interest. With smartphones and/or Internet access, nurses can follow twitter feeds from universities, federal agencies, and well-respected healthcare organizations. From this simplest form to more complex adaptations, IT will remain an important means for nursing collaboration and maintaining continuing education.

SUMMARY

Nurses and other HCPs use health IT in all aspects of providing patient care. There is no choice about being competent with basic computer skills and with information management skills. The nursing informatics competencies are identified in *The Essentials of Baccalaureate Education for Professional Nursing Practice*, by the TIGER Initiative, and revised *Nursing Informatics: Scope and Standards of Practice* are under review at the writing of this book. Informatics competencies are required to improve nursing workflow and care delivery processes. Nurses who are competent users of technology can also keep themselves abreast of changes in practice by engaging in continuing education using interactive Internet- or mobile-based education.

For a full suite of assignments and additional learning activities, use the access code located in the front of your book and visit www.jblearning.com. If you do not have an access code, you can obtain one at the site.

REFERENCES

American Association of Colleges of Nursing. (2008). *The essentials of baccalaureate education for professional nursing practice*. Retrieved from http://www.aacn.nche.edu/education-resources/baccessentials08.pdf

American Nurses Association. (2011). *States which require continuing education for RN licensure*. Retrieved from http://nursingworld.org/MainMenuCategories/Policy-Advocacy/State/Legislative-Agenda-Reports/NursingEducation/CE-Licensure-Chart.pdf

Bartholomew, N. (2011). Is higher education ready for the information revolution? *International Journal of Therapy and Rehabilitation, 18*(10), 558–566.

Campion, J. R., Waitman, L. R., Lorenzi, N. M., May, A. K., & Gadd, C. S. (2011). Barriers and facilitators to the use of computer-based intensive insulin therapy. *Journal of International Medical Informatics, 80*, 863–871.

European Computer Driving License Qualifications. (2013). *About ECDL Foundation*. Retrieved from http://www.ecdl.org/index.jsp?p=93&n=94&a=3235

Gardner, C. L., & Jones, S. J. (2012). Utilization of academic electronic medical record in undergraduate nursing education. *Online Journal of Nursing Informatics (OJNI)*, *16*(2). Retrieved from http://ojni.org/issues/?/p=1702

Graves, J., & Corcoran, S. (1989). The study of nursing informatics. *Journal of Nursing Scholarship*, *21*(4), 227–231.

Hughes, R. G. (2008). Tools and strategies for quality improvement and patient safety. In R. G. Hughes (Ed.), *Patient safety and quality: An evidence-based handbook for nurses*. Rockville, MD: Agency for Healthcare Research and Quality. Retrieved from http://www.ahrq.gov/professionals/clinicians-providers/resources/nursing/resources/nurseshdbk/nurseshdbk.pdf

Institute for Healthcare Improvement. (2012). *How to improve*. Retrieved from http://www.ihi.org/knowledge/Pages/HowtoImprove/default.aspx

Oyler, J., & Vinci, L. (2008). Teaching internal medicine residents quality improvement techniques using the ABIM's practice improvement modules. *Journal of General Internal Medicine*, *23*(7), 927–930.

Technology Informatics Guiding Educational Reform (TIGER). (2009). *Collaborating to integrate evidence and informatics into nursing practice and education: An executive summary*. Retrieved from http://www.tigersummit.com/uploads/TIGER_Collaborative_Exec_Summary_040509.pdf

TIGER Initiative. (2007–2013). About TIGER. Retrieved from http://www.tigersummit.com/About_Us.html

Unertl, K. M., Johnson, K. B., & Lorenzi, N. M. (2012). Health information exchange technology on the frontline of healthcare: Workflow factors and patterns of use. *Journal of the American Medical Informatics Association*, 19, 392–400. doi:10.1136/amiajnl-2011-00043

CHAPTER 3

Informatics and Evidence-Based Practice

Janie T. Best, DNP, RN, ACNS-BC, CNL
Karen H. Frith, PhD, RN, NEA-BC

CHAPTER LEARNING OBJECTIVES

1. Apply knowledge of evidence-based practice (EBP) in patient care.
2. Search library databases efficiently to find current nursing research, systematic reviews, and clinical practice guidelines.
3. Subscribe to electronic resources for EBP including databases, journals, and professional organizations.
4. Understand how EBP can be integrated into electronic health records (EHRs) or other health information technology (health IT).

KEY TERMS

Agency for Healthcare Research and Quality (AHRQ)
Boolean operators
Centers for Disease Control and Prevention (CDC)
Cite while you write
Clinical decision-support systems (CDSS)
Cochrane Library
Cumulative Index to Nursing and Allied Health Literature (CINAHL)
Directory of Open Access Journals (DOAJ)
Evidence-based practice (EBP)
Google Scholar
Interlibrary loan
Literature search

Medical Subject Headings (MeSH)
My National Center for Biotechnology Information (My NCBI)
National Guideline Clearinghouse
National Library of Medicine (NLM)
Open access
Plan-Do-Study-Act (PDSA)
PubMed
PubMed Advanced Search Builder
PubMed Clinical Queries
PubMed LinkOut
PubMed sidebar filters
Rich Site Summary (RSS feeds)
Zotero

CHAPTER OVERVIEW

The skill of finding and appraising current evidence from research, systematic reviews of literature, and clinical practice guidelines can be difficult to transfer from academic to practice settings. However, **evidence-based practice (EBP)** is a core skill necessary to improve nursing care and enhance the safety of patients. This chapter provides a synopsis of EBP, describes the major steps associated with EBP, and supplies readers with resources to make evidence available even after graduation from academic programs. The transfer of EBP skills from academia to practice settings is possible with the aid of IT.

ESSENTIALS OF EVIDENCE-BASED PRACTICE

EBP is a process that has developed from a need to improve the quality and manage the economics of healthcare delivery (Salmond, 2007). The components of EBP include a systematic and critical evaluation of the current literature, the nurse's clinical expertise and available resources, and patients' values and preferences. This information is used to make deliberate clinical decisions based on theory and relevant research that guide patient care (Ahrens & Johnson, 2013; Ingersoll, 2000; Melnyk & Fineout-Overholt, 2011). The expected results of these carefully considered decisions are improved outcomes for patients, efficiency, and cost-effective care delivery for organizations (Melnyk & Fineout-Overholt, 2011; Salmond, 2007).

EBP PROCESS

Cultivating a Spirit of Inquiry

The process of EBP is best learned in sequence with distinct steps. The preliminary step, *cultivating a spirit of inquiry* (Melnyk, Fineout-Overholt, Stillwell, & Williamson, 2010, p. 51), means to be curious about the effectiveness of nursing interventions, to take interest in changing nursing practice or questioning practice, and to try new approaches. Nurses with a spirit of inquiry understand EBP as a way of thinking, not an additional burden to their practice. Nurses who are passionate about EBP will likely become informal leaders or be promoted to leadership positions and can influence others to grow support for EBP. Those who have a spirit of inquiry will have questions and a desire to find the best evidence to support their practice (Melnyk et al., 2010).

Writing the Question

Nurses who use the steps of EBP to formalize their questions about practice should use the PICOT format (Lawson, 2005; Melnyk & Fineout-Overholt, 2011). The term *PICOT* identifies the patient or population (P), issue or intervention (I), what will be compared (C), the expected outcome (O), and the time (T) that it will take to achieve and evaluate the outcome (Melnyk & Fineout-Overholt, 2011). The PICOT format is a systematic method of question writing and helps decrease the time and effort it takes to find evidence specific to the topic being investigated. Consistently using a set format to write the question ensures that all components of the question are addressed before the **literature search** begins (Stillwell, Fineout-Overholt, Melnyk, & Williamson, 2010).

It takes time and practice to learn how to write questions in the PICOT format. Melnyk and Fineout-Overholt (2011) suggest that it takes "practice, practice, practice" to become proficient in writing PICOT questions (p. 31). Questions may be written following a template and may focus on interventions, predictions or prognosis of outcomes for a specific patient population, comparison of diagnosis or diagnostic tests, etiology and associated risk factors for a specific condition, or meaning within a situation (Melnyk & Fineout-Overholt, 2011; Stillwell et al., 2010).

Nurses who embrace EBP may find support in forming groups interested in certain topics. Lawson (2005) suggests that getting other nurses involved helps to clarify clinical issues and to write clear and specific clinical questions. Once a group is assembled and the individuals are comfortable in identifying issues and writing questions, the second step, searching for evidence, can begin.

Finding the Evidence

Conducting a literature search may seem like a daunting task and overwhelming to those who have not had experience with electronic databases. While lack of access to an onsite library or computer database applications can be a major barrier to conducting a search for evidence, the inability of a nurse to effectively use the computer to search the literature adds an additional barrier to embracing EBP (Hoss & Hanson, 2008; Wells, Free, & Adams, 2007). Nurses without computer skills or experience in data searches can seek assistance from a university or hospital librarian, or other experienced professionals (Fain, 2009). Links to tutorials and videos for using commonly accessed databases can be found in the companion website for this text.

Nurses should use databases and websites that have valid and reliable information. **PubMed** and **Cumulative Index to Nursing and Allied Health Literature (CINAHL)** are two databases that index a comprehensive body of healthcare literature. The **Cochrane Library** and the **National Guideline Clearinghouse** support EBP by including systematic reviews and current practice guidelines. Government sources of reliable information include the **Centers for Disease Control and Prevention (CDC)** and the **Agency for Healthcare Research and Quality (AHRQ)**. Many professional organizations make their journals and evidence-based guidelines available electronically for members or individuals who have subscribed online (Fineout-Overholt, Berryman, Hofstetter, & Sollenberger, 2011; Hoss & Hanson, 2008). Guidance about how to use these resources is provided later in the chapter.

To begin the search of PubMed or CINAHL, nurses should select key terms using the PICOT question. These terms are entered into a library database using **Boolean operators** ("and," "or," "not") to combine the terms into phrases. A good search technique is to set limits on the search to improve selection of articles that are specific to the topic. For example, limiting selections to English language, peer-reviewed journals, and articles published within the last 5 years can help in the selection of valid findings that may be applicable to the topic (Hoss & Hanson, 2008; Melnyk & Fineout-Overholt, 2011).

Analyzing the Literature

Not all evidence is equal, nor will all evidence be applicable to a particular clinical setting. When searching for evidence, it is prudent to look for clinical practice guidelines, systematic reviews, meta-analyses of evidence, or randomized controlled trials relevant to the particular clinical question. Single studies or case studies can be used to demonstrate how evidence is put into practice, and textbooks can be used as resources for information on a particular condition. Most nursing research and EBP textbooks will have guides to help evaluate the quality of quantitative and qualitative research studies (Fineout-Overholt et al., 2011; Levin, 2013). The American Nurses Association (ANA) has developed a list of resources to help nurses evaluate the quality of research studies. These tools address the validity of the study, reliability of the results, and the applicability to the particular patient care setting.

Putting the EBP Process into Practice

Once the literature is analyzed using a systematic approach, nurses working on an EBP project will need to decide if a change in practice is needed. If so, then creating enthusiasm for the project and soliciting input from all stakeholders early in the planning stages will be critical. Early and frequent communication by email or other innovative communication strategies such as Twitter, Facebook, or blogging can keep stakeholders involved.

As with any change, a plan needs to be prepared. A theoretical model or process, such as **Plan-Do-Study-Act (PDSA)**, can be used as a framework to plan and implement the project. A timeline for the project is essential to keep it on track. Even strategies to overcome barriers to the planned change need to be included. Selecting an evaluation strategy as part of the initial project plan is also necessary (Melnyk & Fineout-Overholt, 2011). The plan must address any ethical issues and protected health information issues by seeking institutional review board (IRB) approval for the project (Levin, 2013). The project plan can be made using a Microsoft Excel spreadsheet or specific software for project planning such as Microsoft Project. Following the timeline and sharing the project results during implementation will help other nurses and stakeholders remain engaged in the practice change (Lawson, 2005).

Communicating the Findings

Once the practice change is stable, the final step of EBP is to share the result with others. Failure to share the outcomes of EBP projects may lead to unwarranted duplication and delay in getting evidence into practice throughout the practice setting and beyond. Results can be disseminated to the organization at staff meetings, in a nursing newsletter, via a blog post, or as a poster presentation. Findings should be presented at local specialty group meetings or at regional or national conferences (Melnyk et al., 2010). Nurses can also partner with local schools or colleges of nursing to create an Evidence-Based Practice Day, during which nurses from various clinical settings share the results of their projects.

FINDING MORE ABOUT EBP ONLINE _____

Because this chapter provides only a brief overview of EBP, Internet-based resources can be used to supplement knowledge of EBP (see **Table 3-1**). The ANA provides a list of online tutorials that can assist nurses in learning more about EBP, and the University of North Carolina also has free EBP tutorials available for nurses who seek information about the EBP process. These resources can be found on the companion website for this text.

Table 3-1 Resources to Learn About EBP	
Tutorials	**Internet Address**
Appraising the Evidence	http://nursingworld.org/MainMenuCategories/ThePracticeofProfessionalNursing/Improving-Your-Practice/Research-Toolkit/Appraising-the-Evidence
American Nurses Association (ANA) list of online tutorials about EBP	http://ana.nursingworld.org/research-toolkit/Education
University of North Carolina EBP tutorials	http://www.hsl.unc.edu/Services/Tutorials/EBM/welcome.htm
Academic Center for Evidence-Based Practice at the University of Texas Health Science Center at San Antonio	http://acestar.uthscsa.edu/modules/Basic.htm
	http://acestar.uthscsa.edu/modules/Intermediate.htm
Basic Module	
Intermediate Module	

USING LIBRARY SOURCES AFTER GRADUATION

One of the greatest skills that nurses learn in academic programs is the ability to find relevant research on clinical topics. Time spent with a librarian who loves to teach others how to find the treasure troves of information is priceless and will return a lifetime of information power. However, after students leave their colleges and universities, access to databases such as CINAHL depends on the resources available at nurses' places of employment. For those in academic medical centers, access to databases may be assured; those in community hospitals or ambulatory settings will likely find themselves disconnected from the very lifeline of EBP—a library.

PubMed

There are ways to access libraries free or at low costs for individual nurses. The best place to start is a search of PubMed, which is freely available online. As a service of the **National Library of Medicine (NL)**, PubMed is an extensive index of published medical literature with more than 22 million citations. Nursing literature is indexed in this service too.

Most nurses used CINAHL in their undergraduate programs, but PubMed is searched in a different manner from CINAHL. Rather than using key words, PubMed is searched using **Medical Subject Headings (MeSH)**, which are part of a controlled

Previous Indexing:

- Apnea (1966-1979)
- Sleep (1966-1979)
- Sleep Apnea Syndromes (1980-1999)

  All MeSH Categories

  Diseases Category

  Respiratory Tract Diseases

  Respiration Disorders

  Apnea

  Sleep Apnea Syndromes

  Sleep Apnea, Obstructive

  Obesity Hypoventilation Syndrome

All MeSH Categories

Diseases Category

Nervous System Diseases

Sleep Disorders

Dyssomnias

Sleep Disorders, Intrinsic

Sleep Apnea Syndromes

Sleep Apnea, Obstructive

Obesity Hypoventilation Syndrome

FIGURE 3-1   MeSH tree of obstructive sleep apnea produced from search of Pubmed.
Source: http://www.ncbi.nlm.nih.gov/pubmed

vocabulary thesaurus. Once MeSH terms are found for the topic, a more fruitful yield will result from searches of PubMed. **Figure 3-1** shows a MeSH tree for obstructive sleep apnea. Other features of PubMed are the PubMed Advanced Search Builder, sidebar filters, LinkOut, and My NCBI.

The MeSH terms selected should be entered into the **PubMed Advanced Search Builder**, the open boxes in PubMed. The drop-down menus can then be set to MeSH terms, and Boolean operators should be used as needed. If the yield is too high for a reasonable review of articles, then the **PubMed sidebar filters** can be added, including article types (clinical trials, systematic reviews, practice guidelines, etc.), text availability (abstract available, free full text available, or full text available), and publication dates. The filters will limit the search to a number that is more manageable. When the desired articles are selected, some full-text articles may be freely available using the **PubMed LinkOut** service. LinkOut is found in the upper right-hand corner of the screen. To find the desired reference material, the LinkOut icon should be clicked. Icons change depending on the source of the reference material. If the full text is not available, nurses can order it from their hospitals or from public libraries using **interlibrary loan** services. Typically, a public library will have a nominal charge for an interlibrary loan.

Searches of PubMed should be managed well so that the MeSH terms and the yields from searches can be retrieved if needed. PubMed provides a cloud-based folder called **My National Center for Biotechnology Information (My NCBI)** for searching and storing the history of searches. Up to 6 months of search histories can be stored in My NCBI. Registration and use are free. Written tutorials and short videos provide excellent help for nurses who are new to PubMed. Some of the most helpful tutorials and videos are listed in **Table 3-2**.

Google Scholar

Google Scholar is a web-based search engine for scholarly literature across a broad range of disciplines. Its index includes literature from free and paid repositories, professional societies, academic publishers, and other sources across the web. The primary focus is to index all academic papers on the web (via Google). While there is no doubt of the value of the service for researchers of all kinds, it also has its shortcomings. Google takes articles from everywhere it can access them on the web, so users must be careful to vet the articles they find using Google Scholar because the articles may or may not be peer reviewed. One particularly celebrated and useful feature of Google Scholar is the "cited by" feature, which allows users to view the abstracts of papers that have cited the paper they are currently using. This ability to connect literature through citations has historically been available only through paid services. A particularly pervasive shortcoming of the service is that it strengthens the *Matthew Effect*, a term coined by sociologist Robert Merton to refer to the way in which starting advantages tend to build on themselves (Rigney, 2010). With Google Scholar this is seen in the way that articles with more citations are more likely to be at the top of the search results, and newer articles with fewer citations are more likely to be lower on the page and thus less likely to be read and used (Beel & Gipp, 2009). Google Scholar is an unbelievably valuable resource for researchers of all kinds, but as is true with all research tools, it is the responsibility of researchers to verify the veracity of any sources they use.

Table 3-2   PubMed Tutorials and Videos: Learn How to Search Efficiently for Articles

Tutorials	Internet Address
PubMed Tutorial	http://www.nlm.nih.gov/bsd/disted/pubmedtutorial/
Medical Subject Headings (MeSH®) in MEDLINE®/PubMed®: A Tutorial	http://www.nlm.nih.gov/bsd/disted/meshtutorial/introduction/index.html
Branching Out: The MeSH® Vocabulary	http://www.nlm.nih.gov/bsd/disted/video/
Videos	
My NCBI–National Center for Biotechnology Information	http://www.youtube.com/watch?v=ks46w3mNAQE
PubMed Simple Subject Search	http://www.nlm.nih.gov/bsd/viewlet/search/subject/subject.html
PubMed Author Search	http://www.nlm.nih.gov/bsd/viewlet/search/author/author.html
Getting Full-text Articles from PubMed	http://www.youtube.com/watch?v=V0NYKFSphKY
Using Sidebar Filters to Limit Results	http://www.youtube.com/watch?v=696R9GbOyvA&feature=youtu.be
Advanced PubMed Search Builder	http://www.youtube.com/watch?v=dncRQ1cobdc&feature=relmfu
Save Search Results in Collections, including Favorites	http://www.youtube.com/watch?v=iXSttEKntCE
Searching by using the MeSH Database	http://www.youtube.com/watch?v=uyF8uQY9wys
Search for Journal in PubMed	http://www.nlm.nih.gov/bsd/viewlet/search/journal/journal.html
Retrieving Citations from a Journal Issue	http://www.nlm.nih.gov/bsd/viewlet/search/scm/scmissue.html
Selecting Outside Tool Preference	http://www.nlm.nih.gov/bsd/viewlet/myncbi/pref_otool.html

Open Access Journals

Freely available articles are provided by publishers who offer **open access**. The rationale for providing free, online access to scholarly articles and research is to advance scientific thought, particularly for individuals in developing countries who cannot afford the high prices of journal subscriptions (Carroll, 2011). The cost of publication is shifted to authors, rather than readers. While this makes research available, nurses must ensure that they are selecting articles from peer-reviewed journals. Journals that are open access can be found by searching online for the **Directory of Open Access Journals (DOAJ)**. A particular advantage of the DOAJ is that it gives smaller publications a way to expand their reach. Nurses should always be vigilant about the quality of their sources, but they should not neglect open access journals, because they often have research from more varied sources and in smaller research niches.

Systematic Reviews and Clinical Practice Guidelines

Systematic reviews are literature reviews that follow a certain methodology to standardize the critique of research findings. Two excellent sources of systematic reviews are McMaster Plus Nursing + Best Evidence for Nursing Care and the Cochrane Collaboration. McMaster Plus has three functions: It serves as a database of peer-reviewed articles that have been rated by nursing professionals, it provides an email alert system for selected topics of interest, and it provides links to abstracts of systematic reviews of research literature. The Cochrane Collaboration is a library built by healthcare professionals who author Cochrane Reviews, which are the gold standard for pre-appraised research evidence. Only a few Cochrane Reviews are free; most are contained in the Cochrane Database of Systematic Reviews and are available with a subscription. Nurses can join the Cochrane Journal Club and other electronic notifications of systematic reviews and clinical practice guidelines at no cost. **Table 3-3** provides a list of resources and websites.

Table 3-3   Electronic Alerts for Systematic Reviews and Clinical Practice Guidelines

Resource	Internet Address
McMaster Plus, British Medical Journal Updates	http://plus.mcmaster.ca/EvidenceUpdates/
PubMed	http://www.nlm.nih.gov/bsd/viewlet/myncbi/jourup.htm
Knowledge Finder from the National Library of Medicine	http://www1.kfinder.com/newweb/
	https://revolution1.kfinder.com/csnw/register/regform.html
Cochrane Library Journal Club Scroll to bottom to find sign-up form	http://www.cochranejournalclub.com/self-monitoring-and-self-management-oral-anticoagulation-clinical/default.asp?moreinfo=1#moreinformation
National Guideline Clearinghouse Email Alerts	http://www.guideline.gov/subscribe.aspx

Table 3-4 Repositories of Clinical Practice Guidelines	
Resource	**Internet Address**
Agency for Healthcare Research and Quality (AHRQ)	http://www.ahrq.gov/clinic/cpgsix.htm
AHRQ Innovations Exchange	http://www.innovations.ahrq.gov/innovations_qualitytools.aspx
National Guideline Clearinghouse	http://www.guideline.gov/
PubMed Clinical Queries	http://www.ncbi.nlm.nih.gov/entrez/query/static/clinical.shtml
National Institute for Health and Clinical Excellence (NICE) Organization	http://www.nice.org.uk/
McMaster Plus Nursing + Best Evidence for Nursing Care	http://plus.mcmaster.ca/np/Default.aspx

Clinical guidelines are valuable because they contain pre-appraised research. Authors of clinical practice guidelines rate the research for the quality of evidence and the strength of making a recommendation for change based on the findings. The federal government provides at least three sources of free clinical practice guidelines at the AHRQ, the National Guideline Clearinghouse, and the **PubMed Clinical Queries**. **Table 3-4** provides the URLs for the free resources for clinical practice guidelines.

USING REFERENCE MANAGER SOFTWARE TO STORE AND USE SOURCES

Nurses who plan to carry out formal EBP projects need to learn how to manage the results of their searches using software. This is particularly critical if the nurse plans to communicate findings in poster sessions or in published articles. Without software, the research articles, systematic reviews of literature, and clinical practice guidelines can become stacks of paper with little or no organization. Fortunately there are free software solutions: **Zotero** and Mendeley. In order to use Zotero, the Internet browser Mozilla Firefox must first be downloaded and installed. Next, the Zotero add-on will need to be downloaded and installed. Once Zotero is added on to Mozilla Firefox, any results from searches of PubMed, CINAHL, or Google Scholar can be saved. The add-in of Zotero for Microsoft Word (and other word-processing programs) provides the ability to **cite while you write**. This tool is the real magic of reference software. When a reference is selected in Zotero, with the click of one icon, the reference is cited in the narrative and added to a reference list in the word-processing document. Any changes are automatically reflected in the in-text citations and reference list. Finally, references can be shared using a sharing feature in Zotero. This feature is for teams of nurses focused on EBP. Mendeley works in a similar manner, is fully compatible with Windows and Mac operating systems, and can work with any Internet browser.

STAYING CURRENT IN NURSING PRACTICE AND SPECIALTY AREAS _____

Email Notifications

It is impossible to read enough journals to stay current with the short shelf life of most research. Using technology to stay current is a smart decision. With registration at journal publishers' websites, email notifications will be sent when new content is available. Publishers send a table of contents with every issue of the journal. Links from the table of contents often provide an abstract. If an interesting journal article is in the table of contents, then the nurse can order the article using interlibrary loan if it is not available from other sources. **Table 3-5** lists journal publishers who provide free email notifications.

Rich Site Summary (RSS)

Rich Site Summaries (RSS feeds) are simplified summaries of the information provided on whole websites. For example, an RSS feed of the CNN website would show

Table 3-5 Electronic Subscriptions to Journal Email Notifications	
Resource	**Internet Address**
RSS Feeds for Nursing Journals	http://www.nursingcenter.com/rss/rssfeed.asp
Mobile CINAHL	http://www.ebscohost.com/academic/mobile-access
Lippincott Williams & Wilkins Email Alerts	http://journals.lww.com/pages/login.aspx?ContextUrl=%2fsecure%2fpages%2fmyaccount.aspx
Sage Publishers Email Alerts	http://www.sagepub.com/emailAlerts.sp?_DARGS=/common/components/extras_big.jsp.1_A&_DAV=dummy&_dynSess-Conf=1994759084613409176
Springer Publishing Email Alerts	http://www.springerpub.com/products/Journals/Nursing#.UdjEufnVCQo

a list of all the stories on the page. RSS feeds provide a clear and easy way of tracking information from a large number of sources, and nurses should be aware of the wealth of information available to them through RSS feeds. Some notable sources of feeds include the National Institutes of Health, the Food and Drug Administration, the CDC, and the AHRQ. The U.S. government web portal provides a large index of these feeds on its website (http://www.usa.gov).

Social Media

Social media includes Facebook, Twitter, LinkedIn, and all the other similar services. In health care, social media has not been a widely used tool, but that may be starting to change. Social media services help people to connect, share their experiences, develop groups, and communicate more effectively. For a healthcare provider (HCP) that might mean instant-messaging services between patients and nurses or doctors, or video conference–based appointments. It could also mean social networks specific to nurses and doctors where opportunities, research, and wisdom could be shared. A free EHR system called hellohealth (http://hellohealth. com/patients/) is used by a Brooklyn-based practice that provides a model for this type of integration (Hawn, 2009). The practice has developed a patient-management platform where patients can communicate with their HCPs via private instant-messaging, schedule video-chat appointments, renew prescriptions, and access their own personal health record (Hawn, 2009). As the landscape continues to develop and these tools evolve, nurses will have to adapt. By focusing on the improved communication enabled by social media, nurses will be able to build communities and share their experiences and wisdom.

Webinars and Teleconferences

Communication technologies, particularly Internet-based communications, have opened up new ways for nurses to engage with one another to learn about the best practices in patient care. Technologies such as Skype, Google + Hangout, and join. me offer low-cost or free services to connect multiple people via audio, video, and desktop sharing. When used in continuing education or webinars, nurses can participate with experts on clinical topics anywhere Internet service is available. Sortedahl (2012) developed an online journal club for school nurses and assessed nurses' satisfaction with the method after 3 months. Sortedahl found that the nurses valued three key elements: having well-informed, knowledgeable moderators; getting research articles in advance; and discussing the application of findings to nursing practice. The researcher also found that using Internet-based technology allowed the journal club to invite the author of a research article to the club meeting, which benefited the researcher and nurses. There were issues with slow Internet connections, firewalls and other security measures, and operating system incompatibilities. Despite the technical issues, the nurses liked the method and wanted even more interaction with each other between journal club meetings (Sortedahl, 2012).

EVIDENCE-BASED PRACTICE INTEGRATED IN CLINICAL DECISION-SUPPORT SYSTEMS

The most efficient means for integrating EBP into clinical processes is to embed a **clinical decision-support system (CDSS)** in health IT. CDSSs are computer systems designed to impact clinical decision making about individual patients at the moment those decisions are made (Berner & La Jande, 2007) by presenting contextually appropriate information. CDSSs bring the available, applicable knowledge and research together into systems that clinicians can use throughout the decision-making process. The key aspect is that the usefulness comes from the interaction of the human and the computer. Modern CDSSs are not designed as black boxes that interpret information and deliver concrete answers, but as tools to provide the clinician with the best possible evidence relevant to the patient's assessment data and laboratory results to ensure the patient receives the best possible care (Berner & La Jande, 2007).

Most CDSSs are made up of three essential components: the knowledge base, the reasoning engine, and a mechanism to communicate with the user (Berner & La Jande, 2007). The knowledge base contains all the relevant knowledge expressed as if-then rules. The reasoning engine contains a set of instructions that tell the computer how to apply the rules to real patient data. The communication mechanism provides the means for patient data to be entered into the system and for any pertinent findings to be relayed to the user. Many CDSSs rely on the user to input data manually, but the continued acceptance of EHRs and improved interoperability among systems will enable more systems to input data automatically from multidisciplinary team members (Berner & La Jande, 2007).

Commercially available EHRs typically have a CDSS, but the system may need to be customized for use in the particular healthcare setting. Nurses and other healthcare providers need to be involved in the development of CDSSs, because the systems should reflect the best *clinical* decisions, and healthcare providers are equipped to translate clinical research into clinical processes through a reasoning engine in the EHR (Brokel, 2009). In a very basic way, order sets and nursing plans of care in EHRs represent clinical decision support because the predetermined orders are used to simplify the cognitive processes necessary for planning care. When order sets and nursing plans of care are developed, nurses can influence the process by serving on a task force to develop the CDSS by bringing research evidence and clinical practice guidelines to this decision-making group. In this way, nurses contribute to implementation of EBP (Brokel, 2009).

The use of sophisticated CDSSs, developed by multidisciplinary teams, is an efficient way to translate research evidence into everyday practice. However, the steps involved in the appraisal of evidence cannot be missed. It would be irresponsible to take current practice and automate the clinical decisions based on status quo. Likewise, it would be imprudent to base care on a single research article. Nurses and other healthcare providers need to take the time to examine their current practices with respect to best practices when EHRs or other health IT are implemented.

Case Study: Using Technology to Serve Up Best Practices in Transplant Care

Researchers at the University of Alabama in Huntsville developed a web portal and mobile app for HCPs who specialize in transplant (Alexander et al., 2013). Because transplant centers are dispersed across the United States, these HCPs need methods to communicate, collaborate, and learn from one another. The team tested the portal and reported what HCPs liked and what they would suggest for the portal's future development. Using the case in **Box 3-1**, readers can experience some of the tools in the Transplant Professionals' Portal.

Box 3-1   Case Study

A nurse practitioner working in transplantation is preparing for rounds with the surgical team. While seeing Ms. F in clinic, she notices some change in weight. She will need to report BMI at the end of rounds. Ms. F is a 61-year-old who is 61 inches tall and weighs 187 pounds. Her serum creatinine is 2.1.

1. What is her BMI?
2. What is Ms. F's creatinine clearance?

Go to the web portal: http://tpp.uah.edu/
Or download the transplant app for apple or android
Apple http://itunes.apple.com/us/app/transplantpro/id512387289?ls=1&mt=8
Android https://play.google.com/store/apps/details?id=com.itsc.transplantpro

SUMMARY

Nurses learn about EBP while enrolled in nursing programs, but EBP should be used in healthcare settings to transform traditional practices into ones supported by the best scientific evidence. Nurses can get access to primary research, systematic reviews, and clinical practice guidelines by using IT effectively. Information management strategies are essential and include subscribing to RSS feeds, registering for email alerts from journal publishers and from government resources, and purchasing subscriptions to services that provide EBP support. Finally, nurses should advocate for the selection of health IT that has best practices as an integrated feature. Technology can make EBP more seamless for nurses and fulfill the need to improve patient care.

For a full suite of assignments and additional learning activities, use the access code located in the front of your book and visit www.jblearning.com. If you do not have an access code, you can obtain one at the site.

REFERENCES

Ahrens, S., & Johnson, C. S. (2013). Finding the way to evidence-based practice. *Nursing Management, 44*(5), 23–27. doi: 10.1097/01.NUMA.0000429009.93011.ea

Alexander, S., Hoy, H., Maskey, M., Conover, H., Gamble, J., & Fraley, A. M. (2013). Initiating collaboration among organ transplant professionals through web portals and mobile applications. *Online Journal of Issues in Nursing, 18*(3). doi: 10.3912/OJIN.Vol18No02PPT03

Beel, J., & Gipp, B. (2009). Google Scholar's ranking algorithm: An introductory overview. In B. Larse & J. Leta (Eds.), *Proceedings of the 12th International Conference on Scientometrics and Informetrics* (ISSI '09, Vol. 1, pp. 230–241), Rio De Janeiro, Brazil. International Society for Scientometrics and Informetrics. Retrieved from http://www.sciplore.org/publications/2009-Google_Scholar%27s_Ranking_Algorithm_--_An_Introductory_Overview_--_preprint.pdf

Berner, E., & La Jande, T. (2007). Overview of clinical decision support systems. In E. Berner (Ed.), *Clinical decision support systems: Theory and practice* (2nd ed., pp. 4–18). New York, NY: Springer.

Brokel, J. M. (2009). Infusing clinical decision support interventions into electronic health records. *Urologic Nursing, 29*(5), 345–353.

Carroll, M. W. (2011). Why full open access matters. *PLoS Biol, 9*(11), e1001210. doi:10.1371/journal.pbio.1001210

Fain, J. A. (2009). *Reading, understanding, and applying nursing research* (4th ed.). Philadelphia, PA: F. A. Davis.

Fineout-Overholt, F., Berryman, D. R., Hofstetter, S., & Sollenberger, J. (2011). Finding relevant evidence to answer clinical questions. In B. M. Melnyk & E. Fineout-Overholt (Eds.), *Evidence based practice in nursing & healthcare: A guide to best practice* (2nd ed.). Philadelphia, PA: Lippincott Williams & Wilkins.

Hawn, C. (2009). Take two aspirin and Tweet me in the morning: How Twitter, Facebook, and Other social media are reshaping healthcare. *Health Affairs, 28*(2), 361–368. Retrieved from http://content.healthaffairs.org/content/28/2/361.full#sec-6

Hoss, B., & Hanson, D. (2008). Evaluating the evidence: Web sites. *AORN Journal, 87*(1), 124–141.

Ingersole, G. L. (2000). Evidence-based nursing: What it is and what it isn't. *Nursing Outlook, 48*(4), 151–152. doi:10.1067/mno.2000.107690

Lawson, P. (2005). How to bring evidence-based practice to the bedside. *Nursing, 35*(1), 18–19.

Levin, R. F. (2013). Searching the sea of evidence: It takes a library. In R. F. Levin & H. R. Feldman (Eds.), *Teaching evidence-based practice in nursing* (2nd ed., pp. 103–118). New York, NY: Springer.

Melnyk, B. M., & Fineout-Overholt, E. (2011). *Evidence-based practice in nursing and healthcare: A guide to best practice* (2nd ed.). Philadelphia, PA: Lippincott Williams & Wilkins.

Melnyk, B. M., Fineout-Overholt, E., Stillwell, S. B., & Williamson, K. M. (2010). The seven steps of evidence-based practice. *American Journal of Nursing, 10*(1), 51–53.

Rigney, D. (2010). *What is the Matthew effect?* Retrieved from http://cup.columbia.edu/book/978-0-231-14948-8/the-matthew-effect/excerpt

Salmond, S. W. (2007). Advancing evidence-based practice: A primer. *Orthopaedic Nursing, 26*(2), 114–123.

Sortedahl, C. (2012). Effect of online journal club on evidence-based practice knowledge, intent, and utilization in school nurses. *Worldviews on Evidence-Based Nursing, 9*(2), 117–125. doi: 10.1111/j.1741-6787.2012.00249.x

Stillwell, S. B., Fineout-Overholt, E., Melnyk, B. M., & Williamson, K. M. (2010). Asking the clinical question: A key step in evidence-based practice. *American Journal of Nursing, 110*(3), 58–61.

Wells, N., Free, M., & Adams, R. (2007). Nursing research internship: Enhancing evidence-based practice among staff nurses. *Journal of Nursing Administration, 37*(3), 135–143.

Use of Clinical Informatics in Care Support Roles

CHAPTER 4

Human Factors in Computing

Steffi Kreuzfeld, MD
Regina Stoll, MD

CHAPTER LEARNING OBJECTIVES

1. Define ergonomics and associated concepts as applied in healthcare settings.
2. Describe the importance of understanding human factors in healthcare settings.
3. Know the key International Organization for Standardization (ISO) standards for ergonomic principles and design of work settings.
4. Comprehend the influence of work systems on the nurses' physical and psychological health.
5. Analyze information systems and computer applications with regard to human–computer interactions.

KEY TERMS

Anthropometry
Dialogue
Ergonomics
Graphical user interface (GUI)
Hardware ergonomics
Human–computer interaction (HCI)
Information processing
Interactivity
International Organization for
Standardization (ISO)

Natural user interfaces
Selective attention
Software ergonomics
Task design for individuality
User interface
Visual display terminal (VDT)
Voice user interfaces
Workload
Work systems

CHAPTER OVERVIEW

Computer systems and computer applications are used in all areas of life from leisure to work. The systems range from computer workstations, notebooks, and smartphones to networked household appliances and medical devices. To allow humans to comfortably interact with the various applications in a safe and efficient manner, ergonomic principles must be applied. This chapter describes the physiological, psychological, and social aspects of human interaction with computer systems and the effects of computer technology on people at work, particularly in healthcare settings.

INTRODUCTION

Humans and computers form a complex sociotechnical **work system**. If they are to distribute their workloads in a meaningful manner, the different qualities and abilities of human and machine must be considered. The human recognizes problems and can draw on wide-ranging general and specific knowledge in various areas to combine knowledge with experience to creatively apply them to problem solving. The human is capable of complex decisions and accepting the resulting responsibility. For example, nurses have knowledge, skills, and values developed by completing collegiate education in nursing, participating in continuing education, and by practicing in work settings. Nurses, equipped with education and experience, make complex decisions in noisy, fast-paced work environments that have consequences for the safety of patients in their care.

In contrast, computer systems can process huge amounts of data quickly and error free, repeat similar tasks multiple times without fatigue, extract important information, and exclude irrelevant data. Computers can function under extreme conditions and endure factors that would be detrimental to human health (Dul & Weerdenmeester, 2008).

The conditions under which humans work constitute significant factors that influence health and wellbeing as well as productivity and successful outcomes of work. The individual performance of the human is determined, on one hand, by external performance-shaping factors such as work environment, assigned task, technical feasibilities, time constraints, and modes of cooperation. On the other hand, it is also influenced by internal performance-shaping factors such as physical and psychological states of the human. Computer applications that are well suited to humans can ease and enrich human performance. Standards, laws, and recommendations can be used to create a framework to prevent humans from sustaining lasting harm by their work.

HUMAN FACTORS/ERGONOMICS (HFE)

In 2000, the International Ergonomics Association (IEA) defined **ergonomics** as follows:

> Ergonomics (or human factors) is the scientific discipline concerned with the understanding of the interactions among humans and other elements of a system, and the profession that applies theoretical principles, data and methods to design in order to

optimize human well being and overall system performance. Practitioners of ergonomics, ergonomists, contribute to the planning, design and evaluation of tasks, jobs, products, organizations, environments and systems in order to make them compatible with the needs, abilities and limitations of people.

The term *ergonomics* derives from the Greek words *ergon* (work) and *nomos* (law) and describes the systematic study of all aspects of human activity as it relates to work. Ergonomics is a dynamic, interdisciplinary field of study that continuously evolves through new insights into the interaction between humans and work (Wilson, 2000). It differentiates itself from other fields of study through its direct applicability. Ergonomics is central to safety programs in many different fields including manufacturing, aerospace, and health care. The application of ergonomics in health care is gaining attention in the United States as a result of reports by the Institute of Medicine (IOM, 1999, 2004, 2011).

As new knowledge is applied, it should lead to greater humanization of work. This implies that the human is at the center and that the work is being adapted to human needs, not the other way around. Besides increased safety, health, and comfort for the worker, there are also economic considerations included among the target parameters of applied ergonomics. Productivity, quality, and efficiency can be improved by applying ergonomic production processes, and costs can be lowered by decreasing work-related illnesses and illness-related absences from work (Dul et al., 2012). For example, in the United States, the economic influence of properly applied ergonomics can result in better reimbursement from the Centers for Medicare and Medicaid Services (CMS) because adverse events, many of which are caused by mismatch of technology to human factors, can be reduced (Amarasingham, Plantinga, Diener-West, Gaskin, & Powe, 2009; CMS, 2008).

The second part of the IEA definition of ergonomics indicates the breadth of the spectrum of research in ergonomics: It spans from capturing work content and organizational aspects of work, to environmental factors, to consideration of physical and psychological factors and limitations that humans face as they interact with various work equipment. Ergonomics requires specialized education. The disciplines involved are primarily occupational science, human and social sciences, the humanities, computer and design science, and industrial engineering. In the United States, a subspecialty called human factors engineering contributes to knowledge generation through research and improvements in work environments by application of research to healthcare settings.

There are different areas of ergonomics, each with its own focus. For example, in physical ergonomics the health consequences of working posture and repetitive motions are studied as the origins of musculoskeletal disorders. Organizational ergonomics deals with the optimization of work processes and structures, such as time management, teamwork, communication within an organization, telecommuting, and quality control. In contrast, the area of cognitive ergonomics focuses on such issues as cognitive and memory processes in the human brain, decision making, recognition and elimination of work-related stress, reliability of human actions, and human–computer interactions (HCI).

STANDARDS, LAWS, RECOMMENDATIONS, AND STYLE GUIDES

A part of the ergonomic knowledge has been summarized and recorded by way of standards, laws, and recommendations. International standards are issued by the **International Organization for Standardization (ISO)**. They are based on firmly established scientific principles and are determined on an international level, frequently in lengthy discussions and adopted by majority decision. They form the lowest common denominator on which representatives from politics, economics, and science can agree and constitute a framework for their practical application and careful "should do" recommendations. The disadvantage of such generally accepted standards is that they are frequently too nonspecific and new scientific findings are often not considered.

Likewise, laws are frequently nonspecific and provide only minimal standards for occupational safety. They also do not adapt well to the current state of knowledge in the short term. In contrast, recommendations in books or publications incorporate current findings more easily and promote more concrete applications. However, they may be open to interpretation and extensive prior knowledge may be required of the user. Style guides are guidelines for standardizing designs of user interfaces. Generally, they are published by the manufacturer as part of the documentation for computer operating systems (e.g., Microsoft Windows). They frequently are based on the principles of software ergonomics. **Box 4-1** lists pertinent International ISO Standards on Ergonomics.

ISO 6385: Ergonomic Principles in the Design of Work Systems

This international standard contains the significant findings and definitions in ergonomics; it explains relevant basic terms and provides an occupational science framework for all specialists who are involved in the wide-ranging design of work systems. Technical, economic, organizational, and social aspects must all be considered. The standard also applies to the design of products that are not associated with work.

Box 4-1	International ISO Standards on Ergonomics
6385:	Ergonomic principles in the design of work systems
9241-2:	Guidance on task requirements
9241-3:	Visual display requirements
9241-5:	Workstation layout and postural requirements
9241-6:	Environmental requirements
9241-7:	Display requirements with reflections
9241-8:	Requirements for displayed colors
9241-110:	Dialogue principles
61310-1:	Requirements of visual, acoustic, and tactile signals
60601-1-8:	General requirements, tests, and guidance for alarm systems in medical electrical equipment and medical electrical systems
10075-1-3:	Ergonomic principles related to mental workload

A work system provides a super structure for the cooperation of individuals or groups of employees (or users) that allows them to complete their tasks using their tools and equipment within their occupational domain. To create a work system based on ergonomic principles and ISO standards, the following subcategories of the system must be considered: organization of work; task design; design of activity; design of work environment; design of tools and equipment; and design of workplace and work station.

Organization of Work

Organization of work is defined as the systematic organization and design of work-flow under consideration of task-specific, content-specific, and time-specific aspects. It is important to analyze how individual workplaces and activities within a work system (e.g., a hospital) depend on or limit each other, or work synergistically or antagonize each other. A typical organization in an acute care hospital in the United States has functional departments such as nursing, respiratory therapy, physical therapy, laboratory, radiology, surgery, dietary, housekeeping, and administration. However, employees in the distinct departments must work cooperatively to move patients through an inpatient experience. For example, a patient seen in an emergency department is evaluated by a healthcare provider, treated by nurses and other ancillary providers, and admitted for inpatient treatment.

Movement of the patient to a hospital room (task-specific aspects) depends on availability of transfer equipment and personnel, communication between the healthcare providers in the two different treatment areas, and transfer of health information from one area to another (content-specific aspects). The transfer may also be dependent on the availability of a receiving nurse, which can be delayed during change of shifts or when nurses have urgent tasks to complete for other patients (time-specific aspects). The overall workflow in an organization can be improved when ergonomic principles are applied to technologies and the humans who use them.

Contemporary information and telecommunication technologies support and promote cooperation between workers and computers (machines) in different work settings. They guide workers through typical task sequences, monitor error-free completion of work segments, and log outcomes. Frequently, the results achieved by one worker become the basis for additional tasks by other workers.

Task Design

The design of tasks is the second subcategory of ergonomic design of work systems. Important guidelines on task design are listed in Part 2 of ISO 9241. In general, well-designed tasks include the following features:

- They make use of the experience and abilities of the workers.
- They allow the workers to develop their skills and competencies.
- They comprise steps from planning to execution.
- They allow the worker to feel invested in the whole process.
- They afford the worker a certain measure of decision making and autonomy.
- They provide sufficient feedback about the completion of the task.
- They make use of existing abilities and promote development of new skills.

To have an adequate degree of autonomy, the worker should be able to determine such factors as the sequence of tasks, the speed, and manner in which they are executed. The IOM's report, *Keeping Patients Safe: Transforming the Work Environment of Nurses*, called for direct-care nurses to have input into nursing work and workspace design or redesign to improve patient safety (IOM, 2004). Despite the clear recommendation by the IOM, the autonomy of nurses over their own work is not universal. For nurses who work in hospitals that have earned the designation of *Magnet* hospital, perceived autonomy is higher than it is for nurses who work in non-Magnet hospitals (Hess, DesRoches, Donelan, Norman, & Buerhaus, 2011).

When jobs require a high degree of concentration, it is important to make available time segments without interruption. In addition, the work pace varies among workers but also within the same person depending on time of day and current physical state. Rigid workplace rules in regard to work pace or which impose significant restriction of autonomy and excessive dependency on technical systems can create stress and undermine wellbeing. Several research reports illustrate the chaotic and time-pressured nature of nursing work (Cornell et al., 2010; Cornell, Riordan, Townsend-Gervis, & Mobley, 2011; Halbesleben, Savage, Wakefield, & Wakefield, 2010). For example, Cornell and colleagues (2010) reported that 75% of tasks in 98 hours of observations lasted 30 seconds or less. The researchers noted that nurses were constantly shifting between tasks because of time pressures and interruptions. Time pressure is perceived as a stressor by many workers today. Chronic time pressure can promote mental illness, feelings of reduced vitality, and emotional exhaustion (Escribà-Agüir & Pérez-Hoyos, 2007).

The requirement for sufficient feedback regarding the completion of a job includes feedback via software, but also feedback from coworkers and supervisors. Feedback via software needs to be clear and unambiguous. For example, if a nurse enters data outside of acceptable values in an electronic health record (EHR), the software should provide feedback to the user (the nurse) to check the entry to validate the data. Other types of helpful feedback are guided steps for tasks, alerts from clinical decision support, or error messages. Feedback about the quality of the work from supervisors or colleagues is a form of social support. If the feedback is immediate, it can be an effective tool for stress reduction, because the workers receive an affirmation that problems are handled jointly. A prerequisite for well-designed workplaces is the opportunity for social interaction along with a cooperative and communicative office environment (Squires, Tourangeau, Laschinger, & Doran, 2010). Others have described the "culture of safety" as a work environment that encourages all employees to speak up about work conditions that might put the safety of patients or employees at risk (Squires et al., 2010). To have a culture of safety requires supervisors to build relationships with employees by listening, relating, and responding to concerns (Squires et al., 2010).

Design of Activity

Activities should be designed so that they provide an optimal **workload** for the employee, physically and mentally. In ergonomics, the term *workload* has a neutral connotation (ISO 6385) as opposed to its meaning in common usage. Workload includes all external influences acting on humans. This means that degree of difficulty of the task must be considered in addition to the environmental conditions under which the task is being executed.

The total workload can stimulate and challenge workers, promote learning, or fatigue workers. The effect of the workload depends on many factors such as individual preconditions, experience, attitudes, and opinions. The workload that is optimal provides neither too much nor too little challenge. Important elements in avoiding either are appropriate rest periods, job rotation, and job enhancement and job enrichment by assigning multiple sequential tasks rather than repetitive single tasks.

The workload of nurses is measured by counting the number of patients per nurse for inpatient care and the number of patient visits per day in ambulatory settings. There is a body of literature showing that the number of patients per nurse is a significant predictor of inpatient length of stay, medication errors, hospital-acquired conditions, falls, and other adverse outcomes (Frith et al., 2010; Frith, Anderson, Tseng, & Fong, 2012; Kane, Shamliyan, Mueller, Duval, & Wilt, 2007). Technology as a factor in nurse workload has been rarely studied as a predictor of patient outcomes.

Design of the Work Environment

The environment of a workplace includes such external conditions as temperature, noise level, and lighting. Guidelines are listed in the ISO 9241 Part 6: environmental requirements. The ambient conditions are determined by temperature, humidity, air circulation, and heat radiation. What constitutes comfortable ambient conditions is dependent on the individual worker. Surveys of employees show that they are more satisfied when they can choose their ambient conditions. In general, an air temperature of 68–72° F is recommended for visual display terminal workplaces. Drafty conditions or circulating cold air should be avoided because they can promote neck and back pain.

Similarly, noise perception and tolerance are very individual. Noises that are substantially below the danger threshold can still be perceived as annoying. In addition to the volume (noise level measured in decibels), the individual task at hand also influences noise perception. For work requiring intellectual effort and concentration, the ISO 9241 recommends noise levels up to 45 decibels; for simple administrative work requiring communication, it recommends up to 60 decibels. When the ambient noise becomes too loud, errors may increase (e.g., chart entry of patient data) or important signals may be missed. Studies have shown that higher than recommended levels of noise are common in hospitals (McLaren & Maxwell-Armstrong, 2008; Pope, 2010; Zborowsky, Bunker-Hellmich, Morelli, & O'Neill, 2010). For patients who are treated in hospitals, noise can interrupt sleep, lead to delirium, and raise the risk for falls (Tzeng, Hu, & Yin, 2011).

The lighting at a computer terminal workstation must be adapted to the vision of the worker and the specific task to be accomplished. Indirect lighting from the ceiling in combination with adjustable desk lighting is considered optimal. The illumination in the immediate work area should be at least 500 lux. Illumination of 500–1000 lux increases visual acuity and reading becomes more effortless, especially for older workers. The lighting should be even throughout the room so that eyes don't have to continually adjust. To avoid extreme contrasts, glare, and reflections, computer screens should be positioned upright and parallel to the window. If that is not possible, blinds can attenuate incoming sunlight. Evidence-based design of healthcare environments is beginning to appear in the medical and nursing literature. Findings show that patients have better outcomes with natural light from windows with shades or blinds and adjustable lighting levels that patients can control (Bazuin & Cardon, 2011).

Design of Work Equipment (Hardware and Software Ergonomics)

The user-friendly design of computer systems must include elements of hardware and software ergonomics. **Hardware ergonomics** supplies the technical framework and sets the conditions for optimal **human–computer interaction (HCI)**. Input devices (e.g., keyboard or mouse) are differentiated from output devices (e.g., screen, loudspeaker, or printer). Both constitute the operational platform of a computer system and, combined with the software, become the **user interface**.

Software ergonomics deals with the analysis, evaluation, and optimization of user interfaces. By applying various strategies, either the needs of the user can be emphasized or the display of information—the interaction between information and subsequent operations—can be improved. This interaction between display of information and operation is called **dialogue** (refer to the dialogue principles section later in this chapter).

There are various types of user interfaces. The **graphical user interface (GUI)** constitutes a complex platform that allows users to interact with the computer through electronic devices or the computer mouse. Interaction is facilitated by visual elements such as icons (symbols, pictograms). Most modern computers, including laptops and tablets, have graphical user interfaces. EHRs typically look more structured in table formats, and providers uses tab keys or the mouse to move from input field to field. **Voice user interfaces** make human–machine interactions possible through a voice or synthesized speech platform. Input requires a speech recognition system. Voice user interface can be used with EHRs and is commonly called voice recognition (VR) software. In a study of implementation of VR software in a military hospital's on-site and 12 outlying clinics, Hoyt and Yoshihashi (2010) found that the majority of providers persisted in the use of VR. "Compared to clinicians that continued VR, discontinuers generally rated it much lower in helpfulness, accuracy, minutes saved per day, improvement in the quality of EHR notes, and the ability to close the encounter in one day" (Hoyt & Yoshihashi, 2010). **Natural user interfaces** avail themselves of the natural finger and hand movements of the user on a touch screen. They allow intuitive use of the interactive devices.

Interactivity is a key component of computer applications. Depending on user input or given parameters, the flow of information in computer-based applications leads to an output as directed by the application software. Software ergonomics is also dedicated to the question of how to design interactive processes for user friendliness. The usability of systems is determined by the incorporated ergonomic principles. Evaluation methods and design standards have been created to establish the usability of computer-based applications.

Design of the Workplace and Workstation

Anthropometry plays an important role in the design of the workplace in that it allows the worker to assume a comfortable working posture and promotes safety and efficiency as tasks are carried out. The workplace design optimizes visual and tactile human interaction with equipment, allows freedom of leg movement, and promotes support (e.g., seat or auxiliary technical equipment) and optimal arrangement of displays.

The design of the workplace takes into consideration aspects of mobility and stability of posture, sensory requirements and the limits of human perception (e.g., visual or auditory capabilities), and the variation in individual body dimensions. The working height of a table may be ergonomically suitable for an average American male but unsuitable for a small woman. An important characteristic of a well-designed workplace is its capacity to adjust to individual physical requirements, such as the adjustment in table height in the previous example.

When constructing workstations, equipment planners take into consideration the average body size of the population. At intervals the population of a country is measured; various body dimensions are determined for each gender and representative average values (percentiles) are calculated. Generally, an adjustable design is created so that it can serve more than 90% of the population. This range covers body dimensions from the fifth percentile of females (only 5% of women are smaller = small operator) to the 95th percentile of males (only 5% of men are larger = large operator) (Helander, 2006). The 50th percentile represents the population average for a selected physical feature.

For **visual display terminals (VDT)** clear guidelines have been established because of the demands on the musculoskeletal system and the eyes, which take into consideration the dimensions of the workstation and the arrangement of the individual elements (e.g., table, chair, and computer). Guidelines are listed in ISO 9241. The most important elements are summarized in **Figure 4-1**.

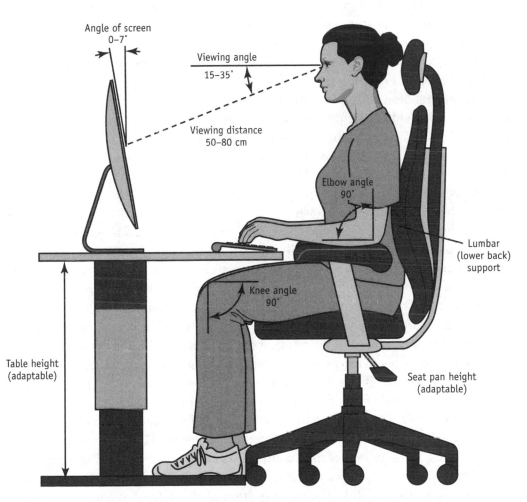

FIGURE 4-1   Posture recommended for visual display terminals (VDT).
Source: Adapted from ISO 9241-5: Workstation layout and postural requirements.

Table and chair height have an impact on the correct posture and must, therefore, be adjustable according to body height. The seat height should be adjusted so that the feet rest on the floor. A footrest may be helpful for short persons. Chairs should pivot and roll to reduce the need of axial body movements. The height of the back support should also be adjustable, and its convex shape should mirror the curvature of the lower back. Correct table height results in an angle of 70 to 90 degrees between upper and lower arms. The height of the keyboard also needs to be considered. Elbow rests of chairs should also be adjustable in height and be short enough to avoid contact with the table. There must be enough room in front of the keyboard to allow support for the wrists. Wrist cushions are optional. There must be sufficient space to allow for changes in working posture and motions. Musculoskeletal problems are frequently the result of prolonged sitting (especially in neck and lower back regions); therefore, standing up at regular intervals is recommended. The creation of workstations that combine sitting and standing tasks is ideal.

The natural head posture results in a gaze that angles down. Therefore, the computer screen should be oriented in such a way that its center is 25–35 degrees below the horizontal visual axis. This position eliminates the need to raise the head while reading and decreases stress on the neck and shoulder musculature. The distance from the eye to the screen should be approximately 50 cm (50–80 cm), depending on screen size. When prescribing appropriate bifocal or multifocal lenses, the exact distance to the screen should be known.

The area that can be seen when the gaze is fixed and the head is held still is called the field of vision. In the horizontal dimension, the field of vision stretches over approximately 180–200 degrees, and in the vertical dimension the field of vision is approximately 130 degrees. Even though humans perceive that everything is in focus within this field, the ability to see details is in reality limited to a small cone (vertex angle 1 degree) around the visual axis (Grandjean, 1979). This is due to the uneven distribution of photo receptors in the retina of the eye. Because the fovea centralis has the greatest number of photo receptors, the visual acuity is greatest there. If one assumes an eye-screen distance of 50 cm, the area of focus is approximately 17 mm in diameter. This equates to a field of about 10 letters that can be visualized simultaneously (Preim & Dachselt, 2010). The eye must continually shift while reading. Toward the periphery, the visual acuity decreases markedly. In the field enclosed in 1–40 degrees around the visual axis, the detection of high contrasts and movements is possible despite the lack of focus. Due to rapid eye movements between discrete objects, the visual perception seems unaffected. In the outer portion of the field of vision (vertex angle between 40 and 70 degrees), movements are still detectable. **Figure 4-2** illustrates the visual fields of a person as he views computer screens.

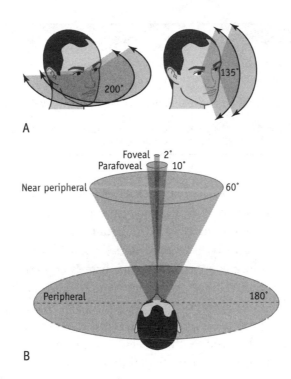

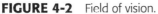

FIGURE 4-2   Field of vision.

Requirements of visual displays Displays must be designed in such a way that information can be acquired quickly, error free, and with little effort. Important factors that influence the acquisition of information are the size of the screen, the quality of the screen, and the recognizability of characters. The following discussion of particulars not only applies to computer screens but also to monitors and other displays of medical devices.

The size of the screen must conform to the task. For office work, the accepted size today is 19 inches (diagonal measurement of the screen = 482.6 mm). The recommended eye-screen distance is approximately 70 cm. The greater the distance, the larger the characters need to be for ease of recognition. At the distance of 70 cm, upper case letters must be at least 4.5 mm in height; at a distance of 60 cm, 3.9 mm in height. At a distance of 50 cm (e.g., 15-inch notebooks), a minimum height of 3.2 mm is recommended (ISO 9241-3). **Box 4-2** shows the calculation of letter height.

Notebooks and tablet-PCs intended for mobile applications are lightweight and reduced in size. To increase the ease of work and data acquisition, the addition of

---

Box 4-2   Calculation of Letter Height

Assignment: Calculate and verify the height of the characters on your computer screen or monitor of a medical device with the following formula:

Minimum upper case letter height (e.g., E, B, H, M, N) in mm = eye-screen distance/155

Source: Adapted from ISO 9241-3: Visual display requirements; Requirements of the German accident insurer (= Berufsgenossenschaften =BG): BG informations number 650.

---

external keyboards and accessory screens of suitable size is recommended. Data acquisition is influenced not only by screen size but also by screen quality. As opposed to the old cathode ray tube (CRT) monitors, the liquid crystal display (LCD) and thin-film transistor (TFT) screens or e-book readers do not flicker and do not have any distortions. Ease of reading is improved by brightness and contrast. A 5:1 ratio of light-dark contrast is required along with crisp edge definition of the characters. The size and number of the pixels determine how well defined the characters are. The smaller the pixels and the denser they are, the more well defined are the characters. The definition is also influenced by the screen resolution, which is variable and, in turn, depends on screen size and the particular application.

Glare and reflections can decrease the quality of the screen image. This can be largely eliminated by matte or anti-glare finishes (see classification of types of reflections). Even for computer housings, matte finishes and light or neutral colors are recommended.

Colors can influence how information is categorized and ranked and how pieces of information relate to each other. Colors can focus the attention of the observer on certain aspects or promote recognition. Colors can negatively influence character recognition; therefore, color is used sparingly in electronic displays.

The human eye perceives color through a type of light-sensitive receptor called the cone, which is located in the retina. These receptors respond to various wavelengths. Some cones are sensitive to red, green, or blue. When light of a certain wavelength enters the eye, different types and numbers of cones are activated to create a subjective color perception after processing by optical neurons. Because there are fewer blue-sensitive cones than red- and green-sensitive cones, the eye perceives blue colors as less intense and cannot distinguish well among shades of blue (Eysel, 2005). In computer applications and electronic displays, this implies that pure blue colors should be avoided for use in text, thin lines, and small formats.

Hue, saturation, and brightness are important factors in the perception of colors. From a psycho-physiological perspective, humans can distinguish about 200 shades of color. Saturation describes how a pure color changes with the addition of grey. Colors with low saturation do not display much color content. Colors with high saturation are similar to pure colors. There are 20 degrees of saturation and 500 degrees of brightness (Eysel, 2005). Saturated colors command our attention and should be used sparingly in software design. They must have a high contrast to be easily distinguishable (ISO 9241-8). Certain color combinations should be avoided.

The highest contrast is created by dark characters on a light background (positive display). However, one cannot easily distinguish among darker colors. The best contrast on a light background is created by black and dark green, red, and magenta.

Certain colors convey specific meanings. Red means imminent danger, stop, or no permission. Yellow signifies alert or caution. Green is linked to safety or lack of danger. Emergency and aid stations and escape routes are symbolized by green color. Color coding needs to consider the conventional meaning of color. Hospital executives and department managers often use dashboard or scorecards that use color to signal performance (Belden, Grayson, & Barnes, 2009).

A typical example is the display of medical devices. Through use of different colors, various states can be indicated such as normal operation (green) or malfunction (red). Optical alerts must be quickly and easily recognizable from a greater distance (4 m). Their luminance should be a minimum of six times greater than the immediate surroundings (ISO 61310-1). Additionally, an indicator for dangerous conditions that require immediate action should flash at a frequency of 2–4 Hz (ISO 60073).

Requirements of acoustic signal devices Acoustic signals and alarms are used as adjuncts when important events take place while executing visual tasks, or when certain conditions occur that require immediate action. However, acoustic signals should be used sparingly because they interrupt the workflow. If several acoustic signals sound simultaneously, a conflict is created for the worker on how to prioritize necessary responses.

For acoustic signals to be recognized with certainty, they need to fulfill certain requirements (ISO 60601-1-8): The sound pressure level (volume) should be at least 5 decibels above the background noise level. Consideration must be given to the environment in which the medical device is used. For warning and alarm signals, 15 decibels above the background noise level are recommended. The minimum recommended sound pressure level for acoustic signal devices is 65 decibels.

In health care, the high number of false-positive alarm signals has been a problem for years. Varpio, Kuziemsky, MacDonald, and King (2012) conducted 49 hours of observations and found that an alarm sounded every 7 seconds. Even though critical states are identified with great certainty, this comes at the cost of a high number of alarms lacking clinical relevancy (Chambrin, 2001). These low-priority alarms deluge healthcare providers, causing high stress levels in personnel and patients. Beyond the strain caused by the flood of acoustic signals, people pay less attention and become desensitized to alarms. Varpio and colleagues (2012) found that 70% of the time, no response to alarms was made. Even more troubling was the finding that 40% of life-threatening alarms were ignored. Conversely, problems arise when alarms fail to sound or are accidentally deactivated in situations requiring action. Critical or life-threatening situations might be overlooked.

Dialogue Principles (ISO 9241-Part 110)

A dialogue is the interaction between a user and an interactive system to achieve a goal that is based on the actions of the user (input) and the reactions of the interactive system (output) (ISO 9241-110). The most common types of health information technology using dialogue are clinical decision support, computerized provider order entry (CPOE), and barcode medication administration systems as stand-alone systems or integrated into EHRs. Well-planned dialogues significantly add to the usability of a product. The dialogue is designed to eliminate typical user problems that cause unnecessary difficulties. These include insufficient or confusing information, unnecessary operational steps, unexpected responses of the interactive system, or the inefficient correction of errors.

Dialogues need to provide relevant, context-specific information for tasks, eliminate the user to search manuals or other external sources of user information, and support the user when learning to navigate the system. Dialogues should conform to generally expected standards and be consistent and predictable to users based on their experience with a system. Even though dialogues may appear automatically, the dialogues should be designed so that users can control the direction or speed of dialogues until the task is completed (ISO 9241-110).

INFORMATION PROCESSING

At the core of HCI are information input, information processing, decision making, and information storage. The starting point is the perception of stimuli from the environment. Of greatest importance in HCI are visual, acoustic, and tactile stimuli.

Rasmussen (1986) assumes that a large part of human **information processing** happens below the threshold of consciousness. Perceived information is subconsciously compared with an inner, dynamic perspective and used to initiate motor processes. This allows automatic actions, such as the automatic limb coordination while walking or the shifting of gears by an experienced driver. From the plethora of perceived information, only few messages emerge into consciousness—those that are needed for conscious action. For example, in a traffic situation, this information would pertain to the current traffic flow, traffic lights, traffic signs, and so on. The ability to concentrate on relevant stimuli and ignore irrelevant information is termed **selective attention**. For an example of this phenomenon, watch Daniel J. Simons' (1999) famous YouTube video (freely available), which has generated millions of views. It can be found using the search terms "selective attention" or "selective awareness" or the following URL: http://www.youtube.com/watch?v=vJG698U2Mvo.

Informational content that otherwise would be ignored can surface into consciousness, especially when mismatches or ambiguities are detected in familiar actions, such as a pedestrian stumbling on uneven pavement or a car not shifting into gear. Such events cause a shift from unconscious to conscious information processing. Human information processing relies on two strategies which, in principle, can also be useful in error avoidance: the focus on essential information and the conscious perception of deviations from the norm.

How much attention is paid to information depends on the manner in which it is presented, on the time available to assimilate the information, and on competing environmental stimuli. Attention is also the key to memory. Perception is the interpretation of certain stimuli (visual, auditory, etc.). Perception aids in the fast grasp of words or sounds, but it can also cause humans to make errors when they "see" what they "expect to see." Medications that have similar spellings or similar sounding names are particularly problematic. A nurse working on a medical unit that specializes in the treatment of respiratory problems might read the brand name drug Advicor (niacin and lovastatin) as Advair (fluticasone and salmeterol) and make a medication error. Attention can be negatively affected by stress, heavy workload, lack of sleep, and interruptions. Added to the stress, poor design of CPOE systems can set up the circumstances for a prescribing order error. **Figure 4-3** shows a CPOE screen with medications presented in a small font size, in long lists, and with little white space.

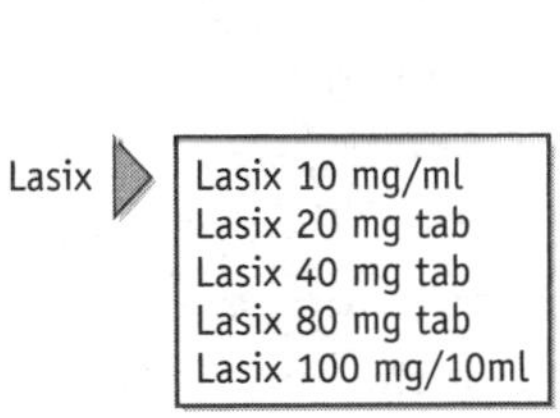

Lasix ▷ Lasix 10 mg/ml
Lasix 20 mg tab
Lasix 40 mg tab
Lasix 80 mg tab
Lasix 100 mg/10ml

FIGURE 4-3 Medication prescription errors occur with selection lists.

In general, memory is defined as the ability of the human nervous system to retain, arrange, and retrieve information. To describe the cognitive processes that enable us to memorize certain information to a greater or lesser extent, sometimes for life, scientists have developed models that show certain similarities to data storage in computers. They greatly simplify the complicated neuronal processes. The multi-store model developed by Atkinson & Shiffrin (1968, 1971) proposes three structures of memory: sensory memory, short-term or working memory, and long-term memory.

The sensory memory acquires stimuli via the sensory organs (e.g., eyes, ears) and retains them in the short-term memory. Visual information is already lost after 0.2 second. Acoustic stimuli can be retained significantly longer (up to 2 seconds). Consciousness and attention play a major role as these data are transferred into the working or long-term memory (Proctor & Vu, 2012).

The expressions "short-term" and "working" memory are used synonymously for memory of limited capacity, where "chunks" of information can be retained for short duration. Repetition can significantly increase and competing stimuli can significantly decrease retention time. Chunks are units of information like numbers, abbreviations, pictograms, words, or complex ideas (e.g., the idea of a person as a whole). Miller (1956) assumed that the short-term memory can store seven chunks. More recent studies point to a storage capacity of three to four chunks (Cowan, 1991). Chunks can be artificially created by grouping information, which allows optimal use of the working memory.

Rouder, a psychologist at the University of Missouri, gave an example in a newspaper interview about how the grouping of information can aid short-term memory. It may be difficult for a person to memorize a sequence of nine letters. However, when the same person is asked to memorize the letters grouped into three acronyms (e.g., IBM-CIA-FBI), the task becomes much easier, and the working memory will need only three slots to retain the information (University of Missouri–Columbia, 2008).

From 1993 to 2003, Baddeley extended and refined the concepts of how working memory functions (Baddeley, 1993, 2002, 2003). It is assumed that the short-term memory is not a single storage unit but a complex aggregate of interacting subsystems that are partially associated with the long-term memory. The data are processed in these subsystems according to their content (e.g., spatial/visual, language).

After processing, storage of information takes place in the long-term memory. Current knowledge seems to indicate that the long-term memory has unlimited storage capacity and duration. The decrease in the ability to memorize new information with increasing age seems to relate less to problems with storage capacity and more to the inability to integrate new information into the long-term memory in a suitable manner to be able to network new with existing information (Herczeg, 2009). Through these associations, various information units are linked, which makes generalizations and comparisons possible, and correlations are established. The counterpoint to the retrieval of information from an arbitrarily distant past is the phenomenon of forgetting. Forgetting, however, is not so much a loss of information as it is a lack of access to the requested information. Linked to this are the entities recall and recognition. Recognition happens much easier than direct access to information by way of association (Herczeg, 2009)

Important conclusions can be drawn about HCIs from knowledge of information-processing theory:

1. Selective grouping of information facilitates retention by the user (Preim & Dachselt, 2010) and assists in the learning process.
2. Tasks should not be too complex due to the limited capacity of the working memory. If the degree of difficulty is high and there is a decision-making requirement, the error rate and the processing time can increase (Jacko & Ward, 1996). Too many possible solutions burden the working memory unnecessarily due to the need for decision making.
3. Due to rapid loss of information from the working memory, complex tasks can be solved only when feedback is received at regular intervals about the status of completion and the attained interim goal, so the next action can be planned (Herczeg, 2009).

A case study demonstrating human factors in complex healthcare settings using health information technology is presented in **Box 4-3**.

SUMMARY

The successful use of interactive systems strongly depends on the physiologic state of the workers in addition to their needs and expectations, which must be matched to the technical capabilities of modern computer technologies. Due to the present extensive knowledge in the area of ergonomics, improper workload can be avoided by the user. Likewise, errors made by users and errors in the execution of tasks can be averted to prevent harm to patients. The changing work environment demands that the organizational framework consider such factors as increasing workload, time pressure, and personnel management.

Box 4-3   Case Study in Human Factors in a Complex Sociotechnical Work System

An important concern for managing patients with complex medical needs in intensive care units (ICUs) is blood glucose control in order to avoid the development of infections and to reduce the chance of longer lengths of stay in ICU. Glucommander, a health information technology (health IT) used in many ICUs, helps physicians make insulin dosing orders through decision support. Glucommander is interactive: It tracks the patient's glucose levels and guides nurses to change intravenous or subcutaneous insulin doses consistent with the physicians' orders.

In an ideal ICU environment, the only persons to interact with the Glucommander are the registered nurses who have been trained on the software and insulin protocol. However, in ICUs with a limited number of computers, other healthcare providers such as occupational therapists, physical therapists, physicians, respiratory therapist, dieticians, unit secretaries, and nurse techs/aids use computers where Glucommander software is running. With so many providers using the same computer, the Glucommander software occasionally gets accidentally closed without the nurse's knowledge. This leads to a potential medication error in the insulin infusion rate, an incorrect lapse of time between blood glucose checks, and a potential loss of the insulin rate infusion history.

The physical environment in the ICU is often hectic and noisy with multiple interruptions from other staff, alarms, other medical devices, portable pagers, telephones, overhead pages, patients' needs, and family members. The computers are located outside of each patient's room in a cubby area that is shared with all providers involved in the patient's care. No defense against the Glucommander's being closed accidentally is present except one confirmation box. A registered nurse, caring for two to three critical patients at various locations in the ICU, may not know if the Glucommander has been turned off. Long lapses can occur before the nurse knows the software is off.

1. What conditions create the potential for medication errors in this situation?
2. What can a registered nurse do to protect patients who are on the Glucommander protocol?
3. What responsibility does a registered nurse have if the software is stopped by accident?
4. What are possible solutions to prevent accidental closing of the software?

---

www   For a full suite of assignments and additional learning activities, use the access code located in the front of your book and visit www.jblearning.com. If you do not have an access code, you can obtain one at the site.

REFERENCES

Amarasingham, R., Plantinga, L., Diener-West, M., Gaskin, D. J., & Powe, N. R. (2009). Clinical information technologies and inpatient outcomes: A multiple hospital study. *Archives of Internal Medicine, 169*(2), 108–114.

Atkinson, R. C., & Shiffrin, R. (1968). Human memory: A proposed system and its control processes. In K. W. Spence & J. T. Spence (Eds.), *The psychology of learning and motivation: Advances in research and memory* (Vol. 2). New York, NY: Academic Press.

Atkinson, R. C., & Shiffrin, R. (1971). The control of short-term memory. *Scientific American, 225*(2), 82–90.

Baddeley, A. D. (1993). *Working memory, thought and action.* Oxford, UK: Oxford University Press.

Baddeley, A. D. (2002). Is working memory still working? *European Psychologist, 7,* 85–97.

Baddeley, A. D. (2003). Working memory. Looking back and looking forward. *Nature Reviews Neuroscience, 4,* 927–839.

Bazuin, D., & Cardon, K. (2011). Creating healing intensive care unit environments: Physical and psychological considerations in designing critical care areas. *Critical Care Nursing Quarterly, 34*(4), 259–267.

Belden, J., Grayson, R., & Barnes, J. (2009). Defining and testing EMR usability: Principles and proposed methods of EMR usability evaluation and rating. Retrieved from http://www.himss.org/files/HIMSSorg/content/files/himss_definingandtestingemrusability.pdf

Centers for Medicare and Medicaid Services. (2008). Hospital-acquired conditions. Retrieved from http://www.cms.hhs.gov/HospitalAcqCond/06_Hospital-Acquired_Conditions.asp

Chambrin, M. C. (2001). Alarms in the intensive care unit: How can the number of false alarms be reduced? *Critical Care, 5,* 184–185.

Cornell, P., Herrin-Griffith, D., Keim, C., Petschonek, S., Sanders, A. M., D'Mello, S., . . . Shepherd, G. (2010). Transforming nursing workflow, part 1: The chaotic nature of nurse activities. *Journal of Nursing Administration, 40*(9), 366–373. doi: 10.1097/NNA.0b013e3181ee4261

Cornell, P., Riordan, M., Townsend-Gervis, M., & Mobley, R. (2011). Barriers to critical thinking workflow interruptions and task switching among nurses. *Journal of Nursing Administration, 41*(10), 407–414. doi: http://dx.doi.org/10.1097/NNA.0b013e31822edd42

Cowan, N. (1991). The magical number 4 in short-term memory: A reconsideration of mental storage capacity. *Behavioral and Brain Sciences, 24,* 87–114.

Dul, J., Bruder, R., Buckle, P., Carayon, P., Falzon, P., Marras, W. S., . . . van der Doelen, B. (2012). A strategy for human factors/ergonomics: Developing the discipline and profession. *Ergonomics, 55*(4), 377–395.

Dul, J., & Weerdenmeester, B. (2008). *Ergonomics for beginners: A quick reference guide.* Boca Raton, FL: CRC Press, Taylor & Francis Group.

Escribà-Agüir, V., & Pérez-Hoyos, S. (2007). Psychological well-being and psychosocial work environment characteristics among emergency medical and nursing staff. *Stress & Health: Journal of the International Society for the Investigation of Stress, 23*(3), 153–160.

Eysel, U. (2005). Visual organ. In R. Klinke, H.- C. Pape & S. Silbernagl (Eds.), *Physiology* (pp. 685–712). New York, NY: Thieme.

Frith, K. H., Anderson, E. F., Caspers, B., Tseng, F., Sanford, K., Hoyt, N. G., & Moore, K. (2010). Effects of nurse staffing on hospital-acquired conditions and length of stay in community hospitals. *Quality Management in Health Care, 19*(2), 147–155. doi: 10.1097/QMH.0b013e3181dafe 3f00019514-201004000-00006 [pii]

Frith, K. H., Anderson, E. F., Tseng, F., & Fong, E. A. (2012). Nurse staffing is an important strategy to prevent medication error in community hospitals. *Nursing Economics, 30*(5), 288–294.

Grandjean, E. (1979). *Physiological work design* (3rd ed.). Thun, Switzerland: Ott.

Halbesleben, J. R., Savage, G. T., Wakefield, D. S., & Wakefield, B. J. (2010). Rework and work-arounds in nurse medication administration process: Implications for work processes and patient safety. *Health Care Management Review, 35*(2), 124–133. doi: 10.1097/HMR.0b013e3 181d116c200004010-201004000-00004 [pii]

Helander, M. (2006). *A guide to human factors and ergonomics* (2nd ed.). Boca Raton, FL: Taylor & Francis Group.

Herczeg, M. (2009). *Software-Ergonomics. Theories, models and kriteria for usable interactive computer systems.* München, Germany: Oldenbourg.

Hess, R., DesRoches, C., Donelan, K., Norman, L., & Buerhaus, P. I. (2011). Perceptions of nurses in Magnet Hospitals, non-Magnet hospitals, and hospitals pursuing Magnet status. *Journal of Nursing Administration, 41*(7/8), 315–323. doi: 10.1097/NNA.0b013e31822509e2

Hoyt, R., & Yoshihashi, A. (2010). Lessons learned from implementation of voice recognition for documentation. *Perspectives in Health Information Management, 7*, 11p.

Institute of Medicine. (1999). *To err is human: Building a safer health system.* Washington, DC: National Academies Press.

Institute of Medicine. (2004). *Keeping patients safe: Transforming the work environment of nurses.* Washington, DC: National Academies Press.

Institute of Medicine. (2011). *Health IT and patient safety: Building safer systems for better care.* Washington, DC: Committee on Patient Safety and Health Information Technology, Board on Health Care Services.

International Ergonomics Association. (2000). Definition of ergonomics. Retrieved from http://www.iea.cc/01_what/What is Ergonomics.html

Jacko, J. A., & Ward, K. G. (1996). Towards establishing a link between psychomotor task complexity and human information processing. *Computers and Industrial Engineering, 31*(1–2), 533–536.

Kane, R., Shamliyan, T., Mueller, C., Duval, S., & Wilt, T. (2007). The association of registered nurse staffing levels and patient outcomes: Systematic review and meta-analysis. *Medical Care, 45*(12), 1195–1204.

McLaren, E., & Maxwell-Armstrong, C. (2008). Noise pollution on an acute surgical ward. *Annals of the Royal College of Surgeons of England, 90*(2), 136–139. doi: 10.1308/003588408x261582

Miller, G. A. (1956). The magical number seven, plus or minus two: Some limits on our capacity for processing information. *Psychological Review, 63*, 81–97.

Pope, D. (2010). Decibel levels and noise generators on four medical/surgical nursing units. *Journal of Clinical Nursing, 19*(17–18), 2463–2470. doi: 10.1111/j.1365-2702.2010.03263.x

Preim, B., & Dachselt, R. (2010). *Interactive systems. Volume 1: Basics, graphical user interfaces, visualization of informations.* New York, NY: Springer.

Proctor, R. W., & Vu, K.-P. L. (2012). Human information processing: An overview for human-computer interaction. In J. A. Jacko (Ed.), *The human-computer interation handbook. Fundamentals, evolving technologies, and emerging applications* (3rd ed., pp. 21–40). Boca Raton, FL: Taylor & Francis Group.

Rasmussen, J. (1986). *Information processing and human-machine interaction, an approach to cognitive engineering* (pp. 74–83). New York, NY: North-Holland.

Simons, D. J. (1999). Selective attention test. Retrieved from http://www.youtube.com/watch?v=vJG698U2Mvo

Squires, M., Tourangeau, A., Laschinger, H. K. S., & Doran, D. (2010). The link between leadership and safety outcomes in hospitals. *Journal of Nursing Management, 18*(8), 914–925. doi: 10.1111/j.1365-2834.2010.01181.x

Tzeng, H.-M., Hu, H. M., & Yin, C.-Y. (2011). The relationship of the hospital-acquired injurious fall rates with the quality profile of a hospital's care delivery and nursing staff patterns. *Nursing Economics, 29*(6), 299–316.

University of Missouri–Columbia. (2008, April 24). Psychologists demonstrate simplicity of working memory. *Science Daily*. Retrieved from http://www.sciencedaily.com/releases/2008/04/080423171519.htm

Varpio, L., Kuziemsky, C., MacDonald, C., & King, W. J. (2012). The helpful or hindering effects of in-hospital patient monitor alarms on nurses: A qualitative analysis. *Computers, Informatics, Nursing, 30*(4), 210–217. doi: 10.1097/NCN.0b013e31823eb581

Wilson, J. R. (2000). Fundamentals of ergonomics in theory and practice. *Applied Ergonomics, 31*(6), 557–567.

Zborowsky, T., Bunker-Hellmich, L., Morelli, A., & O'Neill, M. (2010). Centralized vs. decentralized nursing stations: Effects on nurses' functional use of space and work environment. *HERD, 3*(4), 19–42.

CHAPTER 5

Usability in Health Information Technology

Karen H. Frith, PhD, RN, NEA-BC

CHAPTER LEARNING OBJECTIVES

1. Define user-centered design.
2. Identify the importance of usability testing in health care.
3. Describe the iterative process of design and testing health information technologies.
4. Select among different methods of usability testing.

KEY TERMS

Effectiveness

Efficiency

Health information technology (health IT)

Human–computer interaction

Iterative

Qualitative method

Quantitative method

Satisfaction

System development life cycle

Usability testing

User-centered design (UCD)

User experience (UX)

CHAPTER OVERVIEW

The focus of this chapter is planning and implementing usability tests to study the effects of computer-based technology on the people who use it. Simply put, computers change the way people interact with others at work and with **health information technology (health IT)**. Whether computers are carried in pockets, embedded in medical equipment, or positioned on desks, these systems can lead to fundamental changes in workflow. It is this interaction between humans and computers that is central to **usability testing**.

INTRODUCTION

Usability testing is a "technique used to evaluate a product [or information system] by testing it with representative users" (U.S. Department of Health and Human Services [HHS], 2012). Usability testing is concerned with functionality: It measures users' perceptions about the **effectiveness** and **efficiency** of the product, users' **satisfaction** with the product, and the tendency for errors with the product. To illustrate usability testing, consider two common devices used to control traffic in the United States: traffic lights and four-way stop signs. A traffic light is a device that has three colors—green, yellow, and red. The colors are arranged either from top to bottom or left to right in the same order. Drivers know that green means go, yellow means prepare to stop, and red means stop. Traffic lights work because they are easy for people to understand, are used in a consistent manner, and are effective in controlling traffic. In contrast, four-way stop signs used at intersecting roads are not as effective, because drivers have to make decisions based on the context. Drivers must always stop at the intersection, look at traffic on the other three roads, and go *if they have the right of way*. The right of way is determined by who arrives at the intersection first. This rule is easy if only one car is at the intersection, but if multiple cars arrive at the same time, the car farthermost to the right leaves the intersection first. Using this illustration, usability testing can show that both types of traffic signals are effective—drivers follow consistent rules for stopping at intersections. However, drivers likely find that four-way stop signs are not as efficient, satisfying, or error free as traffic lights because of the multiple decisions about crossing the intersection.

Every piece of technology can be evaluated for its usability and compared to other similar technologies. The goal of usability testing in health care is to develop or purchase electronic health records (EHRs), medical devices, and other health IT that meet users' needs, improve productivity, and safeguard against errors. The need for usability testing is significant, because EHRs and other health IT have been shown to slow workflow, impair performance, and introduce new error-prone processes (Jones, Heaton, Rudin, & Schneider, 2012). Recent participants at the Institute of Medicine's (IOM) workshop on comparative user experiences for health IT called for public reporting of the usability of EHRs (IOM, 2011; Sinsky, Hess, Karsh, Keller, & Koppel, 2012). A panel of experts commissioned by IOM called for public reporting, similar to reviews by *Consumer Reports* of other products to provide essential information to potential purchasers and lead to improvements made by vendors (Sinsky et al., 2012). They further proposed that usability testing of EHRs and other health IT should provide information about cognitive workload, accuracy of decision making, time required to perform tasks, and implementation experience, because these characteristics profoundly affect any healthcare provider's (HCP's) ability to deliver safe patient care.

IMPORTANCE OF USABILITY TESTING

The ideal way to develop EHRs and health IT is to test usability as part of the design project plan. For vendors of EHRs and health IT, usability testing implemented from the beginning of product development is less costly than later changes requiring major revision to code (Shenoy, 2008). Even teamwork is hurt by late usability testing. Any computer programmer will agree that resistance to reworking code is "directly proportional to the number of lines of code that has already been written" (Shenoy, 2008). Usability testing is important enough that the National Institute of Standards and Technology, an agency of the U.S. Department of Commerce, issued a report outlining an EHR usability protocol for vendors to follow in the design of their products (Lowry et al., 2012).

Poor **user experience (UX)** with health IT occurs when the technology is mismatched to the needs of the user. Poor UX is frustrating, dissatisfying, and unlikely to get better without significant redesign of the health IT. Systems with poor UX are costly in terms of dollars, personnel turnover, and unnecessary medical errors. With most EHR systems priced in the millions, selection of a system with poor usability cannot be undone. In other words, once a system has been purchased, the healthcare organization cannot return it for a better system, so the organization is burdened with poor usability for the life of that system. Even admirable efforts to customize the system are typically inadequate to overcome the damage to workflow and the reduced productivity of HCPs. Providers can become so frustrated and dissatisfied that they leave the organization (Kjeldskov, Skov, & Stage, 2010). Poor usability can lead to medical errors and leave the potential for efficiencies and safety as unrealized goals (Horsky et al., 2010).

The federal government has a high stake in adoption of EHR by healthcare organizations and providers. The Health Information Technology for Economic and Clinical Health (HITECH) Act promotes the adoption of EHR by using financial incentives for a period of time, followed by reduced reimbursements for nonadoption of EHRs (Centers for Medicare & Medicaid Services [CMS], 2012). Poor usability means that the goals of ubiquitous adoption of EHRs, easy exchange of health information among HCPs, and improved patient safety could be delayed.

USER-CENTERED DESIGN

User-centered design (UCD) is a method for assessing usability throughout the **system development life cycle** (HHS, 2012). UCD means that the needs, desires, and limitations of users are the driving factors for design, not the technology capabilities. In other words, UCD would require a development team to create features valuable to end users and omit those of little importance, even if the features were technologically challenging or cool to the development team. User-centered design requires developers to understand **human–computer interaction** and to design a natural way for users to interact with the system that satisfies, rather than frustrates, them.

The design of health IT is beyond the scope of this chapter, but readers are encouraged to refer to McGonigle & Mastrian (2012) for discussion of the system development life cycle. Smart design teams employ UCD and usability testing with HCPs throughout the system development life cycle. Testing, when conducted only by health IT designers, will fail to uncover usability issues. When UCD and usability are intertwined and **iterative**, each step informs the next, resulting in health IT that is suited to the needs of HCPs. **Figure 5-1** illustrates the iterative design-test-redesign process. Even after health IT has been implemented, usability testing can uncover problems and frustrations experienced by HCPs that result in potentially unsafe workarounds. When health IT is found to have usability problems, it should be redesigned or retired. Subsequent sections of this chapter present different frameworks for and methods of usability testing.

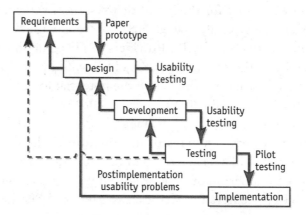

FIGURE 5-1   User-centered design: Iterative process of usability testing and design in system development life cycle.
Source: https://cio.gov/software-development-life-cycle/

DIMENSIONS OF USABILITY

The dimensions examined in most usability tests are effectiveness, efficiency, and satisfaction. The International Organization for Standardization (ISO, 1998) defines effectiveness as the "accuracy and completeness with which users achieve specified goals," efficiency as the "resources expended in relation to the accuracy and completeness with which users achieve goals," and satisfaction as the "freedom from discomfort and positive attitudes towards the user of the product" (p. 2).

Measures of the Three Dimensions of Usability

Since the 1990s, published usability studies and systematic reviews have provided numerous measures appropriate to include in usability evaluations (Hornbæk, 2006; Horsky et al., 2010; Jaspers, 2009; Khajouei, Hasman, & Jaspers, 2011; Kushniruk & Patel, 2004; Park & Hwan Lim, 1999; Zhang & Walji, 2011). Measures can overlap, but most are associated with a particular usability dimension.

Effectiveness

Measures that assess the health IT's fit with the work to be done are typically used in the effectiveness dimension (see **Table 5-1**). Work domain saturation refers to the number of work functions available in the health IT compared to the number of work functions in a job. For example, HCPs could use an information system to manage immunizations. The information system might have functions for documentation, alerts for missed immunizations, a quick reference guide for the immunization schedule, inventory management with alerts, and printable immunization cards. If the HCP

Table 5-1 Effectiveness Measures Used in Usability Studies	
Measures	**Definitions**
Work Domain Saturation	Ratio of work functions in software to work functions in domain
Task Completion	Percentage of tasks completed during a defined session
Accuracy	Percentage of errors in a task
Recall	User's memory of design and content in interface
Quality of Outcome	The extent to which software meets user's goals
Expert Assessment	Usability expert's evaluation of quality of outcomes

only needs to document, use the reference, and print immunization cards, the information system has more functions than are needed by the user. Sometimes the mismatch of the information system to the work results in a more complicated system that reduces the efficiency and satisfaction of users. Other measures in the effectiveness domain are task completion, accuracy, recall, and quality of outcomes. Task completion and accuracy measure the users' interaction with health IT's features to complete work functions. Recall of the interface is also an effectiveness measure, because when users recall the layout or content, the interface can be a good fit with the work domain. The final measures of effectiveness are quality of outcomes. Effective health IT helps users meet their work goals in an acceptable manner.

Efficiency

Measures in the efficiency dimension are designed to assess how easy health IT is to learn and use (see **Table 5-2**). Using specified tasks, the number of trials to completion, time on task, and input rate can be quantified. Success on tasks in short periods of time indicates an efficient system. Efficiency can be assessed by users' mental efforts to interact with health IT; systems that require little thinking to complete tasks are considered efficient. Patterns and numbers of features used in the system can indicate resources users needed to complete tasks. Usage patterns that deviate from ideal patterns or pathways can indicate inefficiencies in the interface. System errors reduce the efficiency of health IT. Measures include the incidence of errors and the percentage of time required by the system to recover from errors. Experts use heuristics or rules of thumb to assess the design of a system's interface. A well-known set of

Table 5-2	Efficiency Measures in Usability Studies
Measures	**Definitions**
Learnability	Number of trials to reach a performance level
Time	Time on task
Input Rate	Rate to add data with a mouse, keyboard, or other input device
Mental Effort	User's cognitive effort to interact with software
Usage Patterns	Count of how much a function in software is used
Error Prevention	Error occurrence rate or error recovery rate
Expert Assessment	Usability expert's evaluation of efficiency using heuristics

Table 5-3 Satisfaction Measures in Usability Studies	
Measures	**Definitions**
Preference	Rank ordering of users' choice of interface features/function
Satisfaction with Interface	Users' overall good experience interacting with software
Users' Attitudes and Perceptions	Users' opinions about content, features, outcomes, or interactions

Source: Reprinted from International Journal of Human-Computer Studies, 64(2), Hornbaek K., Current practice in measuring usability: Challenges to usability studies and research, pp. 79–102, Copyright 2006, with permission from Elsevier.

heuristic assessment of a system was developed by Nielsen (1995) and can be found on the companion website to this text.

Satisfaction

Satisfaction, the third dimension of usability, is a subjective measure of user's approval of health IT. Satisfaction is most commonly assessed with questionnaires (Bangor, Kortum, & Miller, 2008; Chin, Diehl, & Norman, 1988; Davis, 1989; Lewis, 1993; Lund, 2001). These tools can query users on the perceived ease of use, usefulness, ease of learning, satisfaction with work completed, and overall satisfaction (see **Table 5-3**). Most satisfaction questionnaires use a Likert rating scale with five or seven answer options. Semantic differential scales are also used and have a line with bipolar adjectives at each end. Users mark how close they feel with respect to one of the two opposite adjectives (see **Figure 5-2**). Readers who wish to locate satisfaction questionnaires should refer to the references in this chapter.

Usability Methods

Usability studies often employ mixed research methods to understand the effectiveness, efficiency, and satisfaction of users with health IT. **Quantitative methods** produce numbers such as counts, frequencies, and ratios. Quantitative methods might include assessments of tasks, surveys, usage logs, and error logs. **Qualitative methods**

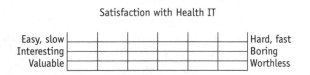

FIGURE 5-2   Example of semantic differential scale.

produce text, video, or audio. Sometimes qualitative data can be converted to quantitative data by counting, for example, instances of users having difficulty finding information on a website. Qualitative methods can include interviews, focus groups, direct or video-recorded observation, "think-aloud" techniques, and task analysis. In simple terms, quantitative methods can show how many usability problems exist, whereas qualitative methods can uncover why usability problems exist and sometimes how to fix them. Because of the complementary nature of the methods, the combination is found to be more successful in the design-redesign cycle (Horsky et al., 2010).

PLANNING USABILITY TESTING

Planning for usability testing is done at the beginning of a project, not after health IT has been fully developed. In fact, it is an iterative process of development-testing-redesign so that results from usability testing serve as feedback into the next steps of development. Most experts advocate for no more than five users in a round of usability testing, because 85% of usability problems can be found with five and having more users simply takes longer and costs more money (Krug, 2010; Nielsen, 2000). Usability testing should be conducted regularly; monthly half-day testing with users is recommended (Krug, 2010). A guide with 234 tips for finding and recruiting participants for usability testing is available for free on the companion website to this text (Sova & Nielsen, 2003).

The design team creates a detailed plan for development and testing, using Gantt charts, flowcharts, and other management tools. The plan includes tasks, start and end dates, milestones, and resources allocated to the various tasks. Because the plan is detailed and shared among team members, specialized project management software is used. Project software can also automate email reminders, calculations of costs associated with tasks, and revisions to the timeline, if milestones are missed. **Figure 5-3** illustrates a typical Gantt chart that design teams use to manage the system development life cycle, including plans for usability testing.

Role of Nurse Informaticist

Nurse informaticists should be on every design team to select or develop usability testing plans. Because the nurse informaticists understand clinical work, they can select usability methods that are most likely to uncover usability problems. Selection should also be guided by the need for user feedback in each step of UCD: planning, designing, testing, and deploying. For example, in the testing phase, a nurse informaticist could develop several case studies to simulate patient care and HCPs' interaction with

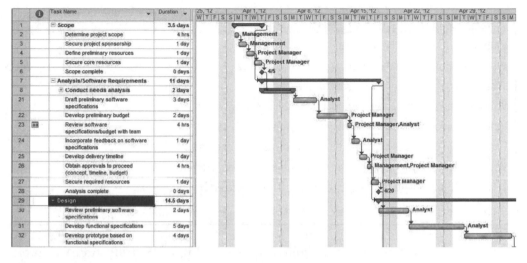

FIGURE 5-3   Example of a gantt chart.
Source: Used with permission from Microsoft.

the target health IT. The case studies could require provider interactions such as finding lab results, documenting interventions, and responding to alerts. Knowledge of the health IT and the nature of clinical work make nurse informaticists essential members of the design team in all phases of usability testing.

Phases of Usability Testing

Planning

In the early stages of UCD, usability is focused on analysis of users' needs and tasks before any design discussions begin. Methods appropriate in the analysis phase to understand users' needs include focus groups, individual interviews, and contextual interviews (HHS, 2012). **Box 5-1** provides a list of questions that the design team could use to develop specific questions for focus groups and interviews. Two other methods used to understand tasks to be implemented in the proposed health IT are task analysis and card sorting (UsabilityNet, 2006).

Designing

In the design phase, the development team changes focus from understanding needs to brainstorming ideas for the health IT solution. Usability experts advocate for extremely early usability testing; one such technique is called napkin testing. While talking with friends, designers can draw some rough ideas about a design and get the

Box 5-1   User-Centered Questions for UCD Planning Phase
Who are the users of the health IT?
Why, when, and where will users access the health IT?
What are the critical needs of users for the health IT?
Which health IT features are important to users?
Which activities are core to the interaction of users with the health IT?
Which activities must be completed quickly by users of the health IT?
What is the level of satisfaction that users can expect from interacting with the health IT?
How much training on use of the health IT can be tolerated by end users?
Source: Adapted from Questions to Ask at Kick-off Meetings found at http://www.usability.gov/basics/ucd/.

immediate impressions of the design (Krug, 2010). **Figure 5-4** illustrates a simple napkin test. Even more formal design work, such as single prototyping, parallel designs, and storyboarding, are still started on paper or using software programs to draw designs (UsabilityNet, 2006). Paper prototyping illustrates the user interface based on a set of requirements for health IT. Parallel designs illustrate more than one design based on the same set of requirements, so users can select among designs. Storyboarding shows the relationships among all screens of health IT. All of the methods bring user feedback to the design team and are important in the early designs to avoid the expense of rewriting code.

Testing

After the team has a working prototype, usability testing involves people outside of the design team: UX experts and actual users. Regardless of the method or the people involved in usability testing, the main point is to understand what users experience and improve health IT. Methods for the testing phase include heuristic evaluation, cognitive walkthroughs, the think-aloud method, user interviews, surveys, critical incident analysis, and satisfaction questionnaires (HHS, 2012; UsabilityNet, 2006). Frith and Anderson (2012) beta-tested nurse staffing decision support software with five nurse managers in a community hospital. Several usability testing methods were used including cognitive walkthroughs, weekly user interviews, daily logs, and user surveys. The beta test was 3 months long, and redesign of software was batched so that users could be kept informed about changes. Users gave valuable feedback about the software. For example, the software was designed to refresh data every 4 hours, but users in the beta test wanted more frequent refresh rates (at least hourly). Usability testing also revealed other needs—nurse managers wanted graphs to trend data over time, to save and print graphs,

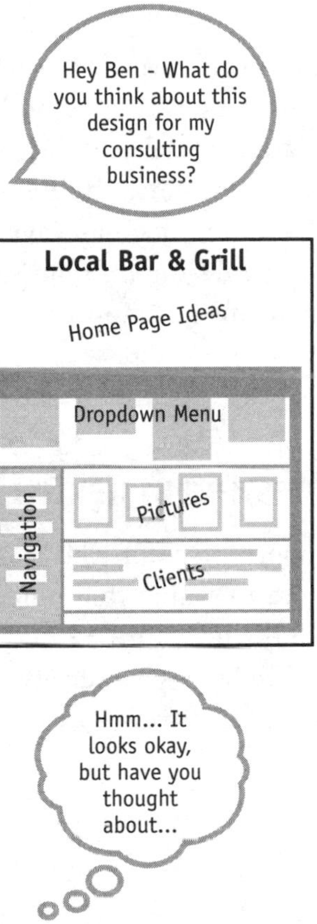

FIGURE 5-4 The napkin test.

and to annotate saved data for productivity reports. These features were not originally planned, but became priorities for redesign (Frith & Anderson, 2012).

Software programs such as Morae can record user mouse actions when users are asked to complete tasks to test the efficiency of health IT (Clearleft, 2013; Tech-Smith, 2013). The design team would develop structured tasks and quantify the time to complete tasks, the number of wrong mouse actions, and the completion rate for tasks by reviewing the software captures. Video cameras can add facial expressions and verbal responses to the usability testing. Specialized hardware can monitor the eye movements of users to determine if they are confused about the layout of health IT. A demo usability test recorded by Krug (2010) is freely available via YouTube, and the link to the video is found on the companion website for this text. It is worth the 25 minutes of time to watch a real usability test!

Deploying

The real test of users' experiences with health IT is when they use it in training or for the first several months. Of course, there are methods to collect data about how well health IT is performing in relation to the usability goals set for it. Usage and error logs can be collected automatically from health IT if the code for logging such activities were designed in health IT. Other manual ways to collect deployment usability data are to note problems with use during training sessions and to log calls to a support center. The usability problems noted in the deployment stage must be fixed quickly to avoid frustrating users.

EXAMPLES OF USABILITY TESTING IN HEALTH CARE

Health IT usability testing is appropriate for EHRs, decision support software, medical devices, and any other health IT–supported functions. The case study presented in this chapter was reported in the literature by Anderson, Willson, Peterson, Murphy, and Kent (2010). The case study shows a variety of usability tests used to improve a clinical decision support system (see **Box 5-2**).

SUMMARY

Usability testing in health care is an integral part of the design of health IT. **Box 5-3** provides helpful links to usability resources available on the Internet. Usability testing should be a regularly scheduled activity in the design plan. When usability is iterative with design, the needs of users become central to the design. The purpose of usability testing is not to prove anything; rather, it is to improve the design and function of health IT. The three dimensions of usability testing—effectiveness, efficiency, and satisfaction—can be measured with a variety of qualitative or quantitative methods. Usability testing should improve health IT so that HCPs can give care in an efficient manner and safeguard against medical errors.

For a full suite of assignments and additional learning activities, use the access code located in the front of your book and visit www.jblearning.com. If you do not have an access code, you can obtain one at the site.

Box 5-2   Usability Case Study

Anderson, Willson, Peterson, Murphy, and Kent (2010) developed a clinical decision support system for Veterans Health Administration's EHRs. The system, called Self-management TO Prevent (STOP) Stroke Tool, was designed to alert providers to clinical indicators for the start of care using clinical guidelines for stroke and associated comorbidities. The design team developed a UCD plan with three major steps that integrated different usability methods. In the first step, the design team translated stroke prevention guidelines to algorithms. Next, the team developed case studies to understand how HCPs would use the algorithms in a clinical context. The design team then used computer programming to develop software that would be used by HCPs. In the second step, the design team asked providers to use a prototype of the software and to think aloud while they completed several tasks. The providers identified confusing instructions in the software; the design team revised the software. In the final step of usability testing, providers were asked to use the software with real patients. The team counted the number of software prompts to initiate clinical guidelines. The design team found that nurses who used the STOP Stroke Tool initiated significantly more clinical guidelines when prompted by the program as compared to the standard system used before the usability testing.

Check Your Understanding

1. What was the benefit of using different usability tests in the three phases of development of the STOP Stroke Tool?
2. What other methods could have been selected to test usability?
3. If you were asked to participate in usability testing and could select only one method, which one would you select and why?

Source: Adapted from Anderson, J. A., Willson, P., Peterson, N. J., Murphy, C., & Kent, T. A. (2010). Prototype to practice: developing and testing a clinical decision support system for secondary stroke prevention in a veterans healthcare facility. CIN: Computers, Informatics, Nursing, 28(6), 353-363. By permission of Lippincott Williams & Wilkins.

Box 5-3   Websites for Usability Testing

Matrix of Usability Methods Based on Their Role in User-Centered Design

- Usability.gov: http://www.usability.gov/methods/index.html
- UsabilityNet: http://www.usabilitynet.org/tools/methods.htm
- Nielsen Norman Group: http://www.nngroup.com/articles/which-ux-research-methods/
- Nielsen Norman Group, "10 Usability Heuristics for User Interface Design": http://www.nngroup.com/articles/ten-usability-heuristics/
- Nielsen Norman Group tips for recruiting users: http://www.nngroup.com/reports/tips/recruiting
- Human Factors International: http://www.humanfactors.com/services/usabilitytestingchart.asp
- Usability Body of Knowledge: http://www.usabilitybok.org/methods

Demo Usability Test

- Steve Krug: http://www.youtube.com/watch?v5QckIzHC99Xc&feature5player_embedded

User Experience

- UX Matters: http://www.uxmatters.com/index.php
- *UX Magazine*: http://uxmag.com/

REFERENCES

Anderson, J. A., Willson, P., Peterson, N. J., Murphy, C., & Kent, T. A. (2010). Prototype to practice: Developing and testing a clinical decision support system for secondary stroke prevention in a veterans health care facility. *CIN: Computers, Informatics, Nursing, 28*(6), 353–363. doi: 10.1097/NCN.0b013e3181f69c5b

Bangor, A., Kortum, P. T., & Miller, J. T. (2008). An empirical evaluation of the system usability scale. *International Journal of Human-Computer Interaction, 24*(6), 574–594. doi: 10.1080/10447310802205776

Centers for Medicare & Medicaid Services (CMS). (2012). *EHR incentive programs.* Retrieved from http://www.cms.gov/Regulations-and-Guidance/Legislation/EHRIncentivePrograms

Chin, J., Diehl, V., & Norman, K. (1988). *Development of an instrument measuring user satisfaction of the human-computer interface.* Paper presented at the Proceedings of ACM CHI'88 Conference on Human Factors in Computing Systems.

Clearleft. (2013). *Silverback.* Retrieved from http://silverbackapp.com/

Davis, F. (1989). Perceived usefulness, perceived ease of use, and user acceptance of information technology. *MIS Quarterly, 13*(3), 319–340.

Frith, K. H., & Anderson, E. F. (2012). Improve care delivery with integrated decision support. *Nursing Management, 43*(12), 52–54. doi: 10.1097/01.NUMA.0000422898.37452.a4

Hornbæk, K. (2006). Current practice in measuring usability: Challenges to usability studies and research. *International Journal of Human-Computer Studies, 64*(2), 79–102. doi: http://dx.doi.org/10.1016/j.ijhcs.2005.06.002

Horsky, J., McColgan, K., Pang, J. E., Melnikas, A. J., Linder, J. A., Schnipper, J. L., & Middleton, B. (2010). Complementary methods of system usability evaluation: Surveys and observations during software design and development cycles. *Journal of Biomedical Informatics, 43*(5), 782–790. doi: http://dx.doi.org/10.1016/j.jbi.2010.05.010

Institute of Medicine (IOM). (2011). *Health IT and patient safety: Building safer systems for better care.* Washington, DC: Committee on Patient Safety and Health Information Technology, Board on Health Care Services.

International Organization for Standardization (ISO). (1998). *Ergonomic requirements for office work with visual display terminals (VDTs)—Part II: Guidance on usability.* 9241-11:1998.

Jaspers, M. W. M. (2009). A comparison of usability methods for testing interactive health technologies: Methodological aspects and empirical evidence. *International Journal of Medical Informatics, 78*(5), 340–353. doi: http://dx.doi.org/10.1016/j.ijmedinf.2008.10.002

Jones, S. S., Heaton, P. S., Rudin, R. S., & Schneider, E. C. (2012). Unraveling the IT productivity paradox—lessons for health care. *New England Journal of Medicine, 366*(24), 2243–2245.

Khajouei, R., Hasman, A., & Jaspers, M. W. M. (2011). Determination of the effectiveness of two methods for usability evaluation using a CPOE medication ordering system. *International Journal of Medical Informatics, 80*(5), 341–350. doi: http://dx.doi.org/10.1016/j.ijmedinf.2011.02.005

Kjeldskov, J., Skov, M. B., & Stage, J. (2010). A longitudinal study of usability in health care: Does time heal? *International Journal of Medical Informatics, 79*(6), e135–e143. doi: http://dx.doi.org/10.1016/j.ijmedinf.2008.07.008

Krug, S. (2010). *Rocket surgery made easy.* Berkeley, CA: New Riders.

Kushniruk, A. W., & Patel, V. L. (2004). Cognitive and usability engineering methods for the evaluation of clinical information systems. *Journal of Biomedical Informatics, 37*(1), 56–76. doi: http://dx.doi.org/10.1016/j.jbi.2004.01.003

Lewis, J. (1993). IBM computer usability satisfaction questionnaires: Psychometric evaluation and instructions for use. *International Journal of Human-Computer Interaction, 7*(1), 57–78.

Lowry, S., Quinn, M., Ramaiah, M., Schumacher, R., Patterson, E., North, R., . . . Abbott, P. (2012). *Technical evaluation, testing, and validation of the usability of electronic health records.* Gaithersburg, MD: National Institute of Standards and Technology.

Lund, A. M. (2001). Measuring usability with the USE questionnaire [Newsletter]. *Usability Interface Newsletter, 8*(2).

McGonigle, D., & Mastrian, K. (2012). *Nursing informatics and the foundation of knowledge.* Burlington, MA: Jones & Bartlett Learning.

Nielsen, J. (1995). *How to conduct a heuristic evaluation.* Retrieved from http://www.nngroup.com/articles/how-to-conduct-a-heuristic-evaluation/

Nielsen, J. (2000). *Why you only need to test with 5 users.* Retrieved from http://www.nngroup.com/articles/why-you-only-need-to-test-with-5-users/

Park, K. S., & Hwan Lim, C. (1999). A structured methodology for comparative evaluation of user interface designs using usability criteria and measures. *International Journal of Industrial Ergonomics, 23*(5–6), 379–389. doi: http://dx.doi.org/10.1016/S0169-8141(97)00059-0

Shenoy, G. (2008). *Benefits of early usability testing.* Retrieved from http://productmanagementtips.com/2008/09/15/product-manager-usability-testing/

Sinsky, C. A., Hess, J., Karsh, B. T., Keller, J. P., & Koppel, R. (2012). *Comparative user experiences of health IT products: How user experiences would be reported and used.* Retrieved from http://www.iom.edu/Global/Perspectives/2012/~/media/Files/Perspectives-Files/2012/Discussion-Papers/comparative-user-experiences.pdf

Sova, D., & Nielsen, J. (2003). *How to recruit participants for usability studies.* Retrieved from http://www.nngroup.com/reports/tips/recruiting

TechSmith. (2013). Morae [Software]. Retrieved from http://www.techsmith.com/morae.html

U.S. Department of Health and Human Services (HHS). (2012). *Usability.gov: How to & tools: Methods.* Retrieved from http://www.usability.gov/methods/test_refine/learnusa/index.html

UsabilityNet. (2006). *Methods table.* Retrieved from http://www.usabilitynet.org/tools/methods.htm

Zhang, J., & Walji, M. F. (2011). TURF: Toward a unified framework of EHR usability. *Journal of Biomedical Informatics, 44*(6), 1056–1067. doi: http://dx.doi.org/10.1016/j.jbi.2011.08.005

CHAPTER 6

Privacy, Security, and Confidentiality

Faye E. Anderson, DSN, RN, NEA-BC
Karen H. Frith, PhD, RN, NEA-BC

CHAPTER LEARNING OBJECTIVES

1. Review the requirements of laws governing protection of personal health information.
2. Describe the actions required of organizations for protecting personal health information.
3. Identify activities of nurses to protect personal health information.
4. Give examples of inappropriate use of protected health information.
5. Analyze clinical situations for compliance with privacy and security regulations.

KEY TERMS

Biometric identifiers
Breach
Business associate
Covered entity
Ethics
Health Insurance Portability and Account-
ability Act of 1996 (HIPAA)
Health Information Technology
for Economic and Clinical Health
(HITECH) Act

Law
Need to know
Notice of Privacy Practices
Patient Safety and Quality Improvement
Act of 2005 (PSQIA)
Patient Safety Organization (PSO)
Privacy
Protected health information (PHI)
Risk assessment
Security

CHAPTER OVERVIEW

This chapter presents the key components of laws governing the **privacy** and **security** of patient health information and contrasts ethical and legal requirements. Components of the **Health Insurance Portability and Accountability Act of 1996 (HIPAA)**, **Health Information Technology for Economic and Clinical Health (HITECH)**

Act, and **Patient Safety and Quality Improvement Act of 2005 (PSQIA)** laws related to protecting health information are presented. Aspects of maintaining the security of electronic forms of health information are discussed and implications for nurses are presented.

INTRODUCTION

Protecting patient information is an ethical and legal responsibility of nurses. Nurses are privy to very personal, intimate information about patients. The health history and physical assessment provide details of a person's life and background, and in the process of providing care, nurses gain even more information about a patient (California Nurses Association [CNA], 2011). If patients fear that health information is shared inappropriately, full disclosure may be compromised. For example, patients may not report a family history of mental illness or chronic disease if they fear the information could be used to deny a job opportunity. A history of sexually transmitted diseases, injuries resulting from violence or abuse, or drug use may be embarrassing. Thus, information needed for appropriate treatment is withheld due to fear of ridicule, judgment, or misuse; such fears may even cause someone to avoid seeking care. Critical information may be withheld that could not only impact quality of care for the individual but could also affect public safety (Rothstein, 2012).

When patients disclose personal information to nurses, they trust that the information will be handled in a professional manner (CNA, 2011). Such trust has been promoted by adherence to basic principles of ethical practice established by professional organizations. The ethical standards for nurses are defined in the American Nurses Association (ANA, 2001) *Code of Ethics for Nurses with Interpretative Statements*, with respect for human dignity as a foundational ethical principle. A component of this respect includes maintaining confidentiality of patient information. Position statements developed by the ANA clearly state the obligation of nurses to maintain privacy and confidentiality of patient information.

Professional healthcare associations and regulatory bodies support the ethical standards of confidentiality and privacy. The American Hospital Association (AHA, 2003) statement of patient rights and responsibilities identifies protection of privacy as a patient's right. Confidentiality is a requirement in accreditation standards, such as those promulgated by The Joint Commission and the Medicare and Medicaid Conditions of Participation (Rinehart-Thompson, 2013).

To comply with ethical and regulatory standards, healthcare organizations develop policies to ensure confidentiality of patient information. These privacy protections typically include restrictions on using patient names or likenesses without

> **Box 6-1   Case Study**
>
> Kandy Brown is a charge nurse on a medical unit. A member of her community garden club, Ms. Smith, is admitted to the unit for treatment of pneumonia. In reviewing the chart, Kandy notices that Ms. Smith is over 65 years old and that she is a Medicare beneficiary. Ms. Smith has never told the club her age but gives the impression that she is much younger than 65. Two weeks later, Kandy shares the information with another member of the club, and they both laugh at the fact they were fooled about Ms. Smith's true age.
>
> • Has Kandy violated any ethical principles?
> • Has she violated any laws?
> • Could her supervisor at the hospital take any actions against Kandy?

permission, disclosing private facts about a patient, providing unfavorable or false statements to the public about a patient, and unreasonable intrusion into a patient's affairs (CNA, 2011).

It is important to remember there is a difference between ethics and law. **Ethics**, a branch of philosopy that is concerned with the values of human behavior, can be subjective; it incorporates moral values and requires examination of the issues involved. Conversely, the **law** is an objective rule. Ethical standards are foundational and rarely change. A law may change or be overturned. A law may incorporate aspects of ethical behavior; so an ethical standard and a law may be essentially the same. Professional ethical codes of conduct are not law; but just as violation of a law can result in penalties, violations of ethical standards can also result in penalties such as termination by an organization or disciplinary action by a state licensing board. **Box 6-1** provides a case study to illustrate nurses' responsibilities.

HISTORY OF LEGAL PROTECTION FOR PRIVACY

Legal protection of personal health information was initially addressed in selected federal laws (Rinehart-Thompson, 2013). The Privacy Act of 1974 required federal agencies to protect personal information but did not specifically address health information and applied only to federal agencies. Federal drug laws of 1970 and 1972 established protection of information related to diagnosis and treatment of substance abuse. The Medicare and Medicaid Conditions of Participation required agencies to maintain confidentiality of patient records, but the scope was limited. The regulation applied only to Medicare and Medicaid patients; other patients were not included (Rinehart-Thompson, 2013).

State laws provide some protection of privacy, but the regulations vary from state to state and are limited in scope (CNA, 2011; Rinehart-Thompson, 2013). States have laws that require protection of sensitive health information such as human immunodeficiency virus (HIV)/acquired immune deficiency syndrome (AIDS) or mental health conditions. State laws also require reporting selected health conditions for public health and safety reasons such as communicable diseases and abuse and neglect of children, elders, and disabled persons. Reporting to maintain vital statistics such as births, deaths, and unnatural causes of death such as homicide or suicide is also required.

Prior to electronic communication, privacy of health information was recognized as an individual's right by federal agencies and professional organizations (Buckovich, Rippen, & Rozen, 1999). However, there was little consensus about some, but not all principles to protect health information. With the adoption of electronic health records (EHRs), new technologies brought the ability to limit access to health information; the same technologies could also make violating health information easier (Rothstein, 2012).

HEALTH INSURANCE PORTABILITY AND ACCOUNTABILITY ACT OF 1996 (HIPAA)

The ethical and regulatory guidelines for confidentiality were codified into federal law in 1996 with the passage of HIPAA (McGowan, 2012). The law covered more than just privacy protections; it included sections promoting continuity of health insurance coverage for employed people, reducing Medicare fraud and abuse, simplifying health insurance administration, as well as a section (Title II) protecting the privacy and security of health information. The passage of the law was significant because it established minimum national standards for protecting health information (McGowan, 2012; U.S. Department of Health and Human Services [HHS], 2005). The privacy section received much public attention; while it was received positively by many, it was also a cause of concern due to the costs of implementation.

Privacy and Security Regulations

The law directed the HHS Secretary to develop privacy and security regulations (CNA, 2011). The privacy rules focused on the rights of the patient; standards were established to protect health information communicated in any manner—verbally, on paper, visually, or electronically. Security rules addressed standards for

Table 6-1 Selected Terms Used in HIPAA Law	
Term	**Definition**
Individual	Person who is subject of protected health information
Personal representative	Person with legal authority to act on behalf of another in making healthcare decisions
Covered entity	One of three categories: healthcare provider, health plan, or health-care clearinghouse
Business associate	Person or organization that performs activities on behalf of covered entity
Designated record set	Records used by covered entities to make decisions about an individual; includes medical, billing, case management, enrollment, payment, and claims records
Breach	Unauthorized acquisition, access, use, or disclosure of PHI

Sources: HHS, 2005; Rinehart-Thompson, 2013.

protecting health information held or transmitted electronically (HHS, 2005). Penalities for failure to protect an individual's identifiable health information were also defined. Regulations to guide implementation of the privacy protection became effective in 2003, and security requirements became effective in 2005. (McGowan, 2012; Rinehart-Thompson, 2013). **Table 6-1** lists definitions of the common terms used in the law.

Privacy

The statute applied to **covered entities** and to **business associates**. Covered entities are defined as: (1) providers (ranging from an individual provider to a large organization) if the provider transmits health information in an electronic form, (2) health plans that provide or pay for health care, and (3) healthcare clearinghouses. A clearinghouse processes billing transactions or processes nonstandard health information received from another entity into a standard format. A business associate is a person or organization that uses protected health information to perform activities on behalf of a covered entity but is not part of the covered entity's workforce (HHS, 2005; Rinehart-Thompson, 2013).

To be considered **protected health information (PHI)**, three criteria must be met. First, PHI includes information that could reasonably identify the person such as name, address, date of birth, and social security number. Second, it includes past, current, or future information about the patient's physical or mental conditions, information about the provision of care, and information about payment for care. Finally, it must be held or transmitted electronically by the covered entity or business associates (McGowan, 2012; Rinehart-Thompson, 2013).

De-identified information does not contain data that could be used to identify an individual. It can be used or disclosed without restrictions. The law specifies two options for de-identification. One option is to use an expert to statistically ensure that any risk of identification is minimal. The other option is to remove the 19 defined identifiers of the individual, household members, or employers. The 19 elements include name; date of birth, admission, discharge, or death; addresses; email addresses; phone and fax numbers; medical record numbers; health plan beneficiary numbers; license and certification numbers; vehicle and device identifiers; **biometric identifiers** such as fingerprints and voice prints; and account numbers (HHS, 2005; Rinehart-Thompson, 2013).

HIPAA has requirements for two privacy documents that must be used to advise patients of how PHI will be protected and obtained from other entities (HHS, 2005). First, the law requires that a **Notice of Privacy Practices** be given to a patient upon the first contact with a covered entity and at other times upon request. The notice must be written in language that is easy for patients to understand and explain how the covered entity will use the patient's PHI. It is not necessary to provide a privacy notice upon subsequent encounters unless there are changes (Rinehart-Thompson, 2013). The second document is the authorization to share PHI. When such an authorization is required or requested by the patient, the law requires that specific components be included (see **Table 6-2**). It must be correct, written in plain language, and contain all the required elements (Rinehart-Thompson, 2013).

Although PHI cannot be shared without authorization to just anyone, HIPAA was not intended to make communication among caregivers difficult. It is important to remember that the intent of the law is to protect an individual's health information. The law requires that access be given only to those with a **need to know**, and that only the minimum amount of information needed to accomplish the purpose be released. A nurse would have a greater need for access to PHI than would a billing clerk. A nurse not involved in an individual's care would *not* have any need to know. Patient care, public safety, or efficient operations should not be compromised by withholding important information (HHS, 2005; McGowan, 2012). **Box 6-2** provides a case study illustrating the concept of need to know.

Table 6-2   Required Components of an Authorization
1. Name and signature of patient or authorized representative (and relationship to patient)
2. Kind of information to be disclosed
3. Individuals authorized to make disclosures
4. Individuals or organizations to whom the protected health information (PHI) will be disclosed
5. Purpose of a disclosure
6. Date of the disclosure authorization and expiration date
7. Statement that authorization can be revoked and how to do so
8. Statement that a copy of disclosed PHI will be provided to the patient
9. Statement that disclosed information may be redisclosed by the recipient and may no longer be protected
10. Statement that disclosure is voluntary and not required for treatment, payment, or eligibility for benefits
11. Statement of any fees for copy services; fees must be reasonable

Source: Reprinted with permission from the American Health Information Management Association. Copyright (c) 2013 by the American Health Information Management Association. All rights reserved. No part of this may be reproduced, reprinted, stored in a retrieval system, or transmitted, in any form or by any means, electronic, photocopying, recording, or otherwise, without the prior written permission of the association.

Box 6-2   Case Study
Joe Kitchens is a senior student in the local baccalaureate nursing program. He is doing a rotation in the surgery center and Mrs. Jones, a member of his church, comes in for the preop visit for a hysterectomy in 2 days. When Joe gets home that night, he tells his wife that Mrs. Jones is having surgery. The next day, his wife attends a prayer meeting and puts Mrs. Jones' name on the prayer lists, stating when and what surgery is scheduled. Later that day, a friend calls Mrs. Jones and asks why she had not told anyone. Mrs. Jones is very upset and calls the dean of the nursing program to complain and ask that Joe be dismissed from the program for violating her rights.
• Did Joe violate Mrs. Jones, PHI even though he didn't share paper or electronic information?
• What are the implications for the surgery center?
• If you were the dean of the nursing program, what action would you take?

HIPAA clearly defines situations when patient information cannot be shared without authorization, situations when information must be provided without authorization, and situations when disclosure is permitted without written authorization (HHS, 2005; McGowan, 2012; Rinehart-Thompson, 2013). Patient authorization is not required or is permitted in situations identified in **Box 6-3** and described in more detail in the paragraphs that follow.

Box 6-3   Sharing of PHI Allowed by HIPAA of 1996

- No authorization is required to disclose information to the patient or to the patient's personal representative (HHS, 2005).
- Providing information in a directory or notification of family and friends is permitted if the patient has an opportunity to informally agree or to object.
- No authorization is needed for sharing of information for purposes of treatment, for conducting the business of the organization, or for billing.
- HIPAA allows for the incidental disclosure of PHI occurring as a routine aspect of doing business.
- PHI may be shared without authorization to public agencies such as the Centers for Disease Control and Prevention (CDC) for surveillance of disease outbreaks.
- No authorization is required for HHS investigative review or enforcement activities. Rather, the information must be provided if requested by HHS (Rinehart-Thompson, 2013).
- Most states require reporting of PHI for vital statistics and public health purposes; HIPAA allows such reporting (CNA, 2011).
- If a state law conflicts with the federal law, the federal law has priority unless the state laws are more stringent (CNA, 2011).

No authorization is required to disclose information to the patient or to the patient's personal representative (HHS, 2005). Patients have a right to inspect and obtain a copy of their own health records (HHS, 2005). A fee may be charged by the covered entity for copying or release of information. The individual may also request that an amendment be made to PHI. Such a request is not automatically approved and may be denied under specific circumstances. For example, denial may be made if the record is already accurate or was not created or is not maintained by the covered entity. An individual may also request a list of disclosures that the covered entity has made. Disclosures that do not have to be included are those for which no authorization is required or those that the individual approved. The individual may request restrictions on uses and disclosures for administrative purposes. Because administrative purposes are a reason for use of PHI without written authorization, these restrictions do not have to be honored; but if the covered entity agrees, the restrictions must be followed (Rinehart-Thompson, 2013).

Providing information in a directory or notification of family and friends is permitted if the patient has an opportunity to informally agree or to object. According to HIPAA, the patient can authorize that information be shared with specified individuals. Permission can be given informally, but the patient must have an opportunity to agree or object. If no objection is raised, permission is implied. This permission enables the facility to maintain a directory of patients being treated and to give the location and general condition of a patient to someone asking for the patient by name. The institution is also allowed to maintain a listing of patients with religious affiliation if no objection is raised, and clergy can be given religious affiliation information. Informal permission is often given for information to be provided to family and friends involved in the person's care. If a patient is not capable of giving permission and is in an emergency situation, PHI can be shared if the healthcare providers (HCPs) determine it is in the best interest of the patient (Rinehart-Thompson, 2013).

No authorization is needed for sharing of information for purposes of treatment, for conducting the business of the organization, or for billing. This includes discussions and consultations among the caregivers, quality assessment and improvement activities, care coordination, compliance programs, fraud and abuse auditing, business planning, and administration of the organization. Information should **not** be shared with HCPs not involved in the care of the patient and who are not involved with administrative functions. Casual conversations and inappropriate disposal of documents containing PHI must be avoided (HHS, 2005).

HIPAA allows for the incidental disclosure of PHI occurring as a routine aspect of doing business—for example, calling a patient's name in a clinic or having patient information on a whiteboard that is in a private area not routinely accessible to the public. The covered entity must have implemented the minimum standards and reasonable safeguards. As long as only minimal information is given and no diagnostic information is provided, disclosure is considered incidental and authorization by the patient is not required (HHS, 2005; Rinehart-Thompson, 2013).

HCPs who are covered by HIPAA and who give care to an employer's employees can release PHI to the employer only for purposes of workplace surveillance and for evaluating an employee's work-related injury or illness, in accordance with other legal requirements (CNA, 2011). The employee must be provided with notice of the release of PHI (CNA, 2011).

PHI may be shared without authorization to public agencies such as the Centers for Disease Control and Prevention (CDC) for surveillance of disease outbreaks. No authorization is required for HHS investigative review or enforcement activities. Rather, the information *must* be provided if requested by HHS (Rinehart-Thompson, 2013).

Most states require reporting of PHI for vital statistics and public health purposes; HIPAA allows such reporting (CNA, 2011). When authorized by state law, PHI may also be shared with individuals who may have been exposed to communicable diseases such as tuberculosis and syphilis. PHI can be shared with appropriate legal entities in cases of suspected abuse and neglect, with other facilities for the donation and transplantation of organs and tissues, with agencies to protect an individual or the public from a serious threat, in worker's compensation cases, in legal proceedings about decedents, and in research (McGowan, 2012). If a state law conflicts with the federal law, the federal law has priority unless the state laws are more stringent. State statutes usually require more restrictions on health information related to a diagnosis of HIV/AIDS, mental illness, or substance abuse (CNA, 2011). The case studies in **Box 6-4** illustrate some of these HIPAA regulations about authorizations.

Security

HIPAA security standards establish the national standards for protection of health information that is held or transferred electronically. It includes all identifiable health information that a covered entity creates, receives, maintains, or transmits in an electronic format (HHS, 2005). It requires covered entities to protect against hazards that might affect the integrity of electronic PHI, protect against inappropriate disclosures of PHI, and ensure compliance by employees.

Karasz, Eiden, and Bogan (2013) note that whether a patient authorizes disclosure or if disclosure is allowed without authorization, transmission of electronic PHI *must* be conducted in accordance with the security rules. The law establishes safeguards to

---

Box 6-4   Case Study

Case Study 1

The surgical unit has a whiteboard in the nursing station listing the patient's last name, age, room number, diagnosis, and important activities for the day such as scheduled x-rays, surgery, or lab tests. The unit is closed to the public, but occasionally a patient's family member enters the unit looking for a specific nurse. Some of the nurses have concerns about the information on the board and question whether it is violating HIPAA regulations.

- As the unit director, what action should you take?
- Should the board be removed?

Case Study 2

The emergency department (ED) in Community Hospital has curtains separating the patients. As the new director, Carl Winslow is concerned about maintaining privacy, especially because many of the patients are elderly and have hearing problems. The caregivers must talk loudly in order for the patients to understand what is said. In addition, patient information is faxed to local nursing homes when a patient is to be transferred.

- Is there a potential HIPAA violation in this ED?
- What actions can be taken to ensure HIPAA privacy protections are met?

minimize the inappropriate use and disclosure as well as the incidental disclosure of PHI. Some standards are required while others are considered addressable, meaning that the organization can implement a reasonable equivalent (Rinehart-Thompson, 2013). Three types of security safeguards are required for electronic records: administrative, physical, and technical. There are requirements for organizational contracts and for policies and procedures (HHS, 2005; Karasz et al., 2013; Rinehart-Thompson, 2013). Organizational safeguards include specific requirements for contracts with business associates and group health plans. The policy, procedure, and documentation safeguards require that policies, procedures, activities to meet standards, and responses to complaints or **breaches** be written (electronic acceptable) and be maintained for 6 years from date of creation or date when last in effect. The policies and procedures must also be available to those who will be required to implement the policies and be reviewed and updated in response to changes that affect PHI (Rinehart-Thompson, 2013).

Administrative Safeguards

Administrative safeguards are the policies, procedures, and actions to protect the electronic PHI and manage the workforce (HHS, 2005; Rinehart-Thompson, 2013). Components of this category are described as follows.

Conduct a Risk Analysis

The risk analysis includes evaluation and impact of potential risks. Security measures to address the identified risks must be implemented with documentation of the measures and the rationale. The risk analysis must be continuous, with regular reporting and review (HHS, 2005; Rinehart-Thompson, 2013).

Develop a Security Management Process

A number of components are required for security management (HHS, 2005; Rinehart-Thompson, 2013). Among the requirements, two are particularly important: having a security officer and developing policies and procedures for access.

Appoint a security officer. The security official is responsible for developing and implementing security policies and procedures. The organization must also appoint someone to receive complaints about privacy policies, noncompliance, and violations of privacy.

Develop policies and procedures for access. Policies and procedures must be developed to ensure compliance with the regulations and limit access to electronic PHI to appropriate users only. Policies must address who has access and the degree of access, how clearance for access is obtained, and how access is terminated if the employee no longer works for the organization. Policies also establish disciplinary action for employees who violate confidentiality policies, including termination, and security incident procedures that describe the actions to respond to and report security issues.

Physical safeguards are required to limit physical access to electronic health information and ensure control (HHS, 2005; Rinehart-Thompson, 2013). Physical safeguards include facility access controls, workstation use and security, and device and media controls. Restrictions must limit unauthorized access and validate appropriate access to all areas and equipment containing electronic PHI. Access may be based on role or on the individual's identity. Use may be restricted such as "read only" or "read, edit, create, and print." Emergency plans must address access and restoration of data following an emergency or disaster. Any repairs or modifications of the physical areas containing PHI are to be documented and retained.

Policies and procedures must specify proper use of workstations and devices including transfer, removal, disposal, and reuse. Workstations in the facility and remote stations should be in secure locations with restricted viewing by the public or those without a need for access. This can be accomplished by privacy shields, automatic logoff, and returns to screensaver mode (HHS, 2005; Rinehart-Thompson, 2013).

The organization must implement policies and procedures to inventory the receipt and removal of devices that contain electronic PHI and for disposal of the devices. These include hard drives, magnetic tapes, disks, memory cards, and flash drives. Information must be deleted from any device that is to be reused. Data backup and storage are required before equipment is moved (HHS, 2005; Rinehart-Thompson, 2013).

Conduct Workforce Training and Management

All employees who have access to electronic PHI must have proper authorization. Training and education of security policies and procedures must be conducted.

Conduct Periodic Evaluations

An assessment must be conducted periodically to determine if the security policies and procedures continue to meet the requirements of the law.

Technical Safeguards

Required technical safeguards are access control, audit controls, integrity, entry authentication, and transmission security (HHS, 2005; Rinehart-Thompson, 2013). Aspects of technical safeguards are described in the following sections.

Implement Controls for Access, Audits, Integrity, and Transmission

Technical procedures must ensure access is proper, and electronic PHI is not altered or destroyed improperly. Hardware and software mechanisms that record access and alterations or destruction must be installed, and technical security measures implemented to prevent unauthorized access for PHI being transmitted electronically.

Access can be controlled through user identification, emergency access procedures, automatic logoff, and encryption. Unique user identification is required in order to identify and track a user and the functions that user is performing. Emergency access enables a user to access records even if controls are in place when an emergency occurs. For example, access may be disrupted if the electrical power is disrupted, or if a user is seeking information for which they normally do not have access. Automatic logoff helps to prevent unauthorized viewing. Encryption or scrambling of data is a way to protect data from being read while in transit. Only the use of user identification and emergency access is required (HHS, 2005; Rinehart-Thompson, 2013).

Policies for disposal of PHI must be developed to ensure that both the patient and the environment are protected. The law requires that a record be maintained of the movements of the hardware and electronic media. When a piece of equipment is disposed of, erasure of the PHI must be documented (Andersen, 2011).

Audit Controls

Mechanisms must be installed to examine and record activity. Audits are done after activity has occurred. There is no requirement for how often audits are conducted or what information is collected. Audits are useful in the investigation of breaches and misuse.

Integrity

Policies must address the unauthorized alteration or destruction of electronic PHI. Such actions may occur by mistake or on purpose. The policies must address all causes.

Entry Authentication

Procedures must be implemented to prevent unauthorized access to PHI. Methods include user or login identification (ID), passwords, key cards, and biometric identifiers such as fingerprints, face prints, or retinal scans. Biometric markers are the most secure means to authenticate users.

Table 6-3   Common Organizational Policies and Practices to Comply with HIPAA

1. Provide HIPAA training during orientation for all new employees.
2. Have employees sign documents acknowledging understanding of privacy requirements.
3. Conduct yearly HIPAA educational reviews and updates for all employees.
4. Require that all paper documents with PHI be shredded.
5. Limit access to areas holding documents with PHI (e.g., by locking doors or cabinets, requiring key cards for access).
6. Require passwords to access computers; require passwords to be changed periodically.
7. Forbid leaving patient information displayed on computers where it can be seen by others; require logging out when leaving the workstation.
8. Forbid sharing of passwords.
9. Install firewalls to protect servers.
10. Forbid access to PHI by caregivers not involved in care.
11. Monitor access to EHRs for inappropriate access.
12. Limit information on whiteboards to minimum necessary.
13. Place general information whiteboards in designated area least accessible to those not involved in care.
14. Install sound-muffling curtains in patient areas divided by curtains.
15. Require incident reporting of all suspected policy violations or unauthorized access, disclosure, transfer, or modifications.

Sources: DHHS, 2005; CNA, 2011.

Transmission Security

Electronic PHI must be protected from unauthorized access when it is transmitted via an electronic network. Firewalls, antivirus software, and encryption may be used to meet this requirement. Common organizational practices to meet the HIPAA regulations are listed in **Table 6-3**.

USE OF PHI IN MARKETING, FUNDRAISING, AND RESEARCH _____

HIPAA requires that authorization be given before PHI can be used in marketing. Marketing is defined as communications that encourage a person to purchase a product or service. Face-to-face communication or gifts of nominal value provided by the covered entity do not require authorization. However, the HITECH Act of 2009 strengthened the marketing restrictions (HHS, 2005; Rinehart-Thompson, 2013).

Disclosure of PHI to a foundation associated with the covered entity for purposes of fundraising is allowed. The privacy notice has to indicate that such use is possible and has to contain an option for the patient to be removed from the solicitation. The HITECH Act also strengthened the provisions related to fundraising (HHS, 2013a; Rinehart-Thompson, 2013).

The HIPAA regulations allow the use of patient information in research under defined conditions. The research must be reviewed by an institutional review board, and informed consent forms should be provided to the research participants. In general, care cannot be contingent upon signing an authorization for research purposes. No authorization is required if the PHI is de-identified or if the research uses a limited data set (Rinehart-Thompson, 2013).

ENFORCEMENT OF PRIVACY AND SECURITY OF PHI

The focus of enforcement is on entities such as healthcare plans and clearinghouses, providers who transmit health data, and Medicare prescription drug card sponsors. Individuals can be liable for conspiracy and aiding or abetting the disclosure of PHI. The HHS can also exclude a provider or entity from participation in Medicare and Medicaid programs for violation of standards. Authority for the enforcement of privacy standards is shared by the HHS Office for Civil Rights and the Centers for Medicare & Medicaid Services (HHS, 2005; CNA, 2011).

The American Recovery and Reinvestment Act of 2009 imposed civil monetary penalties for violations that are not corrected within 30 days, with fines ranging from $100 to $50,000 per violation, with a $1.5 million cap annually (HHS, 2013b). In 2005, the Department of Justice clarified that criminal penalties can be brought against individuals who knowingly (have knowledge of actions that are forbidden) violate, obtain, or disclose identifiable health information. The violator can be fined up to $50,000 and sentenced to 1 year in prison. If someone obtains PHI under false pretense, the fine can be increased up to $100,000, with an accompanying sentence of up to 5 years in prison. If the intent is for commercial purposes or malicious harm, the fine may reach $250,000, accompanied by a 10-year prison sentence (HHS, 2013a; CNA, 2011).

FILING COMPLAINTS

The HIPAA privacy and security provisions are comprehensive; confidentiality of health information is now mandated by federal law. However, the legal requirements do not end with the HIPAA regulations. Two more laws have subsequently been enacted to enhance the protection of an individual's health information.

Patient Safety and Quality Improvement Act of 2005 (PSQIA)

The PSQIA created a voluntary system for reporting medical errors without fear of liability. The patient safety information is considered a "patient safety work product" and can be shared by HCPs and organizations within a protected legal environment, with a common goal of improving patient safety and quality of care. The law contains provisions for the establishment of **Patient Safety Organizations (PSOs)**. A PSO can be public or private, for profit or not for profit. Insurance companies are not eligible to be designated as PSOs. The Agency for Healthcare Research and Quality (AHRQ) is responsible for certifying, listing, and overseeing PSOs (CNA, 2011; HHS, 2008).

PSOs are to receive reports of patients' events and safety concerns from HCPs and organizations, analyze the reports, and provide the results of the analysis to the organization or HCPs who originally reported the safety event or concern. Through analysis of the data, the PSOs can identify trends and patterns and propose measures to reduce risks of adverse events (HHS, 2005).

The PSQIA established civil penalties for knowing or reckless confidentiality violations of patient safety. Enforcement of the act is the responsibility of the HHS Office for Civil Rights. Civil penalties up to $11,000 per violation can be imposed (HHS, 2005).

HEALTH INFORMATION TECHNOLOGY FOR ECONOMIC AND CLINICAL HEALTH (HITECH) ACT

The HITECH Act is a section of the American Recovery and Reinvestment Act of 2009 that was enacted to stimulate the U.S. economy (HHS, 2013a). The health information technology (health IT) industry was identified as an area that could not only stimulate the economy but could also improve healthcare delivery (Gialanella, 2012). The HITECH Act established an Office of the National Coordinator for Health Information Technology (ONC). The ONC is to oversee the development of a national health IT infrastructure that will support the use and exchange of information. The goal of this infrastructure is to improve healthcare quality, reduce costs, promote public health, reduce health disparities, facilitate health research, and secure patient health information. Increasing the availability of health information is clearly related to the stated purposes of the law. Most EHRs enhance the ability to provide care with full knowledge of previous health history. This feature of EHRs can help to minimize duplication and promote care coordination among HCPs and agencies and aid in the development and comparison of performance measures. However, enhanced

---

Box 6-5   Regulations of the HITECH Act

1. Modify HIPAA regulations to make business associates directly liable for compliance with HIPAA regulations, to limit the use of PHI for marketing and fundraising purposes, and to allow individuals to receive electronic copies of PHI.
2. Establish increased, tiered civil money penalties.
3. Establish an objective breach standard.
4. Prohibit health plans from using or disclosing genetic information for underwriting purposes.

Source: Federal Register Vol. 78, No. 17, DHHS, January 25, 2013.

---

access to health records through such a national system also requires additional security to protect the privacy of individuals (Gialanella, 2012).

The HITECH Act establishes two national committees: the Policy Committee and the Standards Committee. The Policy Committee makes recommendations on implementation of the requirements of the law. The Standards Committee is charged with establishing standards for the electronic exchange of health information. The Policy Committee must have two HCPs as members, one of whom is a physician. There is no requirement for a nurse to be a member. There are no specified membership specialties for the Standards Committee (Gialanella, 2012). The regulations of the HITECH Act cover four areas shown in **Box 6-5**.

Under HIPAA business associates were regulated under the agreements with covered entities. After the HITECH Act was passed, business associates and subcontractors to business associates are under the jurisdiction of the HIPAA law and must comply with HIPAA security rules. Patient rights were expanded to include the right to obtain an electronic copy of PHI. If not available, then the individual has a right to a hard copy (Doe, 2009; Freeman, 2013).

The requirements for obtaining authorization for marketing purposes were strengthened. Under HIPAA, the sale of PHI was not specifically prohibited, so provisions in the HITECH Act imposed restrictions on the sale of PHI. If remuneration is received by the covered entity from a manufacturer for use of PHI, authorization is required from the patient. Sharing PHI for fundraising for the covered entity is allowed, but information provided to the patient must clearly state the opt-out option. Treatment cannot be withheld if the authorization is not given or if the patient chooses the op-out option (Doe, 2009; Freeman, 2013).

The law changed the requirement of a reportable breach. Following a breach, a **risk assessment** must be conducted by the covered entity. A breach is presumed unless there is a low probability that PHI has been compromised following a risk assessment. The required risk assessment includes an assessment of the PHI involved, the person who used or to whom the PHI was disclosed, whether the PHI was actually viewed, and the extent of the risk (Freeman, 2013).

Enforcement Activities

The Office for Civil Rights within the HHS has responsibility for enforcement of civil penalties of HIPAA. Under the HITECH Act, state attorneys general now have authority to investigate HIPAA violations and can impose civil penalties of up to $25,000 (Gialanella, 2012; Vanderpool, 2012). Civil actions are most commonly the result of complaints from individuals (Vanderpool, 2012). Examples of civil cases are loss of patient records by an employee taking records home or a health plan failing to honor patient requests for access to their records. The criminal provisions now apply to individuals—not just to a covered entity. Criminal cases may involve accessing PHI for financial gain or for simple snooping. In a recent case, a physician and several hospital employees were individually fined and had to perform community service after inappropriately accessing records of a high-profile patient (Vanderpool, 2012).

Changes to Filing Complaints After Enactment of the HITECH Act

Complaints can be filed by anyone who thinks that a covered entity or a business associate has violated some aspect of the privacy or security rules. The complaint must be submitted to the Office for Civil Rights in writing—paper or electronically. The form and directions for use are available online, and a link can be found on the companion website to this text.

UNRESOLVED ISSUES OF HEALTH INFORMATION _____

Rothstein (2012) notes that concerns about privacy continue to escalate as electronic storage, use, and transmission of health information expand. Individuals give permission to access personal records for many reasons, but individuals may have access to health information that has no relevance to a current condition or situation. For example, Rothstein questions whether an ED physician treating a woman for a broken ankle needs to know her past sexual history. However, an insurance company would want to know her history of cervical cancer. Rothstein suggests that health records be "segmented" to grant appropriate access to a provider or an agency while protecting the privacy of the patient from inappropriate access. However, the technical problems to implement a "segmented" approach are great and the costs are significant.

Concerns have also been identified about the penalties for violations (Sarrico & Hauenstein, 2011). Self-reporting in good faith with actions for improvement may still result in costly fines. This can be especially devastating to individual providers such as physicians and nurse practitioners. Efforts to promote sharing of electronic health information may be hampered by strict enforcement and excessive fines. The unintended consequences of enforcement may be a reluctance to participate in health information exchanges.

Researchers have raised questions about the use of patient data for research purposes while maintaining compliance with privacy regulations (CNA, 2011). Researchers have reported drops in participation rates as a result of the implementation of HIPAA compliance consents and authorizations. Regulations from the HITECH Act have eased some of the requirements for researchers to enable patients to more easily authorize use of PHI for research, but approaches to de-identify data that are effective and low cost are needed when authorization was not obtained or possible.

The use of smartphones and social media (e.g., Facebook, Twitter, YouTube) create new issues with PHI. Not only do covered entities need to have policies that employees follow, but they must also consider what visitors, family members, and students might do to violate the privacy of health information. Ekrem (2011) provides tips to avoid HIPAA violations using social media. The first and most important tip is never to post or tweet about patients, even in general terms. Other helpful tips include: Avoid mixing professional and personal lives in social media; don't complain about work online; and if the information shouldn't be said in an elevator, it shouldn't be posted using social media. Other important confidentiality practices for nurses are described in **Table 6-4**. **Box 6-6** provides a case study about social media and PHI.

Box 6-6   Case Study

Mindy Wheeler is a student nurse in her last semester of nursing school. She is working with a preceptor in a cardiothoracic intensive care unit. One day she has the opportunity to observe coronary bypass grafting from an enclosed theater. During the operation, she was able to take pictures and later she posted them on a social networking website. She did not provide the patient's name but did give age, sex, and details of previous health history leading up to the need for a bypass surgery. She stated she was posting the information to encourage her friends to follow good health habits in order to avoid problems.

- Did Mindy violate ethical standards?
- Did she violate HIPAA regulations? If so, in what way?
- Is it likely there were hospital policies regarding her actions?
- If you were the dean of the school, what would you do?

Table 6-4   Confidentiality Practices for Nurses
1. Do not discuss patient information in public places (hallways, elevators, cafeterias).
2. Keep user names and password secure. Do not share user name or password; do not use another person's password.
3. Log off when leaving a computer; do not leave a computer open for another person to access.
4. Attend educational sessions on updates to confidentiality policies.
5. Do not take or use pictures of patients without permission.
6. Never share patient information with those without a need to know. Only provide information to caregivers involved in care of the patient or to administrative personnel authorized to receive such information.
7. Do not allow observations of care by others not involved in care of patient (such as a student) without the patient's permission.
8. Never post information or pictures of a patient on social media, even if the name of the patient is not used.
9. Dispose of records containing patient information according to policy (such as shredding).
10. Avoid unnecessary printing of PHI.
11. Never transfer PHI to an outside entity unless authorized to do so. Transfer according to policy.
12. Never access records without authorization. This includes own record or records of family members.
13. Follow security requirements for accessing PHI remotely.
14. Report any breaches of privacy immediately.

SUMMARY

Statutes and the associated regulations protecting privacy and confidentiality are detailed and include provisions beyond just the routine delivery of daily care. Organizations establish policies and technology restricting access to PHI to promote compliance with the regulations; however, details of the regulations may not always be covered completely in a policy. It is not a good idea for nurses to assume that they understand procedures for dealing with PHI; instead, questions about unique situations should be directed to the designated experts within the healthcare facility. Failure to adhere to ethical, legal, and policy expectations can result in severe penalties. A nurse may be terminated by the employer, the state board of nursing may take action against the nurse, and the patient may file a lawsuit against the nurse—all are possible negative effects of breaching confidentiality and privacy. The nurse is duty bound, professionally and legally, to know and adhere to confidentiality policies and

Table 6-5 Internet Resources to Understand Laws and Regulations About Protected Health Information	
Resource	**Internet Address**
HHS Health Information Privacy	http://www.hhs.gov/ocr/privacy/index.html
HHS Guide to Privacy and Security of Health Information	http://www.healthit.gov/sites/default/files/pdf/privacy/privacy-and-security-guide.pdf
HHS Health Information Privacy, Security, and Your EHR	http://www.healthit.gov/providers-professionals/ehr-privacy-security
Health Information Privacy Complaint	http://www.hhs.gov/ocr/privacy/hipaa/complaints/hipcomplaintform.pdf
Your Mobile Device and Health Information Privacy and Security	http://www.healthit.gov/providers-professionals/your-mobile-device-and-health-information-privacy-and-security
Seven Tips to Avoid HIPAA Violations in Social Media	http://www.kevinmd.com/blog/2011/06/7-tips-avoid-hipaa-violations-social-media.html

HHS, U.S. Department of Health and Human Services; HIPAA, Health Insurance Portability and Accountability Act of 1996; EHR, electronic health record.

procedures. Nurses must disclose information appropriately to ensure that care and continuity are promoted but should not share information with anyone who does not have a need to know. More information about law and regulations can be found in the companion website and in **Table 6-5**.

The future of privacy protections of health information is unknown. As technology improves, will access be expanded? Will methods be developed to provide enhanced privacy? Today's laws and regulations will evolve and change as the technology changes, but the basic ethical standard for protecting privacy and confidentiality will not change. The challenge for all HCPs, including nurses, is to be aware of the need for privacy, to follow the policies currently in place, to keep abreast of changes, and to lead or participate in developing new approaches and guidelines for protecting privacy.

For a full suite of assignments and additional learning activities, use the access code located in the front of your book and visit www.jblearning.com. If you do not have an access code, you can obtain one at the site.

REFERENCES

American Hospital Association (AHA). (2003). *The patient care partnership: Understanding expectations, rights, and responsibilities.* Retrieved from http://www.aha.org/content/00-10/pcp_english_030730.pdf

American Nurses Association (ANA). (2001). *Code of ethics for nurses with interpretive statements.* Washington, DC: American Nurses Association Publishing. Retrieved from http://nursingworld.org/MainMenuCategories/EthicsStandards/CodeofEthicsforNurses/2110Provisions.html

Andersen, C. M. (2011). A primer for health care managers: Data sanitization, equipment disposal, and electronic waste. *Health Care Manager, 30*(3), 266–270.

Buckovich, S., Rippen, H., & Rozen, M. (1999). Driving toward guiding principles: A goal for privacy, confidentiality, and security of health information. *Journal of the American Medical Informatics Association, 6*, 122–133. doi:10.1136/jamia.1999.0060122

California Nurses Association (CNA). (2011). HIPAA—The Health Insurance Portability and Accountability Act: What RNs need to know about privacy rules and protected electronic health information. *National Nurse, 107*(6), 20–27.

Doe, J. (2009). HITECH meets HIPAA: HITECH Act changes to HIPAA obligations for covered entities and business associates. *Journal of Health Information Management, 23*(4), 15–16.

Ekrem, D. (2011). 7 tips to avoid HIPAA violations in social media. Retrieved from http://www.kevinmd.com/blog/2011/06/7-tips-avoid-hipaa-violations-social-media.html

Freeman, G. (2013). Final HIPAA rule increases penalties, liability for associates. *Healthcare Risk Management, 35*(3), 25–27.

Gialanella, K. M. (2012). Legislative aspects of nursing informatics: HITECH and HIPAA. In D. McGonigle & K. G. Mastrian (Eds), *Nursing informatics and the foundation of knowledge* (2nd ed., pp. 161–184). Burlington, MA: Jones & Barlett Learning.

Karasz, H. N., Eiden, A., & Bogan, S. (2013). Text messaging to communicate with public health audiences: How the HIPAA security rule affects practice. *American Journal of Public Health, 103*(4), e999–e997. doi: http://dx.doi.org/10.2105/10AJPH.2012.300999

McGowan, C. (2012). Patients' confidentiality. *Critical Care Nurse, 32*(5), 61–65. doi: http://dx.doi.org/10.4037/ccn2012135

Rinehart-Thompson, L. A. (2013). *Introduction to health information privacy and security.* Chicago, IL: American Health Information Management Association Press.

Rothstein, M. A. (2012). Currents in contemporary bioethics. *Journal of Law, Medicine & Ethics, 40*(2), 394–400. doi: http://dx.doi.org/10.1111/j.1748-720X.2012.00673.x

Sarrico, C., & Hauenstein, J. (2011). Can EHRs and HIEs get along with HIPAA security requirements? *Healthcare Financial Management, 65*(2), 86–90.

U.S. Department of Health and Human Services (HHS). (2005). *Understanding patient safety confidentiality.* Retrieved from http://www.hhs.gov/ocr/privacy/psa/understanding/index.html

U.S. Department of Health and Human Services (HHS). (2008). *Patient Safety and Quality Improvement Act of 2005, Federal Register, 73*(226). Retrieved from http://www.gpo.gov/fdsys/pkg/FR-2008-11-21/pdf/E8-27475.pdf

U.S. Department of Health and Human Services (HHS). (2013a). *Health information privacy.* Retrieved from http://www.hhs.gov/ocr/privacy/hipaa/enforcement/examples/index.html

U.S. Department of Health and Human Services (HHS). (2013b). *Modifications to the HIPAA Privacy, Security, Enforcement, and Breach Notification Rules Under the Health Information Technology for Economic and Clinical Health Act and the Genetic Information Nondiscrimination Act; other modifications to the HIPAA Rules; Final Rule, Federal Register*, 78(17). Retrieved from http://www.gpo.gov/fdsys/pkg/FR-2013-01-25/pdf/2013-01073.pdf

Vanderpool, D. (2012). Risk management: HIPAA—should I be worried? *Innovations in Clinical Neuroscience, 9*(11/12), 30–55.

CHAPTER 7

Database Systems for Healthcare Applications

Manil Maskey, MS
Susan Alexander, DNP, RN, ANP-BC, ADM-BC
Gennifer Baker, MSN, RN, CCNS

CHAPTER LEARNING OBJECTIVES

1. Review concepts used to describe databases.
2. Describe how databases can be used in healthcare settings.
3. Review tools used to work with databases.
4. Describe examples of how databases can be used in healthcare settings.

KEY TERMS

Data warehouse
Database
Database management system
Embedded relational database
Flat database model
Forms
Integrity rules

Open source relational database
Proprietary relational database
Query
Relational database model
Report
Security
Structured query language (SQL)

CHAPTER OVERVIEW

Databases have become an essential part of everyday life. People constantly interact with databases in some way. Healthcare applications also rely heavily on databases. With the advent of Web 2.0 technologies, improved search and retrieval techniques are being applied for databases. Database technology has made tremendous strides, and in order to understand the technology, a review of the basic concepts used in database systems is needed. This chapter introduces the basics of database systems and their components. Applications of databases in healthcare delivery systems are also reviewed.

USING DATABASES IN HEALTHCARE SETTINGS

Background knowledge relating to the design, implementation, and use of databases is useful, because nurses may interact with databases frequently throughout the course of their daily activities. A **database** is a collection of related data. In healthcare communities, databases may be used by medical personnel for the recording of patient care, patient diagnoses and treatment plans, medications, and for progress toward treatment goals. In assessing the efficacy of drugs and clinical procedures, researchers may also use databases.

A **database management system** (DBMS) is a set of software that enables users to create and maintain a database. **Figure 7-1** depicts a simple DBMS. Consider an example in a healthcare setting: a clinical database for maintaining information concerning patients, medical histories, and medications. **Figure 7-2** illustrates the database structure, along with sample data, that would be used in such a setting. Here, the database is organized using three types of data, on columnar storage: Patient, Medical History, and Medication. Each of the columnar storage levels is called a *table*. Each column in a table defines a *field*. A field describes a particular attribute of a record (a row in a table). Notice that records in the three tables are related. The patient records in the Patient table are related to Medical History and Medication tables. The records in the Patient table are linked to records in the Medical History table using PatientID fields. Similarly, the records

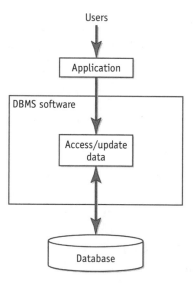

FIGURE 7-1   Elements of database design and management.

Patient

Name	Patient ID	DOB
Jason Smith	12	2012-12-01
Pat Hines	34	1979-02-28

Medical History

Patient ID	Observation ID	Observation Date	Diagnosis
12	3	2013-03-05	Infection
34	5	2012-12-24	Flu

Medication

Patient ID	Observation ID	Prescription
12	3	Amoxicillin
34	5	Tamiflu

FIGURE 7-2 Structure of a database used in a healthcare setting.

in the Medical History table are linked to records in the Medication table using PatientID and ObservationID fields. Database manipulation involves reading and updating the data on the tables. An example read operation may be "all patients and who are older than 4 years old and have been diagnosed with flu." Such read operations can be easily and precisely constructed using **structured query language (SQL)**.

Advantages of Using Databases

There are numerous advantages to using databases. For example, databases can store large amounts of data efficiently, without taking up large amounts of disk space, and data are easily discoverable when stored in a database. Database operations are optimized for fast response. The use of a common language such as SQL makes interacting with data easy, and the data can be imported into and modified by other software applications. In addition, multiple software applications can access the same database simultaneously.

In healthcare settings, other than uses for accounting and billing purposes, databases have other uses such as the long-term storage and maintenance of patient information (histories, medications, and similar items), and for the efficient exchange of patient information between healthcare providers (HCPs). Databases can also be used to develop patient care applications and for research purposes.

Models of Databases Used in Healthcare Settings

Database designs can be classified into two main models: flat and relational. In a **flat database model**, only one table is used, and the attributes are defined as separate columns of the table. In a **relational database model**, a collection of tables is used and linked together by relationship between attributes within the separate tables and/or operations within the tables.

While a flat database can be simple to construct, as a design it is problematic when data from two databases need to be merged. With flat databases, one may add information as necessary without affecting existing data, because there is no relationship between the attributes within the flat database.

Designing a relational database takes more planning than designing a flat database, but there are advantages to the use of relational databases that make these the preferred solution for many settings in which long-term data management is necessary. For example, redundancy of data, or the repetition of a field in two or more places in a database, is a phenomenon that can lead to error and eventual loss of storage space. When a relational database is used, data redundancy is minimized. However, when relational databases are used, one must take care to store data in tables in such a way that the relationships make sense. Building a relational database requires knowledge of the overall schema so that a relational model can be established. The model must fully describe how the data are organized, in terms of data structure, integrity, querying, manipulation, and storage. Because most database design is dominated by the relational model, from here on the chapter will focus on various aspects of the relational database model.

WORKING WITH DATABASES

Types of Relational Databases

There are three primary relational database systems: proprietary, open source, and embedded. **Proprietary relational databases** are licensed by vendors. Frequently, proprietary relational databases provide a robust set of management tools that includes creation of a data warehouse (described later in this chapter). Certain proprietary databases are packaged into software suites, such as Microsoft Office, which can include the Access DBMS. Other proprietary relational database systems include Oracle and Teradata. **Open source relational databases**, such as MySQL (http://www.mySQL.com) and PostGIS (http://postgis.net), are freely available for use. **Embedded relational databases** are packaged as part of other software or hardware applications. For example, local databases used by a mobile application to store phone numbers can be considered an embedded relational database. Application vendors provide packaged databases along with the application that can manipulate the database structure.

Depending on their needs, healthcare applications may use propriety, embedded, or open source relational databases. Large healthcare enterprises tend to use proprietary relational databases due to their needs for customization and support. Smaller healthcare facilities may prefer open source relational databases due to lower cost. However, more and more HCPs are also using the embedded relational databases due to popularity of mobile applications.

Relationships

During the design of a relational database, it is necessary to first create a conceptual model of the data. The Entity-Relationship (ER) Model is frequently used to visually describe the data and their relationships (**Figure 7-3**). The ER model describes data as entities, relationships, and attributes (**Figure 7-4**). An entity is the basic component in an ER model, representing an object or a thing. Properties of the entity are known as attributes. Attributes describe the entity. A patient could be considered an entity, with the patient's name and date of birth as attributes of the patient. In an ER model, attributes from one entity refer to attributes from another entity. Such references are represented as relationships. Knowledge and consideration of these relationships are vital to the design of successful databases and software applications.

Queries

A **query** is an operation that is used to directly retrieve and update data from a database table. SQL standardizes the ways to perform such operations on various implementations of relational databases. Relational databases allow the user to predefine certain record fields as keys or indexes, perform efficient search, join records, and establish integrity constraints. Queries then utilize the predefined record fields, known as the indexes, to perform operations. Search queries are faster and more accurate when based on indexed values. Join queries are used to join records from multiple tables using indexed fields that are common to each table. Think of a query as a tool designed to rapidly retrieve needed data from the database. For example, a basic search query might include a list of pediatric patients who are younger than 6 years old.

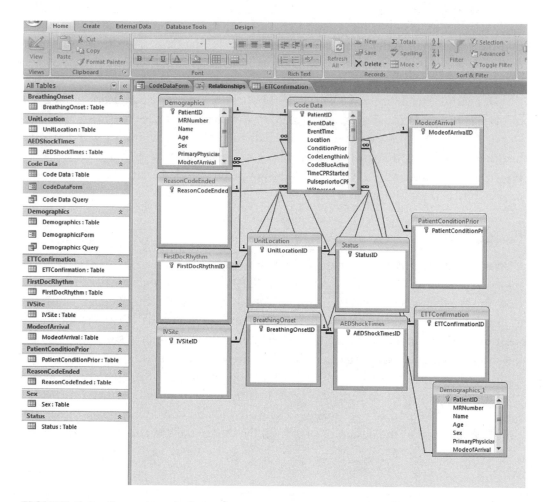

FIGURE 7-3 Illustration of relationships created in a proprietary relational database software application.

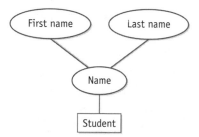

FIGURE 7-4 Entity Relationship Model used to describe relationship between first name, last name, and student in a relational database.

Source: Copyright © 2002, Dr. Angela B. Shiflet. Reprinted by permission.

Reports

Relational databases typically offer a more robust reporting system, when compared to flat database designs, with the use of embedded report generators that can filter and display selected fields. Many applications with embedded relational databases offer the user the capability to build customized reporting modules. A table can be constructed and linked to data sources for multiple reports. Keeping tables up to date in relational databases makes it possible to present well-organized information in attractive formats for quick reporting. Many situations can be identified in healthcare settings in which the need for quick reports exists. For example, it would be useful in a pediatrics office to be able to generate a report illustrating a growth chart for an infant to document whether the infant is following a typical growth pattern.

Forms

Forms are the traditional interface to databases and offer a simple visual mechanism for users to insert new data into relational databases (see **Figure 7-5**). For example, at

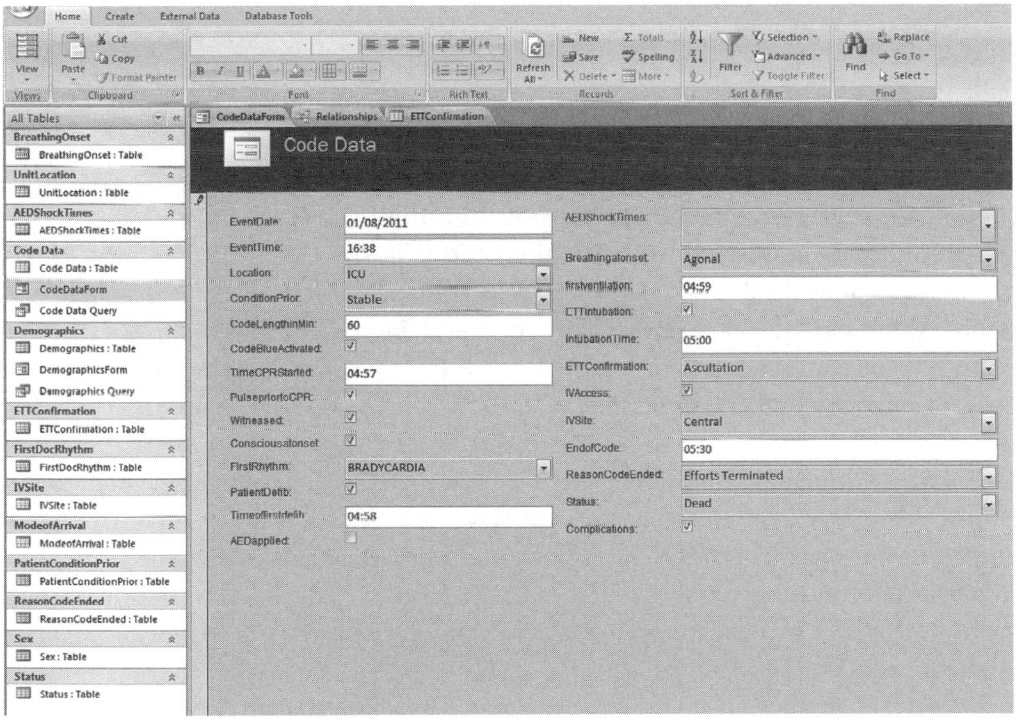

FIGURE 7-5 Example of a form that can be created using a proprietary relational database application.

a clinic, the receptionist fills out the patient information to add a new patient record into the patient database. An advanced form can be constructed that will complete data fields based on historically filled data fields, or drop-down choices can be added. Almost all HCPs use some variation of forms to enter information into their databases.

Integrity and Security

Relational databases allow the enforcement of **integrity rules**. The rules protect the validity of the data. For example, if entity integrity is enforced, then every record will have its own specific identity and there will be no duplicated records. Referential integrity is defined using "primary" and "foreign" keys, which are fields in tables that act as links (relationships) between tables. When properly defined, these keys prevent inconsistent deletions or updates. Healthcare databases require data integrity and **security**. In fact, because healthcare databases store patient information, there is a need for more rigorous protection of the database. Incorrect information presented to clinicians may lead to misdiagnosis, incorrect treatment, and negative outcomes, including the death of patients. Many regulations govern the security of health-related patient information.

DATA WAREHOUSING

Data warehouses have a distinguishing characteristic in that they are designed and optimized with specific applications in mind (Elmasri & Navathe, 2003). A data warehouse consists of several components (**Figure 7-6**). The data source layer includes various databases with which users and applications interact. Implementations of the data warehouse may also contain data sources that include data from external sources. The data that are extracted from various sources are designed to provide specific functionalities and form the structure of the data warehouse. Decision support systems are used in the warehouse to provide specific analyses, reports, mining, and other processing that users seek from the data. In a data warehouse, queries are optimized to provide efficient access to data for analysis, reporting, and mining. Data warehouses designed to store and use data summaries and snapshots are unlike databases that store records in tables. For example, a data warehouse of a healthcare system may keep aggregated data values of all of its patient records.

Often, data warehouses involve executing data analysis queries from various data sources; thus those data analysis queries are optimized for performance and efficiency.

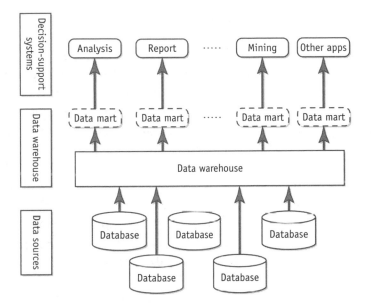

FIGURE 7-6 Elements in a typical data warehouse.

In a healthcare setting, each HCP may store patients' electronic health records in a database. Such a database would be sufficient for the daily business of a small clinic. Imagine that data analysts at the Centers for Disease Control and Prevention (CDC) might want to import information relating to treatment of influenza cases from private HCPs into a data warehouse in order to determine trends or mine for a specific event relating to influenza treatment. A data warehouse would be created, containing aggregated data from many different HCPs, in order to better understand events surrounding an outbreak of influenza.

Designing Data Warehouses

In general, data warehouses consist of several components as depicted in Figure 7-1 (Sen & Sinha, 2005). Operational databases and data sources send data to the warehouse. The design of the data warehouse should always include the flexibility to allow for the inclusion of new databases and data marts that may be available or needed in the future. At the bottom of the data warehouse are operational databases, where data are updated by various sources. From the warehouse itself, specific "views" of the data warehouse are designed to provide the data needed for analyses, reports, and mining activities. Periodic summaries and reports, along with ad hoc analyses, are common functionalities that data warehouse applications provide.

Perhaps one of the great examples to date of construction of an application-driven data warehouse has been a 15-month project involving the tracking of nursing-sensitive care outcomes sponsored by the National Quality Forum (NQF, 2007). The intent of this landmark project was to describe and evaluate the contribution of nurses in acute care hospitals to patient safety, healthcare quality, and professionalism in the work environment. The project used various strategies for data collection, including abstraction from electronic health records directly to the project databases, semi-structured telephone interviews of project participants, and web-based surveys to gather perceptions from hospital nurses and nurse leaders on the contribution of the nursing workforce to patient safety and other outcomes. Despite the obvious importance of the nursing workforce to patient outcomes in hospitals, respondents identified barriers to adoption of NQF standards for the measurement of the quality of nursing care in hospitals, including the lack of a business case for the implementation of measurement and support by hospital administrators (NQF, 2007). Stakeholders hope that ongoing maintenance and updating of the NQF data warehouse will help to determine priorities for future research and priorities for consensus setting to promote widespread adoption of NQF standards.

As analysis of the data in the NQF warehouse continues to progress, other authors hope that this will yield specific recommendations that the nursing profession can adopt to inspire trust in the care that it provides to U.S. citizens. Kurtzman and Jennings (2008, p. 353) have proposed an agenda that includes:

- Identification of measures that quantify nurses' contributions to patient safety and quality outcomes
- Use of performance assessments derived from those measures in daily clinical management
- Regular benchmarking for hospitals' nursing quality goals
- Public reporting of nursing quality measures to key stakeholders and communities

Research in database technology is ongoing. Recent developments include the introduction of NoSQL ("Not only SQL") databases. NoSQL databases come in various flavors, each addressing a particular issue with relational databases. For example, MongoDB (http://www.mongodb.org/) is a document-based database system that is very easy to use and has looser consistency in terms of relations than relational databases do. Cassandra (http://cassandra.apache.org/), a database system that is designed to address performance and scalability, is another example of a new database system.

With the ever-increasing amount of healthcare data and policy changes toward mandating electronic records, scalability and performance of the relational databases will be tested. Furthermore, new and innovative devices that monitor patients' every activity will produce a different set of data relationships that may not be addressed by relational databases.

APPLICATIONS IN HEALTHCARE SETTINGS

While the primary job responsibility of newly graduated nurses may not be to design databases for use in healthcare facilities, it is important to recall that the chances of a nurses interacting with databases in almost any variety of healthcare setting are great. The accurate entry of data into an electronic health record is arguably the most basic responsibility of any nurse and may likely represent the initial exposure of the new graduate to a database. In this section of the chapter, selected models of nurses' utilization of relational databases in aspects of patient care activities are reviewed.

Customizing Relational Databases for the Smaller Practice Setting

The use of relational databases can be customized to meet the needs of healthcare facilities and practices of many sizes. A small, private practice in the Southeastern United States replaced its flat database with a relational database, developed using Microsoft Access, a proprietary software package, for long-term maintenance of patient data in its outpatient diabetes self-management training program (Alexander, Frith, O'Keefe, & Hennigan, 2011). In the diabetes program, retrieval of accurate patient demographic data at 6- and 12-month intervals following initial class attendance was tied to program revenues. Variability and errors contained in the flat database had resulted in reduced revenues for the program. Implementation of the relational database required training for the practice staff, but it resulted in improved accuracy in data entry, when practice staff were surveyed (Alexander et al., 2011). Use of the relational database was reported as an economical solution to meet the long-term data storage needs of the program, because costs for the purchase and installation of the software application, plus staff training, were only slightly more than half of budgeted amounts.

Improving Nurse–Patient Staffing Ratios

Nurse staffing ratios, the number of nurses relative to the number of patients on a given unit, are a source of concern to patients and caregivers. In 2009 the American

Nurses Association acknowledged that "the appropriate skill mix and number of registered nurses engaged in direct patient care is necessary to provide safe nursing care" (p. 4). However, such a determination can be difficult to identify, and it can change on a daily basis as nursing staff fluctuates. Retrospective analysis of data collected over months and years is often insufficient to assist a nursing manager in making real-time staffing decisions. To better characterize the relationships between nursing skill mix, the numbers of registered nurses, and patient data, researchers at an urban hospital in the Northeast United States created the Patient-Nurse Database (Radwin, Cabral, Chen, & Jennings, 2010). Using Microsoft Access, researchers created nine separate databases (five with patient data; four with nurse data) and merged them to form the Patient–Nurse Database, designed to better track patient care processes and outcomes over an 18-month period on a hematology-oncology floor. Researchers found that use of the database was effective in capturing the daily variability unique to the unit's staff and patients, also suggesting that the database and its data-capture protocol could easily be expanded to other units, such as surgical or cardiac floors, where a similar need for real-time staffing management is necessary based on census and nurse skill mix (Radwin et al., 2010).

Using Automated Systems for Nurse Competencies

Learning management systems (LMS) are relational databases that provide educational services for users, including registration, routing, and reporting (Dumpe, Kanyok, & Hill, 2007). Traditionally used in academic settings, the use of LMS has rapidly expanded to fields such as business and health care. In facility-based nursing education, where administrators struggle to maintain the competencies of nurses with variable schedules and needs, LMS can offer an economical and easily accessible solution for employers and employees. In 2003, the Cleveland Clinic Foundation partnered with the Division of Education at the Foundation in order to create an online curriculum, delivered via an LMS, that would educate all employees on the Health Insurance Portability and Accountability Act (HIPAA) and patient confidentiality. The LMS was subsequently expanded to include options such as customized assignments based on job functions, staff surveys, reporting to supervisors and human resource personnel, and automatic scoring of quizzes for tracking of progress. Use of the LMS represented a cost savings for the Division of Nursing due to a reduction in overtime related to competency assessments for personnel and the use of nursing education personnel needed to complete the competency assessments (Dumpe et al., 2007).

The Virtual Dashboard

The Collaborative Alliance for Nursing Outcomes (CALNOC) is a coalition of acute care hospitals and is the largest nurse quality reporting network in the United States (Aydin, Bolton, Donaldson, Brown, & Mukerji, 2008). To date, CALNOC has 15 years of data from more than 1,700 nursing units in nine states. The CALNOC system is a secure, multi-tier, web-based system that consists of two major subsystems: a membership-management application containing demographic information for member hospitals and employees and a data-analysis application where data are stored, analyzed, and reported to CALNOC members. Member facilities submit data in spreadsheets using applications such as Microsoft Excel. Various types of reports can subsequently be generated from CALNOC data, and the reports can be drilled down to specific hospitals or units for benchmarking of performance. This reporting capacity is unique in that member hospitals can create their own virtual dashboards containing selected performance measures to meet their needs for projects such as performance initiatives, goal setting, or root cause analysis (Aydin et al., 2008).

Nursing Quality Benchmarks as Clinical Dashboards

The power of databases can truly be demonstrated when used to improve care for patients. Pressure ulcers and patient falls are two conditions that have been identified as key indicators of nursing care quality in hospitals by the NQF. In further study of the potential utility of the CALNOC databases, Donaldson, Brown, Aydin, Bolton, and Rutledge (2005) reported on a project designed to transform data analysis into useful information. Pressure ulcers and patient falls are examples of nurse-sensitive quality measures; NQF has recommended that all hospitals collect data on these measures (NQF, 2007). One CALNOC site decided to transform its own data on patient falls and pressure ulcers into an internal performance improvement project by adding these clinical benchmarks to its virtual dashboard. The addition of data on these indicators aided the facility in quickly evaluating baseline performance measurement across its specific units. In subsequent data analysis, Donaldson and colleagues (2005) found that half of the patients who developed pressure ulcers during inpatient stays at the facility were found to be "at risk" upon admission. The authors further noted that a quarter of the patient falls in the facilities occurred in critical care/step-down units, which are areas traditionally associated with closer patient monitoring and reduced fall risk. The facility was able to implement highly specific performance-improvement activities and use the clinical dashboards in ongoing follow up of the activities.

Box 7-1   Case Study

Brian has worked for the past 7 years on a medical-surgical floor. Because of his exceptional skills in initiating intravenous access (IVs), Brian is often called upon to assist in situations when patients have experienced multiple failed attempts by other staff members to start IVs. Brian's skills, and those of other nurses in the facility, have been noted by nurse leaders, and efforts to create an IV team have started. Because charting in the facility is hybrid (a mix of paper and electronic methods), documentation of the workflow surrounding IV requires thoughtful attention to user experiences and workflow. Brian is appointed to participate in a team that is designated to create a new electronic IV charting pathway that will reflect desired outcomes. A flow form, or an electronic template used to chart data and clinical findings, would be used as the basis of the IV charting pathway.

Brian understands the need to collect and aggregate data on multiple elements per patient, such as advanced techniques used in the placement of difficult IV starts and the size and length of IV catheters used to access deeper veins. Using a proprietary relational database, an IV charting pathway is designed for efficient capture of the IV team's activities. Fields in the database have pre-programmed entries, appearing as drop-down boxes, preventing the entry of free text and minimizing error, while increasing the charting speed by the staff. For example, one field contains all possibilities of IV catheter sizes, while another contains anatomical sites for IV starts. The IV team enters data into the fields by using a form, which is often visually easier to manipulate than the data tables.

Other embedded capabilities of the relational database make the IV charting pathway useful for nurse leaders. For example, the reporting or query function can be used to generate data on specific team members, such as in validating the daily activities of the team member. Effects on outcomes are reflected in continuity of care, provider satisfaction, patient satisfaction, and financial outcomes. The electronic charting coupled with a handoff communication report at shift change ensures the continuity of care for the patients who receive services of the IV team.

Information collected in the database, which occurs with consistent use of the IV charting pathway, can be important in planning for future patient care. Data trends can be identified and proactively used to address patient needs. Reports may validate the decreased utilization of more invasive infusion catheters, which in turn can minimize the occurrence of catheter-related bloodstream infections. Outcomes include lower overall cost to the organization, increased patient satisfaction, increased employee satisfaction, and validation of the IV team's worth in its role with value-based purchasing.

SUMMARY

Nurses, as part of the larger healthcare community, can realize benefits from learning how to use relational databases as opposed to flat databases or spreadsheets that are commonly used in healthcare settings. Though there is a learning curve in adopting the relational databases into practice, many common software applications that use relational databases hide complicated steps and make it easier for HCPs to use these types of databases. Although relational databases and data warehouses seem to be the ideal solution for healthcare applications, the increasing amounts of healthcare data that are collected will influence the needs for new types of applications and analyses of such data. To support these new applications and analyses, systems that complement relational databases will need to be developed.

> (WWW) For a full suite of assignments and additional learning activities, use the access code located in the front of your book and visit www.jblearning.com. If you do not have an access code, you can obtain one at the site.

REFERENCES

Alexander, S., Frith, K. H., O'Keefe, L., & Hennigan, M. A. (2011). Implementation of customized health information technology in diabetes self management programs. *Clinical Nurse Specialist*, *25*(2), 63–70. doi: 10.1097/NUR.0b013e31820aefd600002800-201103000-00005 [pii]

American Nurses Association. (2009). *Position statement: Rights of registered nurses when considering a patient assignment*. Retrieved from http://nursingworld.org/rnrightsps

Aydin, C., Bolton, L., Donaldson, N., Brown, D., & Mukerji, A. (2008). Beyond nursing quality measurement: The nation's first regional nursing virtual dashboard. In R. Hughes (Ed.), *Patient safety and quality: An evidence-based handbook for nurses*. Rockville, MD: Agency for Healthcare Research and Quality. Retrieved from http://www.ahrq.gov/qual/nurseshdbk/

Donaldson, N., Brown, D., Aydin, C., Bolton, M., & Rutledge, D. (2005). Leveraging nurse-related dashboard benchmarks to expedite performance improvement and document excellence. *Journal of Nursing Administration*, *35*(4), 163–172.

Dumpe, M. L., Kanyok, N., & Hill, K. (2007). Use of an automated learning management system to validate nursing competencies. *Journal for Nurses in Staff Development*, *23*(4), 183–185. doi: 10.1097/01.NND.0000281418.50472.2e

Elmasri, R., & Navathe, S. (2003). *Fundamentals of database systems* (4th ed.). Boston, MA: Addison-Wesley Longman.

Kurtzman, E., & Jennings, B. M. (2008). Trends in transparency: Nursing performance measurement and reporting. *Journal of Nursing Administration*, *38*(7/8), 349–354.

National Quality Forum. (2007). Tracking NQF-endorsed consensus standards for nursing-sensitive care: A 15-month study. Retrieved from http://www.qualityforum.org/pdf/reports/Nursing70907.pdf

Radwin, L. E., Cabral, H. J., Chen, L., & Jennings, B. M. (2010). A protocol for capturing daily variability in nursing care. *Nursing Economics*, *28*(2), 95–105.

Sen, A., & Sinha, A. (2005). A comparison of data warehousing methodologies. *Communications of the ACM*, *48*(3), 79–84.

CHAPTER 8

Adapting Business Intelligence for Health Care

Rahul Ramachandran, PhD
Diana Hankey-Underwood, MS, WHNP-BC

CHAPTER LEARNING OBJECTIVES

1. Describe basic principles of analytics for answering healthcare questions.
2. Review types of descriptive and predictive algorithms generated by data-mining methods.
3. Discuss how algorithms are created in health care to address clinical questions.

KEY TERMS

Artificial neural network
Association rules
Bayesian modeling
Business intelligence
Data mining
Decision tree
Descriptive algorithm
Index patient

Information gain
Instance-based learning classifiers
K-means
Modeling
Predictive algorithm
Simulation
Support vector machine modeling

CHAPTER OVERVIEW

The field of business has long been interested in using data to understand why buyers make purchasing decisions and developing well-defined techniques that increase its ability to understand what makes a business successful. This practice can also be referred to as **business intelligence**. The field of health care is increasingly using similar techniques of data analysis to describe past trends and predict future trends in ways that support decision making for increased performance in healthcare organizations and improved safety for patients and communities.

Using data to predict the future is often done with techniques such as **modeling** and **simulation**. Modeling can be used in many fields, from forecasting the track of a hurricane to predicting sports championship winners. A model is simply a set of mathematical terms used to create a computer application capable of anticipating a response to a situation. In simulation, reality is imitated for purposes such as training or entertainment. In some cases, artificial environments are used to mimic real-world experiences. For example, a Wii game entitled "Hysteria Hospital Emergency Ward" is now available, in which players attempt to manage the constant flow of people into an emergency department. The game is structured so that no matter how good the "nurse" player becomes at carrying out the order of nursing tasks, the patients will come faster and some will turn green for lack of care. While the scenarios are carried out in a comical manner, for the sake of entertainment, the game is an effective example of the possibilities of both modeling and simulation in health care. In this chapter, examples of applications of data analytics, which incorporate modeling and simulation, adapted from the field of business intelligence and applied to health care are presented. A review of different techniques of basic data mining, networks, and algorithms is also presented.

BASIC PRINCIPLES OF DATA ANALYTICS

The term *analytics* is often used interchangeably with data mining or knowledge discovery in databases (Fayyad, Piatetsky-Shapiro, & Smyth, 1996). There are slight, but important differences between data mining and analytics. Fayyad, an accomplished researcher in the field, defined data mining as the process of identifying valid, and likely useful, patterns in data. Analytics is a more-focused process, concentrating on the customization of data mining in response to the specific needs of end users or those who seek to gain knowledge from manipulation of the data or application (Kohavi, Rothleder, & Simoudis, 2002). Such customization should enable an end user to use the results of an analysis in a way that is meaningful or that produces a positive impact.

Businesses commonly apply principles of analytics to data that are gathered in order to seek competitive advantages. Analytics concepts are used to examine questions ranging from personnel performance to business processes for improving efficiencies, lowering costs, and improving hiring strategies to retain new employees (Walker, 2012). In many instances, data are used as the basis for the quantitative evaluation of decisions, on small and grand scales, that affect the performance of the organization. Since the early 2000s, federally funded large-scale projects involving the application of data analytics have been conducted. Examples of results from these projects, which are discussed later in this chapter, now shape the nature of healthcare delivery across the nation.

Analytics components consist of descriptive and predictive models for analyzing data. Data-mining algorithms are sets of mathematical rules and are often used in combinations for building predictive and descriptive models. An example of a simple algorithm could use responses to a picture or numerical scale commonly used to measure subjective phenomena such as customer satisfaction or pain (**Figure 8-1**). Perhaps a nurse wishes to compare the difference between the pain that patients experience after cholecystectomy with the pain that patients experience after cardiac bypass surgery. A data-mining algorithm could be constructed. The algorithm, which would instruct a computer to average the pain scores of a specified number of patients who had undergone cholecystectomy and compare it with the average pain scores of a similar number of patients who had undergone coronary bypass surgery, would be a simple mathematical calculation that would yield a ratio. Would the ratio be significantly valuable information? Would gathering data on a specified number of patients who had experienced each surgery be sufficient to draw useful conclusions?

0	1	2	3	4	5
No hurt	Hurts little bit	Hurts little more	Hurts even more	Hurts whole lot	Hurts worst

Brief word instructions: Point to each face using the words to describe the pain intensity. Ask the child to choose the face that best describes own pain and record the appropriate number.

Original instructions: Explain to the person that each face is for a person who feels happy because he has no pain (hurt) or sad because he has some or a lot of pain. **Face 0** is very happy because he doesn't hurt at all. **Face 1** hurts just a little bit. **Face 2** hurts a little more. **Face 3** hurts even more. **Face 4** hurts a whole lot. **Face 5** hurts as much as you can imagine, although you don't have to be crying to feel this bad. Ask the person to choose the face that describes how he is feeling.

FIGURE 8-1   Wong-Baker FACES Pain Rating Scale.

Source: From Hockenberry MJ, Wilson D: Wong's essentials of pediatric nursing, ed. 8, St. Louis, 2009, Mosby. Used with permission. Copyright Mosby.

In this example, it is not likely that useful conclusions can be made. In actual practice, data-mining algorithms are typically much more complex. To obtain a more detailed picture of the differences in pain between patients who undergo the different surgical procedures would require collection of descriptive data, such as ages and gender of the patients and more frequent measurements of pain from the patients. Though humans can intuitively understand the need for collection of multiple data points to illustrate differences, mathematical models exist that offer insight into the appropriate numbers of variables to use in specific types of equations. In the pain sample, a larger number of data points and sample patients used in each group would help create a better "model" of pain; therefore, it could predict a typical course of pain in a patient, providing a warning if a particular patient is far from the "normal" range. In the next section an overview of the analytics process and discussion of data-mining algorithm concepts that are used in analytics are presented.

ANALYTICS IN USE

Before describing the analytics process, it is important to understand some basic definitions. Specific uses of the terms have been updated to address the emerging paradigms of data-intensive science and big data (Bell, Hay, & Szalay, 2009) (**Box 8-1**). Recall that data are used to derive information needed to support or negate a hypothesis. Data alone cannot formulate a hypothesis; however, new patterns discovered in data combined with knowledge about a particular domain of interest can be used to formulate new hypotheses. Analytics, therefore, is the toolbox that allows for data management and discovery of new knowledge within an organization, such as a healthcare organization.

Analytics is an interactive process composed of multiple, sequential steps. **Data mining** is an important component within the process of analytics, in which a particular mining algorithm is used to extract patterns from the dataset. The first step requires the user to closely define the objective of analysis and select the correct dataset. The second step consists of data preparation, which involves cleaning and preprocessing of the target data. Very often, data preparation represents the most time-consuming step of the process. The final step is manipulation and analysis of the dataset to identify patterns, which may be used for descriptive and predictive purposes.

Consider the extraction of data from the electronic health record (EHR). While the removal of personal identification information from the EHR should be fairly simple if the dataset is limited to a single provider or small office, the process can be

---

Box 8-1 Types of Data

Data are observable and therefore measurable and factual. It is sometimes a significant challenge to convert subjective information into objective data.

Knowledge is a statement about a hypothesis, and science is organized knowledge, that is, a collection of one or more hypotheses in some logical order. Consider the statement, "A nurse, Susan, knows that women experience pain 24 hours after a C-section." Susan has experience with previous patients, so she has confidence in her prediction of future patients reacting in the same way. Because we do not have data on the future, Susan is predicting based on previous data, which in science is termed a *hypothesis*. Nursing knowledge is gained by testing a hypothesis based on suitably organized data.

Information is a measure of uncertainty about a hypothesis; the role of data is to change the amount of information.

Knowledge management and discovery are the systematic use of data to test a hypothesis and/or help formulate new hypotheses.

Analytics dashboards, or simply "dashboards," are used as visualization components to effectively communicate and display analysis results, usually to end users. Much like the dashboard of a car provides information on the operating condition of the car and the driver's speed, analytics dashboards provide information in usable picture-like illustrations so that adjustments can be made as appropriate.

---

more complex if the record contains information generated by multiple healthcare providers (HCPs). In addition, if the data abstraction requires the retrieval of data from multiple EHR systems, considerable preprocessing effort would be required to generate a usable dataset. When manipulating multiple datasets, the discovery of relevant patterns from the data often requires the use of term definitions. One of the best examples of the application of term definitions used in health care would be in the use of the *International Classification of Diseases, 10th Revision, Clinical Modification* (ICD-10-CM). ICD-10-CM codes are lists of terms used to identify diagnoses and are commonly used in billing. Widespread use of ICD-10-CM codes makes these data retrievable for many patient visits, even though use of a particular ICD-10-DM code may not contain all of the information needed for accurate data processing. For instance, there are many ICD-10-CM codes that could be applied to a patient who has a diagnosis of back pain (**Box 8-2**). If a program were designed to identify patients who visited an HCP with a complaint of back pain, could those visits be isolated by using only one ICD-10-CM code, or term, to describe back pain? The answer is no— many term definitions would be needed to accurately capture all patients with the similar complaint.

Box 8-2   ICD-10-CM Codes That Can Be Used to Describe the Diagnosis of Back Pain

Lumbosacral spondylosis without myelopathy

- M47.26–M47.28
- M47.816–M47.818
- M47.896–M47.898

Spondylosis of unspecified site without mention of myelopathy

- M47.20
- M47.819
- M47.899–M47.9

Displacement of lumbar intervertebral disc without myelopathy

- M51.26
- M51.27

Degeneration of lumbar or lumbosacral intervertebral disc

- M51.36–M51.37

Degeneration of intervertebral disc, site unspecified

- M51.34–M51.37
- M51.9

Other unspecified disc disorder of lumbar region

- M46.46–M46.47
- M51.86–M51.87

Spinal stenosis of lumbar region

- M48.06–M48.07
- M99.23, M99.33
- M99.43, M99.53
- M99.63
- M99.73

Lumbago

- M54.5

Sciatica

- M54.30–M54.42

OVERVIEW OF ALGORITHMS GENERATED BY DATA-MINING METHODS ___

In 1990, it was likely that the skill set of an experienced and educated nurse did not include the ability to create a presentation using Microsoft PowerPoint. However, within only a few years' time, familiarity with the use of Microsoft Office programs, including PowerPoint, became a standard skill for many nurses. Similarly, many algorithms, both predictive and descriptive, exist today to analyze and manage data-sets. Data-mining algorithms can be categorized based on their purpose as either predictive or descriptive mining algorithms (Dunham, 2003). **Descriptive algorithms** are generally used to explore data and identify patterns or relationships within them. Examples of descriptive algorithms include clustering, summarization, and association rules. **Predictive algorithms** make predictions about values of data using a set of known results. Though the baccalaureate-prepared nurse may not be expected to design and implement such algorithms, a familiarity with these concepts will likely prove useful as data analytics tools continue to permeate healthcare delivery systems. The following sections present a brief overview and examples of algorithms that are commonly used in health care.

EXAMPLES OF PREDICTIVE ALGORITHMS

Decision Trees

Decision trees are often used for patient protocols as an aid to decision making, and they are used in analytical research. Often represented as a tree-shaped diagram, each branch may be used to represent a possible decision or occurrence. The structure of the branches can illustrate how one decision may lead to another. Because the branches are separate, each choice can be seen as a stand-alone decision. The following example of a decision tree and how it could be used to help make intelligent business decisions may be helpful.

Envision the trunk of the decision tree as including all patients having avian flu at Hospital X (**Figure 8-2**). On the trunk are three branches designating patients who were born in 1900–1960 (65 patients), 1960–2000 (7 patients), and 2001–2014 (38 patients). Under each of the branches are three leaves that separately designate patients who received immediate antiviral medications (costing $150), patients who received antiviral medications by day 3 of symptom onset, and patients who did not receive antiviral medications until post-laboratory confirmation of diagnosis. Below each of the leaves are designations for patients whose lengths of hospital stay were 1–14 days, 14–45 days, and those patients who died during their hospital stays. Hospital reimbursement is assigned to each leaf as a total of the patients within that leaf. Analysis reveals that patients who received antiviral medications had a length of stay that was one-third less than those who did not receive antiviral medications. Their hospital bills were less than half of those patients who did not receive antiviral medications, regardless of the age range. Does this mean that all patients should receive antiviral medications immediately? Would the answer change if only one patient died

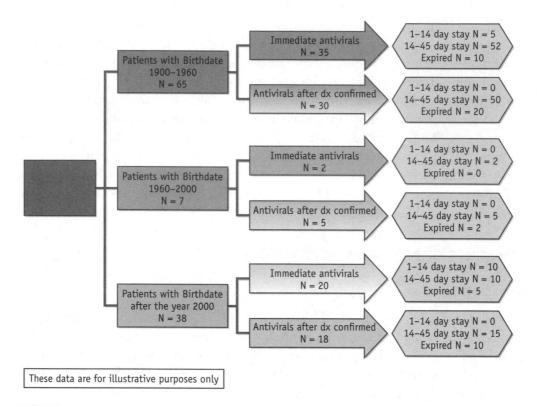

FIGURE 8-2   Decision tree applied to treatment of avian influenza.

and the patient was in the group that received antiviral medications immediately? What other leaves should be on the decision tree to help decide for whom antiviral medications are the best choice? Would analysis of a larger data pool help? Would dividing the groups into male and female patients make a difference? Use of an algorithm such as the decision tree can help to inform HCPs of the important leaves and enable more effective decisions.

Another important concept used in the evaluation process is a statistical property known as **information gain**. Information gain is a measure of how well a given attribute separates a subset of the whole dataset (also known as training sample data) to achieve the target classification. The best attribute is selected and is used as the root node of the tree. Descendant nodes are created for all possible values of the root node. The entire process is repeated with more data to create the tree using the training samples. This program might inform us that patients are likely to benefit most from the antiviral based on month of admission, weight of 50 pounds or more or over

BMI of 24, and a cough when entering the hospital. It might inform us that patient sex and smoking status are irrelevant—in other words those data were found to be a poor fit to the model of the tree that it created. Based on the decision tree formulated, the best time to use the antiviral would be in January and February, making sure to dose larger patients and all of those with a cough of any kind upon entering the hospital to achieve the target classification of a shorter hospital stay.

Artificial Neural Networks

An **artificial neural network** is an information-processing system that is based on biological neural networks such as are present in the human nervous system. These networks have been developed as mathematical models of human cognition. Artificial neural networks are most useful when pattern recognition or prediction is necessary or when it is not possible to create a conventional, straightforward algorithm that could be used to answer a problem. An artificial neural network is constructed upon the assumptions that information processing involves many simple elements, called neurons, and that signals are passed between these neurons over connection links (Fausett, 1994). These connection links have associated weights that influence how quickly the signal is transmitted, similar to the transmission of signals along axons in the human nervous system. Artificial neural networks can also be classified according to the direction in which the signal is transmitted across the connection links, as either forward or backward. The back propagation neural network (BPNN) is a commonly used artificial neural network algorithm in data mining.

In health care, artificial neural networks are used in clinical diagnosis, image and signal analysis, and drug development. Using an artificial neural network, Jiang and colleagues (2013) identified a group of five serum protein markers that could be used to detect early stage ovarian cancer, a disease for which there is presently no screening protocol and is commonly undiagnosed until it reaches an advanced stage. Artificial neural networks have also been used to examine functional magnetic resonance images (fMRI) of the brains of adult patients with attention deficit disorder, supporting researchers' hypothesis that the disorder is associated with maturational deficits in the brain that persist throughout life (Sato, Hoexter, Castellanos, & Rohde, 2012). Image analysis can be enhanced with the use of these networks. Borujeny, Yazdi, Keshavarz-Haddad, and Borujeny (2013) used wireless sensors attached to the arms and thighs of epileptic patients to collect data used in creating an automatic detection algorithm for the onset of epileptic seizures. Results of the project yielded important information for the patients' HCPs on the nuances of behavioral changes that preceded the onset of seizures and for improving the safety of patients in the post-seizure period. Artificial neural networks have even been used to improve the quality of tablet design in drug manufacturing (Aksu et al., 2012).

Other Types of Algorithms

Instance-Based Learning Classifiers

Instance-based learning classifiers store labeled training data. As a new sample is presented to these classifiers, it is matched against a set of similar stored instances in order to assign a classification label. This is similar to a computerized scholastic test with which many students may be familiar. The answers are given to the program, and when a new "sample" is presented, the program can correctly detect and classify "fail" and "pass." If a test contained only 25 items, it is likely that a human could do the work almost as fast, but comparing various complex genetic codes to ascertain "easily transmissible" or "poorly transmissible" traits, for example, can be done only by using computer analysis.

Support Vector Machines

Classifiers use many different methods. **Support vector machine modeling** informs the program to learn from the data. Support vector analysis has been used recently in analyses of healthcare coverage in large populations of people. In addition, this modeling technique has been used to identify those people who are without health insurance in the populations that were studied, and to offer explanations for the lack of healthcare coverage in the groups (Delen & Fuller, 2013).

Bayes Classifiers/Bayesian Modeling

Bayes' theorem is the underpinning of the **Bayesian modeling** classifier. Bayes' theorem is used to estimate the conditional probability of a given data point belonging to a particular class. Bayesian classifiers use a probabilistic approach for data classification and are based on the assumption that attributes in the training examples are governed by probability distributions. Classification decisions can be made by using these collective probabilities. Bayesian classifiers allow prior knowledge, also known as initial probability, to be combined with observed data to determine conditional probability. When predicting influenza outbreaks, the aspect of numbers, such as the sheer amount of contagious people present in the population, is important. The probability of an individual becoming ill after exposure, however, is gained from analysis of past epidemics. This information can also be used in predicting pandemics, though the numbers may not always be accurate.

When initial probabilities are unavailable, assumptions have to be made regarding the underlying distribution. Sometimes assumptions are made that the attribute values are conditionally independent. When three cases of a new respiratory ailment arrive and two of the three people die within days or weeks, there can be no way to know immediately if these cases have any relationship, but there will be intense scrutiny to determine ways that the cases may be related, which is also known as conditional dependence. For example, perhaps the patients all became ill after sharing a pizza at the same restaurant. To find out more about the potential need to prepare for extensive outbreaks of illness in a community, it is important to discover if a common source of infection is present. Even if the cases appear at first glance to be conditionally independent, meaning that they do not share obvious history, characteristics, or other connecting conditions, detailed assessments are often helpful. Bayesian computer modeling can use known data to "fill in the blanks" and to provide models with "created" missing data. As data on new cases are loaded into the application, the models and projections continuously change, which can be helpful in a situation where some or many of the "knowns" are not known.

DESCRIPTIVE ALGORITHMS

Descriptive algorithms can be broadly divided into rules of clustering and association. Examples of clustering rules used in descriptive algorithms include single-link clustering, density-based spatial clustering of application with noise, and K-means clustering. The clustering algorithm discovers the groupings in the data based on similarities in the attributes of the data. These types of algorithms are often useful as exploratory tools, where the general behavior of the data can be observed by the cluster results and can also be used to summarize the data.

When outbreaks of disease occur, epidemiologists gather large amounts of data on many aspects related to the first known case of the disease, or the **index patient**, and subsequent cases in an attempt to identify the origin of the disease and its associated exposure risks. In the Guangdong province of China, a rural area bordering Hong Kong and eastern China, health officials noted an outbreak of serious avian influenza A (H7N9) infections in March through April 2013 (Cowling et al., 2013). Officials further noted that the initial cases occurred in older men, many of whom had been in close contact with unvaccinated sick or dead poultry found in small, backyard farms. Viral samples from the index patients were analyzed, with results suggesting that the virus likely emerged from "reassortment," a process in which two or more influenza viruses co-infect a single host and exchange genes (Cowling et al., 2013). Descriptive algorithms were used to help in identifying the genetic changes found in the H7N9 virus causing infection in the index cases. These algorithms are helpful, because they can also identify outlier data points that vary substantially from the rest of the data. If all the patients have a virus that is genetically identical, it suggests a simultaneous exposure, but as the virus proceeds through patients, it acquires subtle changes, which can be identified with descriptive algorithms. These changes provide clues about the age and source of the new viral illness.

Association Rules

Association rules are designed to capture information about items that are frequently associated with each other. Association rules have been used in business applications such as market-basket analysis to find relationships present among attributes in large datasets. Companies may review credit card receipts, for instance, and find that if someone buys peanut butter, they are more likely to buy jelly. Analyzing the increase in sales of over-the-counter medications for influenza or cold symptoms and related products can use association rules and clustering to visualize movement of an influenza epidemic across the nation.

K-Means

K-means is an example of a partitional clustering algorithm where the desired number of clusters to partition the data is specified. Initial cluster means are randomly selected and patterns are assigned to these closest cluster means. New cluster means, referred to as K, are then calculated. K-means is one of the most widely used clustering algorithms and has been utilized in several different science applications. Sometimes the assigned K will be assigned colors so that data can be visually separated. Using the K-means algorithm, investigators can assign case numbers and ages of patients affected with influenza-like illnesses across a specified region, such as a state, so that flu activity surveillance can be quickly visualized.

While the examples described in the previous paragraphs may seem complex, in the business world, it is common for analytics projects to compare several factors simultaneously. For instance, much information is needed to reliably forecast the spread of influenza. The migratory pathways of birds (because droppings are contaminated with influenza viruses), human traffic patterns, the temporal distribution of influenza cases in patients, data on the rapidity of human-to-human transmission, and even weather patterns are all needed to improve predictions of influenza outbreaks and to target efforts to control those outbreaks. These data can be used to improve planning and surveillance efforts, such as the purchase of adequate amounts of protective equipment and vaccinations. Modeling can even be used to calculate what occurs when the population is vaccinated at different rates and to predict the method of social distancing (quarantine) that will work best in epidemics.

TRACKING TRENDS IN DATA

Using data analytics techniques borrowed from business intelligence can have implications for real-world healthcare settings. By using data from radio frequency identification (RFID) device tags, researchers tracked the movements of nurses throughout a unit, documenting the time spent with patients and performing other tasks within the unit. Hendrich, Chow, Skierczynski, and Zhengiang (2008) combined the data gathered from use of the RFID tags with modeling and simulation techniques to better describe the movements of nurses over architectural and unit layout schematics. Techniques such as these can improve the design of units, or even entire hospitals, and maximize efficiency. This is an example of evidence-based architecture—one form of business intelligence and use of technology in the world of health care.

Computer scientists and statisticians can create avatars and analyze real and projected data to visibly demonstrate consequences of various business decisions. Yet, it is the responsibility of the current generation of nurses and other HCPs to help ensure that quality data exist, to use creativity in devising methods to apply data, and to use the information that is produced with data analytics tools in a constructive manner. The idea that tracking and monitoring can be conducted may be uncomfortable, and some nurses object to a perceived intrusion upon privacy (AbdelMalik, Boulos, & Jones, 2008). Nurses can feel that data collection is burdensome, even with the knowledge that the data could have some importance to someone else or have significance in the future. These discomforts are important because nurses need to be sensitive to the great potential for use and the great potential for abuse that come with almost all great inventions. Just as narcotics can make lengthy surgeries possible and thereby save millions of lives, they can also be abused and have destroyed many peoples' lives. Understanding the dichotomy can aid nurses in protecting patients while gaining huge advantages. Many articles have been written about the potential abuses of large datasets in the media, but few nurses have great acquaintance with the ways large datasets are created, used, or provide the amazing possibilities for the improvement of health care for mankind, or for their individual patients and even for their own safety. With this in mind, a review of the ways in which large datasets might have an impact on nursing safety, community planning, and hospital management in the near future is needed.

Global Tracking of Avian Flu

In May 2013, the World Health Organization (WHO) reported the diagnoses of three cases of H7N9, a highly pathogenic avian flu, in China (Centers for Disease Control and Prevention, 2013). All three cases presented with respiratory tract infection with progression to severe pneumonia and breathing difficulties, resulting in two deaths and one patient in critical condition. Three months later, there were 132 lab-confirmed cases of influenza A H7N9, which included 127 (96%) hospitalized, 78 (59%) recovered, and 39 (30%) dead (**Figure 8-3**). Only 77% of patients remembered any exposure to live animals, mostly chickens and ducks. Analysis revealed that the median age of onset for H7N9 was 61 years. This was concerning

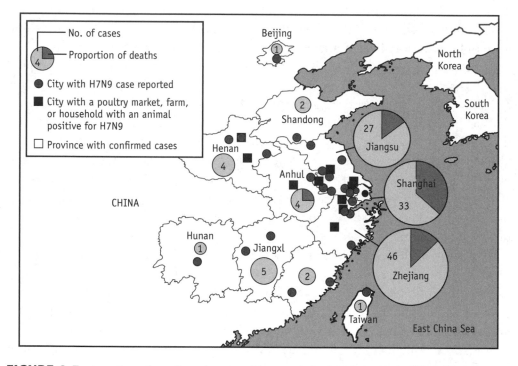

FIGURE 8-3   Location of confirmed cases of human infection (n = 126) with avian influenza A(H7N9) virus and deaths (n = 24) — China, February 19–April 29, 2013.

Source: Centers for Disease Control and Prevention (CDC) (2013, May 10). Emergence of Avian Influenza A(H7N9) Virus Causing Severe Human Illness — China, February–April 2013. Morbidity and Mortality Weekly Reports (MMWR). Retrieved from http://www.cdc.gov/mmwr/preview/mmwrhtml/mm6218a6.htm?s_cid=mm6218a6_w

because preliminary results of sera collected from the general population suggested little pre-existing cross-reactive antibodies against H7N9 in all age groups tested (6–80+ years). The virus has also demonstrated resistance to amantadine and rimantadine, commonly used antiviral medications in the United States. Resistance to oseltamivir and zanamivir, other antiviral medications, was demonstrated in at least one other viral sample.

Once it was discovered that the virus had emerged with two deaths, it was imperative to try to find hospital personnel who might have been exposed to the three patients. Perhaps if treatment could have been started earlier, their lives might have been spared. If the people with possible exposure could not be found, but instead spread the new disease broadly, the risk of a ghastly pandemic would be increased. Efficient use of RFID could have identified in a matter of minutes, not only who was in the room, but what equipment was in the room. Like many hospitals in the United States, the hospital in China was not that advanced, so a search for those in need of quarantine was not as expedient. It is quite possible that the use of business intelligence might mitigate a pandemic in the future.

Predicting the spread of a disease is the first, and arguably most important, step in designing effective and efficient mitigation strategies. For many years, the most common form of disease-spread model was a homogeneous mixing model, which is based on the premise that all members of a population can be treated identically, and everyone is equally likely to come into contact with anyone else. Each infected person in the population will infect the same number of people; this number is called the basic reproduction number (R).

In real life, some people live much more isolated lives than others. A school teacher will be exposed to more sneezes on an average day than an astronaut. Some researchers are trying to use social media to calculate more accurate predictions about viral spread by analyzing vast amounts of data.

Monitoring of Adverse Drug Events

Over the course of a nurse's career, it is likely that he or she will administer thousands of medications to patients, representing classes of drugs used to treat everything from the pain of a myocardial infarction to infection in a wound. While it is likely that many patients will be given medications with no ill effects, some will experience severe adverse reactions that should be reported. Healthcare professionals and consumers (or their family members) can voluntarily report adverse occurrences to pharmaceutical manufacturers or directly to the U.S. Food and Drug Administration (FDA). If a pharmaceutical manufacturer receives a report of an adverse drug event, it

> **Box 8-3   Case Study**
>
> Teri, the new nursing informatics officer of a large urban hospital, is asked to help prepare for the chief executive officer's meeting with several division directors, including the pharmacy director. Preparation for the meeting necessitated the analysis of large datasets containing details on the types and amounts of medications purchased by the hospital over past years. After the analysis was complete, Teri discovered that the purchase of opiate medications increased by 25% last year. The nursing counts for opiate medication use on each floor were consistent with the main pharmacy counts, with zero discrepancies, yet the pharmacy count revealed a decrease of 3,000 doses of oxycodone from the total purchased this year. Costs per pill rose 29.3%.
>
> Teri needs to know which nursing unit had significantly higher rates of oxycodone use when compared to the unit's past use and to use in other units. Should Teri be concerned about possible misuses of the oxycodone medication? Could employees in the pharmacy be involved?
>
> Teri understands that data can be misused, and interpretation of analysis of large datasets can be skewed. In this case, fortunately for the pharmacy director, Teri was wise enough to look at additional data before speaking to anyone about this. The new orthopedic center, which opened 10 months ago, increased revenue by $6 million, and the cost of extra pain medications as part of the increased operating costs was $500,000. All other units are within 5% of the trends from previous years. When Teri's hospital bought out the nearby smaller hospital in an adjacent county, they asked to "borrow" several sets of medications that were in short supply nationally. Teri went into the meeting and congratulated the pharmacy director on his amazing competence at overseeing his pharmacy and the merger with all the extra work that entailed. Arrangements were made to complete the return of medications to normalized counts and also to work on surge management in case of community disasters or pandemics. Data can harm others even when there is no malicious intent. Nurses must be prepared to research carefully and fully before assuming or repeating any harmful conclusions based on data analysis.

is required to then forward this information to the FDA. Reports of adverse drug events are maintained in a database known as the FDA Adverse Event Reporting System (FAERS). Because it contains data contributed by pharmaceutical manufacturers, healthcare professionals, and consumers, the FAERS database is considered to be quite robust. FAERS data are available to the public for retrieval, in the form of statistics, files of raw data, or case study reports (FDA, 2012).

The FAERS database is an excellent resource for research in pharmacoepidemiology, the study of the effects of drugs in populations. Pharmacovigilance, which is defined as the use of scientific methods to study and maintain the quality of medications (Partnership for Safe Medicines, 2002–2011), is a process that requires early detection of adverse drug events. Despite the wealth of information contained in the FAERs database, there are deficiencies that make the rapid recognition of adverse drug events difficult. The lag between the time data are reported to FAERs and released to the public, file types in which data are released, and duplication of data in files or reports have been cited as examples of difficulties in manipulating the FAERs database to yield relevant clinical information (Bate & Evans, 2009; Böhm, Höcker, Cascorbi, & Herdegen, 2012; "Making a Difference," 2009; Pratt & Danese, 2009). To examine the utility of the FAERs database in detecting adverse drug events, Sakaeda, Tamon, Kadoyama, and Okuno (2013) created four data-mining algorithms designed to analyze reports of hemorrhage, hematemesis, melena, and hematochezia associated with use of common anticoagulants (aspirin, warfarin, and clopidogrel). In the analysis, higher numbers of adverse events were detected as "signals." Statistically significant associations, meaning that the adverse events were detected as signals, were found between the use of warfarin and hematemesis, consistent with reports elsewhere in published literature of adverse reactions associated with the drugs (Sakaeda et al., 2013).

Sakaeda and colleagues (2013) acknowledge that there are advantages and limitations related to data mining of the FAERs database. The existence of the database is not well publicized, which leads to underreporting of adverse events by healthcare professionals and consumers, and the numbers of adverse events may be increasingly reported on two separate occasions: in the first 2 years after a drug is launched and immediately after an adverse event receives wide publicity (Hauben, Reich, & Gerrits, 2006; Pariente, Gregoire, Fourrier-Reglat, Haramburu, & Moore, 2007; Raschi, Piccinni, Poluzzi, Marschesini, & De Ponti, 2013; Sakaeda et al., 2013). Yet, potential advantages related to data mining of the FAERS database remain. While the preferable method to determine the risks of adverse reactions associated with a drug is with a randomized, controlled trial, this method is not always feasible due to financial and temporal constraints, particularly when the event is rare. Regular mining of the database could offer insight into important associations between the uses of drugs and adverse events, and serve as a mechanism of directing further clinical investigation of those relationships (Sakaeda et al., 2013).

SUMMARY

Every nurse is responsible for collecting the most accurate data possible. Patient privacy and data security are sensitive and critical components of good nursing care. A team approach is needed to design healthcare delivery systems that can reduce danger to patients, families, communities, and even nations. An understanding of the concepts of advanced data analytics techniques, including the algorithms used to generate various models used in health care, can assist the generalist nurse who may work in tandem with informatics specialists or computer analysts. Nurses can assist in designing ways to eliminate time wasters and work in teams to discover which treatments work best for patients based on genetic composition, age, gender, and weight. These methods may benefit every member of the healthcare team.

> (www) For a full suite of assignments and additional learning activities, use the access code located in the front of your book and visit www.jblearning.com. If you do not have an access code, you can obtain one at the site.

REFERENCES

AbdelMalik, P., Boulos, M. N. K., & Jones, R. (2008). The perceived impact of location privacy: A web-based survey of public health perspectives and requirements in the UK and Canada. *BMC Public Health, 8*, 156. doi: 10.1186/1471-2458-8-156

Aksu, B., Paradkar, A., de Matas, M., Ozer, O., Guneri, T., & York, P. (2012). Quality by design approach: Application of artificial intelligence techniques of tablets manufactured by direct compression. *AAPS PharmSciTech, 13*(4), 1138–1146. doi: 10.1208/s12249-012-9836-x

Bate, A., & Evans, S. J. (2009). Quantitative signal detection using spontaneous ADR reporting. *Pharmacoepidemiology and Drug Safety, 18*, 427–436.

Bell, G., Hey, T., & Szalay, A. (2009). Beyond the data deluge. *Science, 323*.

Böhm, R., Höcker, J., Cascorbi, I., & Herdegen, T. (2012). OpenVigil—free eyeballs on AERS pharmacovigilance data. *Nature Biotechnology, 30*, 137–138.

Borujeny, G. T., Yazdi, M., Keshavarz-Haddad, A., & Borujeny, A. R. (2013). Detection of epileptic seizure using wireless sensor networks. *Journal of Medical Signals and Sensors, 3*(2), 63–68.

Centers for Disease Control and Prevention. (2013). Emergence of avian influenza A(H7N9) virus causing severe human illness—China, February–April 2013. *Morbidity and Mortality Weekly Reports, 62*(18), 366–371. Retrieved from http://www.cdc.gov/mmwr/preview/mmwrhtml/mm6218a6.htm?s_cid=mm6218a6_w

Cowling, B. J., Freeman, G., Wong, J. Y, Wu, P., Liao, Q., Lau, E. H., . . . Leung, M. (2013). Preliminary inferences on the age-specific seriousness of human disease caused by avian influenza A(H7N9) infections in China, March to April 2013. *EuroSurveillance, 18*(19), 1–6. Retrieved from http://www.eurosurveillance.org/ViewArticle.aspx?ArticleId=20475

Delen, D., & Fuller, C. (2013). An analytic approach to understanding and predicting healthcare coverage. *Studies in Health Technology and Informatics, 190*, 198–200.

Dunham, M. H. (2003). *Data mining: Introduction and advanced topics.* Boston, MA: Pearson Education.

Fausett, L. (1994). *Fundamentals of neural networks.* Englewood Cliffs, NJ: Prentice Hall.

Fayyad, U. M., Piatetsky-Shapiro, G., & Smyth, P. (1996). From data mining to knowledge discovery: An overview. In U. M. Fayyad, G. Piatetsky-Shapiro, & P. Smyth (Eds.), *Advances in knowledge discovery and data mining.* Cambridge, MA: MIT Press.

Hauben, M., Reich, L., & Gerrits, C. M. (2006). Reports of hyperkalemia after publication of RALES—a pharmacovigilance study. *Pharmacoepidemiology and Drug Safety, 15*, 775–783.

Hendrich, A., Chow, M. P., Skierczynski, B. A., & Zhengiang, L. (2008). A 36-hospital time and motion study: How do medical-surgical nurses spend their time? *Nevada RNformation, 12*(3), 25–34.

Jiang, W., Huang, R., Duan, C., Fu, L., Xi, Y., Yang, Y., . . . Huang, R.-P. (2013). Identification of five serum protein markers for detection of ovarian cancer by antibody arrays. *PLoS One, 8*(10), e76795. doi: 10.1371/journal.pone.0076795

Kohavi, R., Rothleder, N. J., & Simoudis, E. (2002). Emerging trends in business analytics. *Communications of the ACM, 45*(8), 45–48.

Making a difference. (2009). [Editorial]. *Nature Biotechnology, 27*, 297.

Pariente, A., Gregoire, F., Fourrier-Reglat, A., Haramburu, F., & Moore, N. (2007). Impact of safety alerts on measures of disproportionality in spontaneous reporting databases: The notoriety bias. *Drug Safety, 30*, 891–898.

Partnership for Safe Medicines. (2002–2011). What is pharmacovigilance? Retrieved from http://www.safemedicines.org/what-is-pharmacovigilance.html

Pratt, L. A., & Danese, P. N. (2009). More eyeballs on AERS. *Nature Biotechnology, 27*, 601–602.

Raschi, E., Piccinni, C., Poluzzi, E., Marschesini, G., & De Ponti, F. (2013). The association of pancreatitis with antidiabetic drug use: Gaining insight through the FDA pharmacovigilance database. *Acta Diabetologica, 50*(4), 569–577. doi: 10.1007/s00592-011-0340-7

Sakaeda, T., Tamon, A., Kadoyama, K., & Okuno, Y. (2013). Data mining of the public version of the FDA adverse event reporting system. *International Journal of Medical Sciences, 10*(7), 796–803. doi: 10.7150/ijms.6048

Sato, J. R., Hoexter, M. Q., Castellanos, X. F., & Rohde, L. A. (2012). Abnormal brain connectivity patterns in adults with ADHD: A coherence study. *PLoS ONE, 7*(9), e45671. doi: 10.1371/journal.pone.0045671

U.S. Food and Drug Administration. (2012). Protecting and monitoring your health. Retrieved from http://www.fda.gov/Drugs/GuidanceComplianceRegulatoryInformation/Surveillance/AdverseDrugEffects/default.htm

Walker, J. (2012). Meet the new boss: Big data. *Wall Street Journal.* Retrieved from http://online.wsj.com/news/articles/SB10000872396390443890304578006252019616768

Wong, D. L., Hackenberry-Eato, M., Wilson, D., Winkelstein, M. L., & Schwartz, P. (2008). Wong-Baker FACES Rating Scale. In *Wong's essentials of pediatric nursing* (6th ed.). St. Louis, MI: Mosby.

CHAPTER 9

Workflow Support

Karen H. Frith, PhD, RN, NEA-BC

CHAPTER LEARNING OBJECTIVES

1. Define workflow in a healthcare delivery system.
2. Identify appropriate methods for workflow analysis.
3. Select charts, tables, or other tools to display workflow data.
4. Describe the rationale for workflow redesign after implementation of health IT.
5. Identify technology that automates workflow.

KEY TERMS

Clinical decision support systems
Data display
Defects
Effectiveness
Efficiency
Flowchart
Gap analysis
Inefficiency
Nursing intelligence data warehouse

Process mapping
Productivity
Satisfaction
Task analysis
Workarounds
Workflow
Workflow analysis
Workflow redesign

CHAPTER OVERVIEW

Healthcare providers (HCPs) need to be involved in the planning and implementation of health information technologies (health IT) so that clinical processes (**workflow**) can be supported instead of hampered by health IT. This chapter outlines **workflow analysis** in a health IT planning framework as a method to avoid the consequences of poorly designed health IT and its impact on workflow. Nurse informaticists need to examine workflow prior to implementation of health IT, measure **productivity** after health IT implementation, and redesign workflow when needed. The chapter concludes with a discussion of using health IT to automate workflow for clinical and business processes.

INTRODUCTION

A primary innovation in health care during the early part of the 21st century has been the rapid implementation of health IT. Proponents of health IT believe its use can transform health care from a fragmented, error-prone system to an integrated system capable of consistently delivering high-quality, low-cost care (Bowens & Jones, 2010). However, early research shows mixed results about time and cost savings, patient safety, and consumer satisfaction (Jones, Heaton, Rudin, & Schneider, 2012).

Because the nature of health IT is radically different from the paper systems it replaces, implementation of health IT causes big changes in the way things get done. In other words, health IT affects workflow—the sequence of tasks, communications, and interactions needed to accomplish desired work (McGonigle & Mastrian, 2012). Depending on how well the health IT is implemented, changes in workflow ripple or rip through every part of a healthcare organization and can cause substantial problems for continuity of care.

THE PROMISE OF HEALTH IT

Throughout the beginning of the 21st century, reports about patient safety and escalating costs of medical care in the United States have resulted in a call for more efficiency in health care (Institute of Medicine [IOM], 1999, 2011; Page, 2004). Believing that health IT can bring about the needed changes, the federal government used its power to induce hospitals and HCPs to adopt health IT. Under the Health Information Technology for Economic and Clinical Health (HITECH) Act of 2009, the federal government will have invested $27 billion dollars in health IT by the year 2015 by providing incentive payments to hospitals and providers for adopting health IT and meeting "meaningful use" criteria (U.S. Department of Health and Human Services [HHS], 2009). This large investment has provided the needed incentive for widespread adoption of health IT in the U.S. healthcare system.

Health IT plays an integral part of any healthcare system because it is used to store, process, and aggregate healthcare data. Widespread use of health IT is believed to improve communication between healthcare organizations, leading to more integration and reducing fragmentation of care for patients (IOM, 2011). Improved communication among providers in a healthcare organization is also possible with health IT when documentation from one provider is accessible and can be reused by others in their clinical processes. When designed properly, health IT can shorten time for delivery of medications, supplies, and equipment using supply chain management and make patient movement through the system more efficient, particularly in areas such as surgery, imaging, and procedures. These processes are termed *workflow*, and are the focus of this chapter (IOM, 2011).

Negative Consequences of Health IT

Although the promise of health IT is positive, its delivery on that promise is not guaranteed. Two major factors influence the outcomes: the usability of the health IT and the plan for implementation, also called the system development life cycle. Problems with usability affect every part of human interaction with health IT from training sessions to long-term use in a healthcare facility (Boone, 2010). In order to achieve maximum **effectiveness**, **efficiency**, and provider **satisfaction** with health IT, the user interface should be designed with a simple and consistent appearance so that the provider does not have to remember a series of steps to complete a task or to search the interface for needed information (Boone, 2010). The health IT needs to allow efficient interactions, allow for corrections, provide immediate cues if information entered by providers is outside normal ranges, and use language that is understood by providers (Boone, 2010). For example, health IT that requires a provider to enter medication information on six different screens is not as usable as one that requires the same input on one screen. Health IT that fails to automatically fill data-entry fields with information collected from other providers requires duplicate documentation and can lead to errors.

Failures in health IT design and implementation to support workflow and practice patterns of providers will decrease the efficiency of HCPs and increase costs associated with clinical processes. For example, the number of nonproductive hours paid for providers to learn new health IT will be higher with a system that is poorly matched to provider roles and responsibilities (Lee & McElmurry, 2010). When unexpected workflow issues surface during the initial "go live" period, additional providers may be necessary to continue giving care during the initial months of health IT implementation. An even more severe problem occurs when there is a failure to understand provider workflow and a failure to bridge the gap to the desired future state of workflow with health IT (Kohle-Ersher, Chatterjee, Osmanbeyoglu,

Hochheiser, & Bartos, 2012; Unertl, Johnson, & Lorenzi, 2012). Poor design for the workflow and practice patterns cannot be reconciled to a new health IT with more practice (Kjeldskov, Skov, & Stage, 2010), and lost productivity of providers becomes integrated into the healthcare delivery system. Health IT that is poorly matched to workflow can even introduce new errors into care processes (Helmons, Wargel, & Daniels, 2009).

PLANNING FOR HEALTH IT

The adoption of health IT can be planned to avoid many problems, but understanding workflow must be a primary driver of which system is selected and how it is implemented in a healthcare-delivery system. A workflow-oriented framework developed by Choi and Kim (2012) illustrates the importance of workflow analysis (see **Figure 9-1**). The framework shows that workflow analysis precedes health IT configuration. An adaptation process follows where members of the health IT implementation team test the system with a small group of providers to decide if it performs as expected. If it does not, then adaptation continues. If the system is satisfactory, then full implementation occurs. The health IT system continues to be adjusted as more providers use the system. If the system meets the needs of providers, then it is maintained by an IT department. If the system is not satisfactory to providers, adjustments to the system continue until providers can use the system without sacrificing satisfaction, productivity, and patient safety.

Role of Nurse Informaticist

One of the responsibilities of nurse informaticists is workflow analysis and process redesign for health IT implementation. Nurse informaticists are members of process redesign teams and have the requisite clinical and analytical knowledge to map workflow successfully. Other skills of nurse informaticists are the ability to lead or moderate groups, organize concepts, manage details, and generate solutions in consultation with HCPs.

Nurse informaticists should work closely with executive leadership to develop a **nursing intelligence data warehouse**, which is analogous to business intelligence. Nursing intelligence is a collection of nursing-relevant data elements that can be mined to answer clinical questions, examine results of practice changes, and compare the effectiveness of different nursing interventions

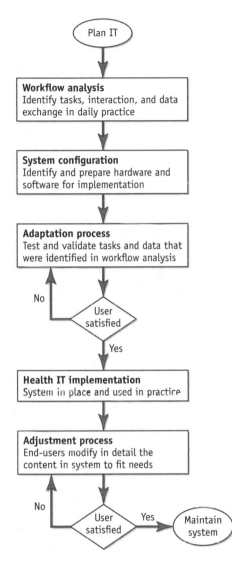

FIGURE 9-1 Workflow-oriented framework of health IT implementation.

Source: Choi, J., & Kim, H. (2012). A workflow-oriented framework-driven implementation and local adaptation of clinical information systems: A case study of nursing documentation system implementation at a tertiary rehabilitation hospital. *Computers, Informatics, Nursing, 30*(8), 409–414. Reprinted by permission of Lippincott Williams & Wilkins.

on patient outcomes. In addition to clinical data, nurse informaticists should work to integrate data from financial, human resources, and other administrative information systems into the nursing intelligence data warehouse (Thomas, 2006). Integrating data from these different systems can give nurse informaticists and nurse leaders the capability to apply analytics to clinical and business goals of the healthcare organization.

WORKFLOW ANALYSIS

Definition of Workflow

Workflow is any process that occurs in a healthcare system. Workflow is not a linear process (although it is often depicted as such); rather, it is dynamic, moving between different levels of the organization. Workflow is defined as:

> The flow of people, equipment (including machines and tools), information, and physical and mental tasks, in different places, at different levels, at different timescales continuously and discontinuously, that are used or required to support the goals of the clinical work domain. Workflow also includes communication, coordination, searching for information, interacting with information, problem solving, and planning. (Carayon, 2012, pp. 509–510)

Workflow analysis is the assessment of workflow using specific tools for health IT planning, implementation, and continuous improvement. The analysis should be led by a health IT core team (including a nurse informaticist) with representatives from clinical disciplines in the healthcare system.

Nature of Healthcare Provider Workflow

Workflow of HCPs varies widely based on the discipline (nursing, medicine, physical therapy, etc.) and setting (inpatient or outpatient). The most chaotic workflow is experienced by nurses in inpatient hospitals (Buchini & Quattrin, 2012; Cornell, Riordan, Townsend-Gervis, & Mobley, 2011; Holden et al., 2011; Varpio, Kuziemsky, MacDonald, & King, 2012). The workflow is characterized as having a rapid pace with abrupt switching between tasks (Cornell et al., 2010). For example, Cornell and colleagues (2010) reported that 40% of observations of nursing tasks lasted only 10 seconds, and the majority of tasks were interrupted by a switch.

Interruptions are a type of switch that is not initiated by the HCP. Interruptions are reported in the literature describing medication errors because an interruption during medication calculation or other cognitive processes of a nurse is particularly risky (Buchini & Quattrin, 2012; Elganzouri, Standish, & Androwich, 2009). Interruptions during medication administration in a rehabilitation unit were studied to count the number of interruptions. Observers watched 29 nurses as they administered medications to 250 patients. During 3,000 hours of observation, there were 1,170 documented interruptions, representing one interruption every 3 minutes. Another study found that nurses were interrupted on average 1.2 times per medication pass (Elganzouri et al., 2009).

Another unique aspect of HCP workflow is the amount of walking involved in patient care. Researchers have reported that nurses who work in hospitals routinely walk 5 miles in a 12-hour shift due to supplies and equipment being stored away from patient rooms (Elganzouri et al., 2009). In another study, observers recorded activities of nurses and found that walking represented 20% of the activities. Walking was common to administer medications, seek supplies and equipment, and respond to calls from patients (Cornell et al., 2010).

Interruptions, switching, and walking are just a few human factors to be considered in workflow. A nurse informaticist with education about human factors will understand that the HCP's knowledge, skills, experience, attention, stress, and physical capabilities influence the workflow (Carayon, 2012). Other relevant factors in workflow include the HCP's tasks, the physical environment (lighting, noise, and physical layout), and the organizational characteristics (teamwork, scheduling, culture of safety, and management style). The factors of person, task, technology, physical environment, and organization interact and influence the clinical workflow (Carayon, 2012). A thorough workflow analysis will include as many of these factors as possible so that the proposed health IT is suited to conditions in which it will be used.

Methods of Workflow Analysis

Workflow analysis is the examination of tasks, interactions among providers and between providers and patients, and the exchange of information using quantitative and qualitative methods (National Institute for Health Care Management Foundation, 2005). Workflow analysis should start before discussions with vendors commence because healthcare organizations and their providers first need to understand their own care processes and then design ways that health IT can bridge the gap between the current and desired workflow. The analysis should include representatives from all stakeholders who share the responsibility for setting goals for the health IT implementation process and outcome. Products of workflow analysis should include written requirements for the proposed health IT, including all tasks that the health IT must support or achieve (that is, the cognitive processes, communication exchanges, and procedures or actions). Each requirement should be analyzed for its utility in achieving the overall goal. Any redundant and unnecessary tasks should not be included in requirements. All requirements that are retained should have time and cost estimates associated with them. After completing an extensive workflow analysis, nurses and other decision makers can make more informed choices about selecting the health IT. As described previously, workflow analysis is appropriate when planning for health IT but it is also useful after health IT has been implemented. Workflow analysis methods include observing providers as they work, interviewing providers, and collecting structured data with questionnaires. The Agency for Healthcare Quality and Research (AHRQ) and the Health Resources and Services Administration provide free guides, toolkits, and other resources to support workflow analysis.

A study conducted by Watkins and colleagues (2012) illustrates the use of mixed methods in workflow analysis. The researchers examined the physical layout of nursing units and nurse workflow patterns in three phases before the implementation of new health IT (Watkins et al., 2012). In Phase 1 the researchers gave questionnaires to nurse–patient pairs to examine perceptions of workflow and patient-centered care. In Phase 2, each nurse was given a personal digital assistant (PDA) that automatically queried nurses about their activity 30 times in a 12-hour shift. Nurses also wore pedometers to measure the number of steps in a 12-hour shift. In this way, the researchers gathered data that were representative of nurses' activities during their shifts. This method is called work sampling. In the final phase of the research, nurses participated in focus groups to discuss the results of the first two phases and to provide feedback on their perceptions of the "best" fit of the health IT with their current unit layout and workflow. Nurses suggested several changes in the physical environment, including decentralization of medications, supplies, equipment, and computer access to reduce inefficiencies, reduce walking distances, and keep nurses closer to their patients.

Tools for workflow analysis are classified into 11 categories of workflow tools that can be used in specific phases of health IT from planning through continuous improvement (Carayon, 2012). The tool categories are **task analysis**, **process mapping**, **data display**, data collection, idea creation, problem solving, project planning, risk assessment, statistical analysis, and usability. For the purposes of this chapter, three categories of workflow analysis tools will be discussed: task analysis, process mapping, and data display.

Task Analysis

Task analysis is a qualitative and quantitative method for understanding the activities associated with a particular goal of patient care. A common method to conduct a task analysis is to start with a detailed list of activities and then observe providers as they perform the tasks to measure time to completion and incidence of interruptions. In a study by Dasgupta and colleagues (2011), task analysis was conducted on medication administration with barcode technology to understand its effects on quality of care and time spent in direct patient care. The data collector observed eight nurses as they treated 29 patients on the dayshift for a total of 20 hours. The data collector used a stopwatch to measure time associated with each part of medication administration. The analysis revealed the most frequently occurring tasks were medication preparation, giving medications, and documenting medications. Of the three, documenting medications took the longest time. There were few interruptions, but telephone calls and delivery of meals to patients were the causes of the interruptions.

Work can be cognitive in nature, making it difficult to analyze using customary task analysis methods. In this case, interviews are an effective method to understand the thinking processes required by providers (Effken, Brewer, Logue, Gephart, & Verran, 2011). Effken and colleagues interviewed nurse managers, directors of nursing, IT managers, and quality managers in three acute care hospitals. These managers revealed an overall cognitive goal of "efficient, safe, high-quality patient care in context of nursing shortage, organizational culture, census variation, public opinion, regulations, and budget limits" (p. 702). Based on the goal, the managers had values and priorities, purpose-related functions (e.g., communication and quality improvement), and object-related processes (information management and care coordination). Using a cognitive work analysis, the researchers were better able to understand managers' needs for decision support tools.

Process Mapping

Workflow is often mapped using **flowchart** tools to show documents, tasks, decisions, and interactions associated with care delivery. A flowchart that shows work across time and roles is called a swimlane chart. Such a flowchart is helpful for illustrating the relationship of tasks among providers (see **Figure 9-2**).

Diagraming workflow with a flowchart follows a certain convention: Movement forward in time can either be diagramed from left to right or top to bottom. Symbols on flowcharts have specific meanings to improve understanding of workflow. The symbols are not interchangeable. For example, a diamond shape is always used to

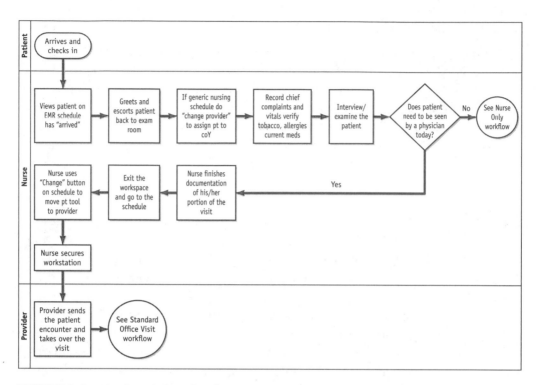

FIGURE 9-2   Simple swimlane flowchart.

document a decision point. **Figure 9-3** shows the customary symbols to document workflow.

Data Display

Data collected from observations of workflow and from interviews with providers need to be presented in an understandable manner. Common methods include flowcharts (previously discussed), Pareto charts, Gantt charts, run charts, control charts, scatterplots, force field analysis, and fishbone charts. Each of the presentation methods has a particular purpose.

A Pareto chart is useful for displaying the most important areas for **workflow redesign** or safety improvement activities. The principle behind a Pareto chart is that improvement activities should focus on 80% of problem areas, not the less frequently occurring problems. **Figure 9-4** shows a Pareto chart with medication errors. Based on the results illustrated in the Pareto chart, safety improvement should focus on administering and transcribing medications.

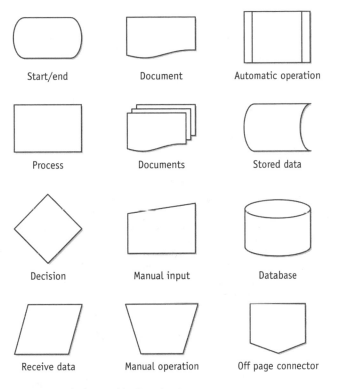

FIGURE 9-3 Common symbols used in flowcharts.

Gantt charts are used primarily for project management. For example, workflow analysis before implementation of health IT requires a review of all other technologies and processes in a health system before the introduction of a new information system. **Figure 9-5** shows a Gantt chart illustrating tasks, duration of tasks, start and end dates of tasks, persons responsible for tasks, and a graphical display of duration of tasks. The Gantt chart keeps the health IT implementation team informed about the progress toward task completion.

Run charts and control charts display change in data over time. These charts are important to use when monitoring a process for quality improvement. For example, if a nursing unit were trying to reduce the time from request of pain medication to administration time, a run chart can be used to show the average number of minutes per day that it took patients to receive pain medication after the request was made. Control charts are run charts with three additional lines: center line (CL), upper control limit (UCL), and lower control limit (LCL). These lines provide a "window" of

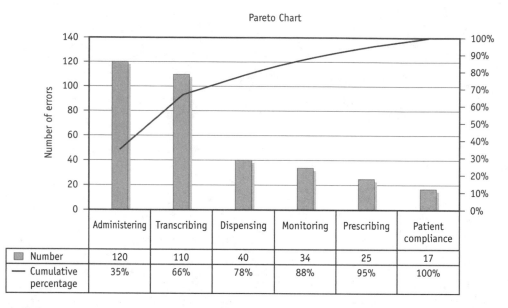

FIGURE 9-4   Pareto chart.

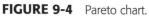

FIGURE 9-5   Gantt chart.

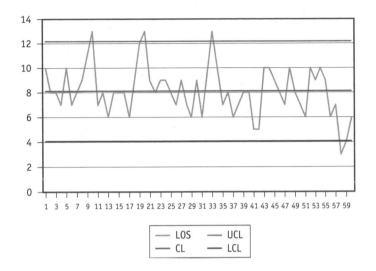

FIGURE 9-6   Control chart.

acceptable performance. **Figure 9-6** shows a control chart for a 60-day period of time. The CL is a horizontal line representing the average for a day. The UCL and LCL are placed 2 or 3 standard deviations above or below the average to create the window. Any point above the UCL or below the LCL would be considered outside of the acceptable limits for the process. In the case of promptness of pain medications, a point below the LCL is actually good.

Scatterplots demonstrate the relationship of two points to one another. Scatterplots are useful when looking for an association or correlation. **Figure 9-7** illustrates a scatterplot of patient age and the length of hospital stay. This relationship is positive—in other words, as the age of a person increases, the length of hospital stay increases too. Scatterplots can show an inverse or negative relationship. For example, as a person's age increases, the muscle strength decreases.

A force field analysis is used to analyze the issues surrounding change. Implementation of an electronic health record (EHR) represents a large departure from paper systems. When conducting a force field analysis, the health IT team examines the forces driving change and forces restraining the change. If the team can increase the driving forces, change is more likely to occur. A force field analysis is shown in **Figure 9-8**. The driving forces are the factors that are likely to move an exercise program for patients with cancer forward, whereas the restraining forces are likely to reduce the chances of the exercise program being successful.

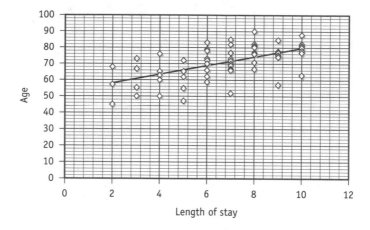
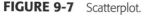

FIGURE 9-7   Scatterplot.

A tool that works well for brainstorming and illustrating workflow problems is a cause and effect chart, commonly called a fishbone chart. The problem is illustrated as the head of the fish, and each spine represents a category of causes. In **Figure 9-9**, communication with patients who have limited English proficiency is the problem. The causes are identified as time constraints, patient education, hospital interpreter list, Health Insurance Portability and Accountability Act of 1996 (HIPAA) compliance, economics, documentation, health literacy, and telephone language line. Each cause has multiple contributing issues. This data display tool is effective because it conveys a great deal of information in an understandable manner.

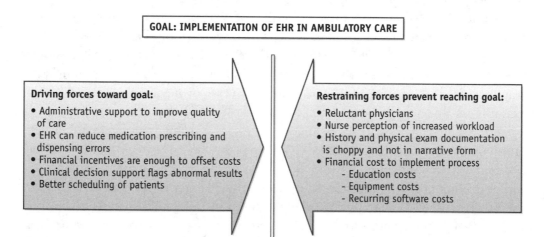

FIGURE 9-8   Force field analysis.

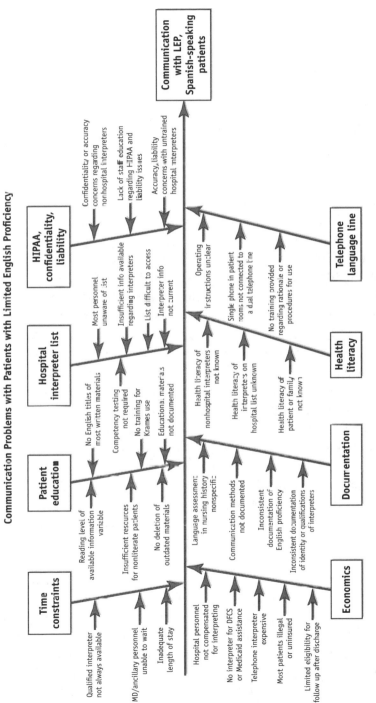

Communication Problems with Patients with Limited English Proficiency

FIGURE 9-9 Cause and effect chart.

167

GAP ANALYSIS AND WORKFLOW REDESIGN _____

An initial workflow analysis conducted before health IT is implemented will likely reveal **inefficiencies** that can be improved with workflow redesign. For example, a workflow study of vital sign assessment and documentation in three hospitals demonstrated differences in time based on the type of documentation system in use (Yeung, Lapinsky, Granton, Doran, & Cafazzo, 2012). In hospitals with paper-based systems, nurses documented vital signs immediately on bedside flowsheets, whereas nurses in hospitals with EHRs wrote vital signs on notepaper and later documented them in the patient record. This transcription of vital signs in hospitals with EHRs was redundant and inefficient with regard to time. The delay in documenting in the EHR also made vital signs unavailable to other HCPs. Finally, the transcription of vital signs from paper notes to the electronic record could have introduced errors (also called **defects** in the workflow literature).

The inefficiencies discovered in a workflow analysis could be used as a starting point for redesign (Bowens & Jones, 2010). The inefficiencies represent a gap between the current, inefficient workflow and the future, desired workflow with health IT. A formal report of the gap is called a **gap analysis**. Using the results described earlier (Yeung et al., 2012), a health IT design team would readily understand the need for bedside documentation capabilities in an EHR. The documentation of vital signs needs to be fast and error free, so one solution could be mobile electronic vital sign monitors with wireless communication to a mobile vital sign documentation module in the EHR. This solution would eliminate the need to remember vital signs, write them down, and transcribe them later into an EHR. Having identified the gap between current and future workflow, the health IT team can select products that meet the requirements. It is through analysis of workflow that real return on health IT investment can be achieved (Jones et al., 2012).

An area of workflow inefficiency many nurses experience is searching for medication, supplies, and equipment. Health IT systems can be used to maintain appropriate inventory levels of frequently used medications and supplies. Medication systems that store, count, track use, and automatically generate messages for inventory restocking are particularly efficient because the systems remove the requirement for redundant work such as counting narcotics and calling for supplies to be restocked. Systems can reduce the time nurses wait for deliveries of newly ordered medications and supplies. When supplies and medications are readily available via a health IT system, it can reduce the tendency for nurses to stash supplies, a costly practice, in terms of inventory.

Nurses and other HCPs who experience workflow problems after implementation of health IT will often develop **workarounds**, which are unauthorized ways to use health IT (Miller, Fortier, & Garrison, 2011). Miller and colleagues conducted a study of medication administration after implementation of a bar code medication administration system. The approved workflow had eight steps, including review of medication order, bar scan of patient wrist band, review of electronic medication administration record (e-MAR), bar scan of medication, resolution of any system alert, administration of medications, confirmation of administration in e-MAR, and review of documentation in charting session. The researchers found that 20% of medications generated alerts requiring additional steps by nurses. Of the medications with alerts, 97% were administered with an override of the system, most of the time without a documented reason. This behavior of administering when alerts were generated without documenting a reason for administration may represent "alert fatigue," a dangerous consequence of an improperly calibrated alert system. In addition to alert overrides, the researchers found other workarounds categorized as "omission of a process step, performance of an unauthorized step, or performance of steps in improper sequence" (p. 164). These workarounds represent defects in the health IT implementation and should be corrected because of the risk for medication errors (Miller et al., 2011).

Studies of nursing efficiency following implementation of health IT indicate that several work processes can become more efficient: handoffs at the change of shift, medication reconciliation, order processing, and follow up on new orders (Thompson, Johnston, & Spurr, 2009). Processes that can be automated greatly add to nursing efficiency including automatic flow of data from medical devices into the EHR; automated lists of tasks generated from orders; documentation that auto-populates fields with previous entries from the EHR, with options to edit or enter new information; decision support alerts; auto-calculation of medications and intravenous fluids; and auto-fill of documentation from dietary, respiratory, physical therapy, and creation of discharge instructions from physician orders and nursing care plans (Thompson et al., 2009).

TECHNOLOGY TO AUTOMATE WORKFLOW

Technology can be deployed to automate clinical and business workflow in healthcare organizations. For clinical workflow, the most common type of technology is **clinical decision support systems (CDSS)** integrated as part of an EHR. The Office of the National Coordinator for Health Information Technology (2013) provides the following definition of CDSS:

> Clinical decision support provides clinicians, staff, patients or other individuals with knowledge and person-specific information, intelligently filtered or presented at appropriate times, to enhance health and health care. CDS [clinical decision support]

encompasses a variety of tools to enhance decision-making in the clinical workflow. These tools include computerized alerts and reminders to care providers and patients; clinical guidelines; condition-specific order sets; focused patient data reports and summaries; documentation templates; diagnostic support, and contextually relevant reference information, among other tools.

Clinical decision support is developed by understanding clinical workflow at a very granular level. The workflow is mapped using flowcharts and sophisticated logic that continuously monitors and moves workflow based on definitions and preset conditions. To understand CDSS, watch a short YouTube video on the Soarian Workflow Engine Congestive Heart Failure on the companion website for this text.

Business process automation in healthcare organizations is most often used for inventory management, billing, patient throughput, human resource management, and other business processes. Two of these functions are most pertinent to HCPs: patient throughput and human resource management. Patient throughput is the movement of patients from one part of a healthcare delivery system to another. For example, the movement of patients from an emergency department to an inpatient unit is a critical process because emergency departments need to see patients quickly to reduce wait times. Vendors of software provide many different types of solutions to track patients and provide automatic prompts to housekeeping to clean rooms from newly discharged patients. There are many different human resource management software solutions that are aimed at managing workflow. For example, the assignment of newly admitted patients to nurses on a particular unit of a hospital can be calculated based on a nurse's workload for the past 15 minutes to estimate an anticipated workload for an entire shift (Sundaramoorthi, Chen, Rosenberger, Kim, & Buckley-Behan, 2010).

HEALTHCARE PROVIDER ROLES IN WORKFLOW ANALYSIS

Providers who worked with paper systems are likely to experience the profound changes in the clinical processes after health IT is implemented, because they are inexperienced with systems such as EHRs. However, even nurses and other providers who enter the workforce after the implementation of EHRs is widespread will be involved in continuous improvements to health IT and implementation of cutting edge technology. It is important for nurses to participate in workflow studies by participating in a design team or by being observed and interviewed. Participation in a health IT implementation team represents an opportunity to understand clinical processes and the fit with health IT. **Box 9-1** provides a case study of workflow analysis involving nurses.

Box 9-1   Workflow Analysis After Implementation of Computer Provider Order Entry y

A study of medication administration workflow was conducted after implementation of Computer Provider Order Entry (CPOE) by Tschannen, Talsma, Reinemeyer, Belt, and Schoville (2011). The researchers used mixed methods to gather data about workflow of nurses. The first step of the analysis was to map the process of medication administration. Tschannen and colleagues interviewed nurses who worked in the target hospital and found that the process had 17 distinct steps.

Next, Tschannen and colleagues observed nurses as medications were being administered, and they timed each step with a stopwatch. The researchers observed 86 medication administrations for 32 hours over a 30-day period in an adult intensive care unit (ICU) and a pediatric unit. The researchers found the mean time for medication administration in the adult ICU was 8.45 minutes and in the pediatric unit it was 9.92 minutes. Nurses who worked in the pediatric unit spent more time preparing medications because they had to crush or dilute medications for children.

The researchers interviewed nurses to better understand workflow issues. They found four main concerns: "systems issues, variations in standards of care, workflow variability, and changes in communication practices" (p. 407). System issues were related to the screen layout in the e-MAR. The print was small, and nurses had to scroll and click more often than they liked. The computers were also slow and at times would not function. Variations in standards of care concerned the lack of a designated time to check for new medication orders. If a stat dose had been entered by a provider in the CPOE, nurses might not know, and the system did not provide an alert. Duplicate orders were problematic for nurses in the system. The nurses also reported that medication reconciliation was more difficult to perform with CPOE than with paper orders. The most profound change was communication between physicians and nurses. Because physicians entered their own orders, there was little need for discussion. Nurses did find the organization of medications in the CPOE to be better than paper orders because the medications could be grouped by name or route, making review much faster. Observations by researchers corroborated the concerns nurses expressed in interviews.

Check Your Understanding

1. What other data-collection methods could have been used to analyze workflow of medication administration after implementation of CPOE?
2. What charts or graphs could be used to illustrate nurses' workflow or concerns with altered workflow?
3. Which changes in workflow after implementation of CPOE could result in medication errors?
4. Could any of the workflow be automated? If so, which processes would benefit from automation?

SUMMARY

Implementation of health IT requires analysis of workflow, which is a detailed examination of the care processes. Analysis of workflow should be directed by an implementation team that includes a nurse informaticist. The implementation team uses many methods to study workflow and communicate the results of the analysis. The most common of these are task analysis, interviews, flowcharts, and process mapping (see **Table 9-1**). After understanding current workflow and finding gaps to the future, desired workflow, product review, and selection can be targeted to health IT that fill the workflow gaps. High priority should be given to health IT that automates clinical or business processes to improve efficiency and productivity.

Table 9-1	Workflow Tools found Online	
Source	**Website**	**Description**
U.S. Department of Health and Human Services	http://www.hrsa.gov/healthit/ toolbox/HealthITadoptiontoolbox/ SystemImplementation/ workflowanalysis.html	Guide and tools for workflow analysis
Agency for Healthcare Research and Quality (AHRQ)	http://healthit.ahrq.gov/portal/ server.pt/community/health_it_ tools_and_resources/919/ workflow_assessment_for_ health_it_toolkit/27865	Workflow Assessment for Health IT Toolkit
AHRQ	http://healthit.ahrq.gov/portal/ server.pt/community/health_it_ tools_and_resources/919/ time_and_motion_studies_ database/27878	Time and Motion Studies Database. Formatted, blank access database available for free download. User manual is provided.
AHRQ	http://healthit.ahrq.gov/health- it-tools-and-resources/health-it- evaluation-measures-quick- reference-guides	Health IT Evaluation Measures: Quick Reference Guides. This is a collection of tools with advice about methods of data collection that can be used to assess and then compare performance and outcomes before and after implementation of health IT.
AHRQ	http://healthit.ahrq.gov/portal/ server.pt/community/health_ it_tools_and_resources/919/ health_it_survey_ compendium/27874	Health IT Survey Compendium. This is a searchable database of survey tools for use in the preliminary stage of health IT adoption through reevaluations of health IT impact.
Soarian Workflow Engine	http://www.youtube.com/ watch?feature5player_ embedded&v=ZC4b4dEusEY	Video demonstrating clinical decision support workflow with congestive heart failure.

For a full suite of assignments and additional learning activities, use the access code located in the front of your book and visit www.jblearning.com. If you do not have an access code, you can obtain one at the site.

REFERENCES

Boone, E. (2010). EMR usability: Bridging the gap between nurse and computer. *Nursing Management*, *41*(3), 14–16.

Bowens, F. M. A., & Jones, W. A. (2010). Health information technology: Integration of clinical workflow into meaningful use of electronic health. *Perspectives in Health Information Management*, 7, 1–15.

Buchini, S., & Quattrin, R. (2012). Avoidable interruptions during drug administration in an intensive rehabilitation ward: Improvement project. *Journal of Nursing Management, 20*(3), 326–334. doi: http://dx.doi.org/10.1111/j.1365-2834.2011.01323.x

Carayon, P. (Ed.). (2012). *Handbook of human factors and ergonomics in health care and patient safety* (2nd ed.). Boca Raton, FL: CRC Press, Taylor & Francis Group.

Choi, J., & Kim, H. (2012). A workflow-oriented framework-driven implementation and local adaptation of clinical information systems: A case study of nursing documentation system implementation at a tertiary rehabilitation hospital. *CIN: Computers, Informatics, Nursing, 30*(8), 409–414; quiz 415-406. doi: 10.1097/NXN.0b013e3182512ffd

Cornell, P., Herrin-Griffith, D., Keim, C., Petschonek, S., Sanders, A. M., D'Mello, S., . . . Shepherd, G. (2010). Transforming nursing workflow, part 1. *Journal of Nursing Administration, 40*(9), 366–373. doi: http://dx.doi.org/10.1097/NNA.0b013e3181ee4261

Cornell, P., Riordan, M., Townsend-Gervis, M., & Mobley, R. (2011). Barriers to critical thinking workflow interruptions and task switching among nurses. *Journal of Nursing Administration, 41*(10), 407–414. doi: http://dx.doi.org/10.1097/NNA.0b013e31822edd42

Dasgupta, A., Sansgiry, S. S., Jacob, S. M., Frost, C. P., Dwibedi, N., & Tipton, J. (2011). Descriptive analysis of workflow variables associated with barcode-based approach to medication administration. *Journal of Nursing Care Quality, 26*(4), 377–384.

Effken, J. A., Brewer, B. B., Logue, M. D., Gephart, S. M., & Verran, J. A. (2011). Using cognitive work analysis to fit decision support tools to nurse managers' work flow. *International Journal of Medical Informatics, 80*(10), 698–707. doi: 10.1016/j.ijmedinf.2011.07.003

Elganzouri, E. S., Standish, C. A., & Androwich, I. (2009). Medication administration time study (MATS): Nursing staff performance of medication administration. *Journal of Nursing Administration, 39*(5), 204–210.

Helmons, P. J., Wargel, L. N., & Daniels, C. E. (2009). Effect of bar-code-assisted medication administration on medication administration errors and accuracy in multiple patient care areas. *American Journal of Health-System Pharmacy, 66*(13), 1202–1210. doi: 10.2146/ajhp080357

Holden, R. J., Scanlon, M. C., Patel, N. R., Kaushal, R., Escoto, K. H., Brown, R. L., . . . Karsh, B.-T. (2011). A human factors framework and study of the effect of nursing workload on patient safety and employee quality of working life. *BMJ Quality & Safety, 20*(1), 15–24. doi: 10.1136/bmjqs.2008.028381

Institute of Medicine. (1999). *To err is human: Building a safer health system*. Washington, DC: National Academies Press.

Institute of Medicine. (2011). *Health IT and patient safety: Building safer systems for better care*. Washington, DC: Committee on Patient Safety and Health Information Technology, Board on Health Care Services.

Jones, S. S., Heaton, P. S., Rudin, R. S., & Schneider, E. C. (2012). Unraveling the IT productivity paradox—lessons for health care. *New England Journal of Medicine, 366*(24), 2243–2245.

Kjeldskov, J., Skov, M. B., & Stage, J. (2010). A longitudinal study of usability in health care: Does time heal? *International Journal of Medical Informatics, 79*(6), e135–e143. doi: http://dx.doi.org/10.1016/j.ijmedinf.2008.07.008

Kohle-Ersher, A., Chatterjee, P., Osmanbeyoglu, H. U., Hochheiser, H., & Bartos, C. (2012). Evaluating the barriers to point-of-care documentation for nursing staff. *CIN: Computers, Informatics, Nursing, 30*(3), 126–133.

Lee, S., & McElmurry, B. (2010). Capturing nursing care workflow disruptions: Comparison between nursing and physician workflows. *CIN: Computers, Informatics, Nursing, 28*(3), 151–161.

McGonigle, D., & Mastrian, K. (2012). *Nursing informatics and the foundation of knowledge*. Burlington, MA: Jones & Bartlett Learning.

Miller, D. F., Fortier, C. R., & Garrison, K. L. (2011). Bar code medication administration technology: Characterization of high-alert medication triggers and clinician workarounds. *Annals of Pharmacotherapy*. doi: 10.1345/aph.1P262

National Institute for Health Care Management Foundation. (2005). *Steps in a basic workflow analysis*. Retrieved from http://nihcm.org/pdf/AHRQ-QandA.pdf

Office of the National Coordinator for Health Information Technology. (2013). *Clinical decision support*. Retrieved from http://www.healthit.gov/policy-researchers-implementers/clinical-decision-support-cds

Page, A. (Ed.), Committee on the Work Environment for Nurses and Patient Safety, Board on Health Care Services. (2004). *Keeping patients safe: Transforming the work environment of nurses*. Washington, DC: National Academies Press.

Sundaramoorthi, D., Chen, V. C., Rosenberger, J. M., Kim, S. B., & Buckley-Behan, D. F. (2010). A data-integrated simulation-based optimization for assigning nurses to patient admissions. *Health Care Management Science, 13*(3), 210–221.

Thomas, R. (2006). Information-based transformation: The need for integrated, enterprisewide informatics. *Healthcare Financial Management, 60*(9), 140–142.

Thompson, D., Johnston, P., & Spurr, C. (2009). The impact of electronic medical records on nursing efficiency. *Journal of Nursing Administration, 39*(10), 444–451. doi: 10.1097/NNA.0b013e3181b9209c

Tschannen, D., Talsma, A., Reinemeyer, N., Belt, C., & Schoville, R. (2011). Nursing medication administration and workflow using computerized physician order entry. *CIN: Computers, Informatics, Nursing, 29*(7), 401–410. doi: 10.1097/NCN.0b013e318205e510

Unertl, K. M., Johnson, K. B., & Lorenzi, N. M. (2012). Health information exchange technology on the front lines of healthcare: Workflow factors and patterns of use. *Journal of the American Medical Informatics Association, 19*(3), 392–400. doi: 10.1136/amiajnl-2011-000432

U.S. Department of Health and Human Services. (2009). HITECH Act. Retrieved from http://www.healthit.gov/policy-researchers-implementers/hitech-act-0

Varpio, L., Kuziemsky, C., MacDonald, C., & King, W. J. (2012). The helpful or hindering effects of in-hospital patient monitor alarms on nurses: A qualitative analysis. *CIN: Computers, Informatics, Nursing, 30*(4), 210–217. doi: 10.1097/NCN.0b013e31823eb581

Watkins, N., Kennedy, M., Lee, N., O'Neill, M., Peavey, E., Ducharme, M., & Padula, C. (2012). Destination bedside: Using research findings to visualize optimal unit layouts and health information technology in support of bedside care. *Journal of Nursing Administration, 42*(5), 256–265. doi: 10.1097/NNA.0b013e3182480918

Yeung, M. S., Lapinsky, S. E., Granton, J. T., Doran, D. M., & Cafazzo, J. A. (2012). Examining nursing vital signs documentation workflow: Barriers and opportunities in general internal medicine units. *Journal of Clinical Nursing, 21*(7/8), 975–982. doi: http://dx.doi.org/10.1111/j.1365-2702.2011.03937.x

CHAPTER 10

Promoting Patient Safety with the Use of Information Technology

Stephanie Lenz-Norman, BSN, RN
Crayton Fargason, Jr., MD, MBA
Mariah Strickland, BSN, RN
Elizabeth Clark, BA, BSN, RN

CHAPTER LEARNING OBJECTIVES

1. Provide an overview of the major information technologies (ITs) that have the potential to impact the safety of care.
2. Describe the manner in which these technologies are deployed in order to improve patient safety.
3. Review the nursing impact of such technology deployments.
4. Describe data and connectivity requirements that are needed to implement these safety strategies.
5. Discuss common points of failure experienced when these technologies are implemented.

KEY TERMS

Alert fatigue

Clinical decision-support systems

Clinical microsystem

Commission

Errors

Knowledge-based error

Omission

Out-of-range alarms

Patient safety

Point of care

Rule-based error

Slip

System fault alarms

CHAPTER OVERVIEW

The focus of this chapter is the use of health information technology (health IT) deployed to improve the safety of patient care. More specifically, the primary focus is on technologies that directly impact nursing workflow and practice. The need for improvement in health IT is not a new issue, but it has gained national attention because of reports by the Institute of Medicine in 1999 and 2011.

The Healthcare Information and Management Systems Society (HIMSS) defines information as "data to which meaning has been assigned, according to context and assumed conventions" (HIMSS, 2010, p. 62). Furthermore, it defines an information system as one that "takes input data, processes it, and provides information as output" (HIMSS, p. 63). Using these definitions, one can see that the information infrastructure at a patient's bedside is a more sophisticated environment than it was a generation ago. While many new tools are available to address the healthcare needs of patients, not all advances in health care have improved outcomes, and many have resulted in increased healthcare costs (Lighter, 2013). Likewise, many of the promised patient safety benefits of health IT are yet to be completely realized.

HEALTH IT USED IN PATIENT CARE

The area where changes in health IT are most visible is at the sharp end of care, the **point of care**, whether the location is an inpatient room or an exam room in a clinic. The point of care (shown in Level 1 of **Figure 10-1**) can contain a vast array of medical devices and technology to manage and properly document patient care. The electronic health record (EHR) has evolved over time to include electronic processing of orders and results, maintaining the electronic medication administration record (eMAR), and healthcare provider (HCP) documentation. The EHR has further developed with the concept of computerized provider order entry. With this advancement, the recent versions of EHRs have been developed to be more comprehensive, impacting many aspects of workflow for HCPs. Moving from the point of care, the next area of consideration is the hospital unit or clinic (Zone 2 in Figure 10-1). The first and second zones establish a **clinical microsystem**, which is considered to be a small group of people who work to provide care to a group of patients (The Dartmouth Institute, 2013). These clinical microsystems are often embedded in larger organizations such as hospitals, multispecialty practices, or other outpatient settings, which form the third level of the diagram. The fourth level of the diagram shows the information exchange across organizations such as a health system with hospitals, clinics, home health, and outpatient services. This fourth level also includes communication with patients using portals and other care providers through the use of a health information exchange. At each of these levels, specific IT tools are used to improve patient safety. The tools employed at different levels often have different connectivity and data infrastructure requirements associated with them and varying levels of influence on nursing workflow.

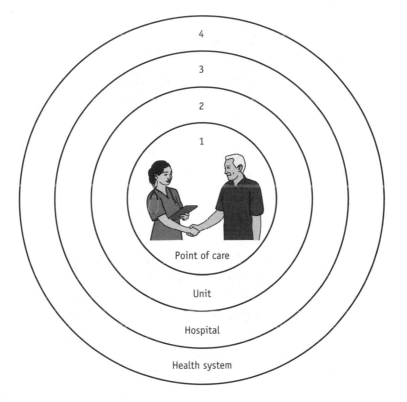

FIGURE 10-1 Zones in health care.

BEGINNING AT THE POINT OF CARE

For HCPs, errors are not intentional; however, errors may equate to individuals being harmed in the course of receiving care. HIMSS defines **patient safety** as "freedom from unacceptable risk of harm" (HIMSS, 2013, p. 89). Most errors result from deficiencies in systems of care, and the generation of errors in general can be conceptualized using Reason's Swiss Cheese Model (Reason, 2000). Reason defines **errors** as risks that pass through gaps in protective barriers that normally defend patients from harm. The model also asserts that errors can occur when too few barriers to harm exist (Reason, 1990). In this model, the probability of errors is reduced by adding protective barriers (adding additional slices of cheese to the process), or by minimizing the safety gaps (holes in the cheese) at a given layer (see **Figure 10-2**). New ITs are often envisioned to provide new protective barriers; however, achieving such benefits depends on far more than technology.

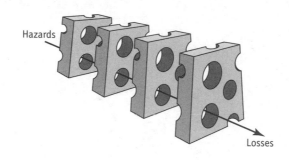

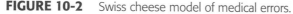

FIGURE 10-2   Swiss cheese model of medical errors.

Source: Adapted by permission from BMJ Publishing Group Limited. British Medical Journal, 320, Reason, J., Human Error: models and management, p. 768, 1990.

Healthcare services are ultimately delivered by people, and the delivery of care is therefore influenced by the limitations of humans. Reason's (1990) model recognizes several human sources of error that have implications for the safety of care delivered to patients. One type of error, a **slip**, is an instance in which a person knows the correct actions, yet at the time care is delivered, an incorrect action is taken (Reason, 1990). An example of this would be placing a carton of milk in the kitchen cabinet instead of the refrigerator or grabbing the wrong breastmilk from a refrigerator and giving it to a patient. A second type of error is a **rule-based error**. This is when a good rule is applied in the wrong situation. Making a right turn when the traffic light is red after a complete stop is a good rule but should not be applied if it leads to driving the wrong direction on a one-way street. Likewise, while penicillin may be the antibiotic of choice in the treatment of streptococcal pharyngitis, it is not appropriate if the patient is allergic to penicillin. Finally, **knowledge-based errors** occur when an individual does not possess the information needed to determine the appropriate action. An example of this might be the simultaneous administration of two intravenous (IV) medications that are chemically incompatible. Information systems and the rules built into the framework known as **clinical decision-support systems** are often deployed in an attempt to minimize the risk of these types of errors.

Other concepts that help in discussions of safety are **commission** and **omission**. HIMSS defines error as: "An act of commission (doing something wrong) or omission (failing to do the right thing) that leads to an undesirable outcome or significant potential for such an outcome" (HIMSS, 2013). An act of commission would be administering penicillin to a patient with a known allergy to penicillin. When an opportunity to perform an action that could benefit a patient is missed, an error of omission has occurred. For example, failure to rescue a patient in septic shock because of delayed recognition is an example of an error of omission (Schmid, Hoffman, Happ, Wolf, & DeVita, 2007). Each of the human vulnerabilities identified by Reason (1990) can lead to acts of commission or acts of omission.

Additional layers of protection and checks within each layer aid HCPs to help guard against slips, rule-based errors, and knowledge-based errors. These systems serve as reminders when action is necessary (preventing acts of omission) in addition to lending warning in the instances that prevent inappropriate actions (preventing acts of commission). Indeed, nurses may view such health IT aides as essential, yet they are often unaware of the limitations and risks associated with the adoption and implementation of such tools. The discussion that follows focuses on how failure can occur despite the use of health IT and then how improvements in patient care can be made possible with the use of ITs.

There have been many technological advances to improve patient safety at the point of care. Physiologic monitors and the alarms associated with them, smart medication pumps, electronic handheld communication devices, barcode medication administration, radiofrequency identification (RFID), and varying uses of clinical decision support within the EHR are examples that are discussed in the sections that follow.

Using Reason's Swiss Cheese Model framework, consider the technologies available to add layers or barriers to the delivery process. These technologies are reflected in **Table 10-1**.

Table 10-1	**Devices at the Bedside**		
Device	**Location**	**Minimal Level of Data Integration**	**Type of Error Addressed**
Physiologic monitors	Bedside	Device/unit centric	Omission: inattentive slips
Smart pumps	Bedside	Local datasets residing in device "brain"	Commission: slips, rule-based errors, knowledge-based errors
Location monitoring	Unit or institution	Unit-based or centrally integrated information	Omission: inattentive slips
Bar coding devices	Unit	Centrally integrated with eMAR	Commission: slips
Embedded sensors	Institution	Centrally integrated information	Omission: inattentive slips

eMAR, electronic medication administration record.

Many of the devices utilized in the care of patients are physiologic monitors designed to prevent errors of omission that may result if staff do not respond promptly to significant changes in a patient's physiologic condition. These technologies do, however, offer other advantages. For example, electronic capture of bedside parameters linked to the EHR allow for immediate access to information for multiple providers in various locations (even away from the bedside), which may improve the safety and efficiency of patient care.

Physiologic Monitoring

The patient's physiologic condition can be monitored noninvasively and invasively. Noninvasive outputs of the bedside monitors can generate graphical (waveforms) and numeric displays by means of leads or probes attached to the patient. Examples of noninvasive parameters that can be monitored are blood pressure, heart rate, respiratory rate, body temperature, and pulse oximetry. Before the implementation of electronic physiologic monitoring, many of these parameters were determined manually. Consider pulse oximetry, for example: Prior to the advancement of pulse oximetry, oxygen saturation was monitored directly by staff, which had to be vigilant and also skilled in estimating oxygen levels based on observation. Even skilled observers may have disagreed (O'Donnell, Kamlin, Davis, Carlin, & Morley, 2007). More widely used presently, pulse oximetry eliminates problems with observer error. However, accurate pulse oximetry readings require the presence of quality pulsations. In the absence of quality pulsations, erroneous readings can occur. This can be a challenge for the critically ill patient with poor perfusion. Active patients (children, for example) can also disrupt the quality of the signal received by the device, leading to false alerts. When these false alerts occur frequently, staff members experience **alert fatigue**. This fatigue introduces a "cry wolf" bias in staff: Pulse oximeter alarms in the absence of any problem with oxygen saturation are ignored. Errors of omission can occur when meaningful alerts are ignored.

Similar to pulse oximeters, most monitoring technologies have basic requirements for successful use. When these conditions are not met (such as in the case of a poorly perfused patient with pulse oximetry monitoring), more sophisticated, noninvasive technologies are sometimes available. For example, staff might use near-infrared spectroscopy (NIRS) to monitor tissue oxygenation in the cases where patients have decreased pulsatile flow. NIRS can be more accurate to evaluate oxygen status even when a pulsatile waveform is not present (Boas et al., 2001).

In some cases, limitations of noninvasive approaches necessitate the use of invasive monitoring tools. In complex cases, providers rely on information from more invasive types of monitoring such as intracranial pressure (ICP), cerebral perfusion pressure (CPP), central venous pressure (CVP), invasive blood pressure (IBP), or invasive cardiac monitoring. While invasive monitoring provides valuable information, its use directly increases the risk of harming patients. For example, insertion of a central line to monitor CVP could increase the risk of a catheter-associated bloodstream infection.

Most bedside physiologic monitoring devices produce nearly continuous streams of information, which remain in the local monitor during the patient's stay. In addition, the bedside nurse can pull samples of this continuous information into nursing computerized documentation on a regular basis (depending on orders). These bedside monitors can also generate alarms and alerts by comparing the input received from the patient with predefined parameters that are either manually entered by the caregiver or derived from algorithms in the device. Such algorithms often correct for factors such as the patient's age. Examples of additional alerts often encountered by nursing staff are **out-of-range alarms** and **system fault alarms**:

- *Out-of-range alarms* are triggered when a patient's value is above or below a set parameter. These high and low limits can be set manually by the nursing staff or can be set to a default determined by the institution.
- *System fault alarms* are triggered when there is an ineffective reading potentially due to displaced leads or other system malfunction(s).

As with any technology, alarms should not take the place of the licensed caregivers who care for the patient, but rather aid in the decision-making process. Indeed, overreliance on such devices often contributes to errors of omission. Physiologic monitoring must be validated with the physical assessment of the patient. This type of monitoring depends on many factors, including proper placement of electrodes for noninvasive monitoring and accurate calibration of devices, proper setup, and maintenance for invasive monitoring.

BEYOND THE POINT OF CARE

When signals are produced by manual documentation at the point of care, there is usually an interest in propagating this information beyond the bedside. For information generated by medical devices to be meaningful beyond the point of care, there must be some connection to a larger information network. Connection to a larger information infrastructure also allows more sophisticated modulation of the information that is returned to the provider at the point of care. This connection can be accomplished by hardwired or wireless connections. The hardwired connections are generally more reliable, but less portable. Wireless connections offer portability and connection to devices on the network. One downside to wireless connections is the potential for disruption by interference, or by simple signal decay.

The benefits of connectivity are typically realized initially within the clinical microsystem. Central monitoring stations for the management of cardiac rhythms is one example of such connectivity. Generally, these central stations are hardwired to bedside devices. Central monitoring stations receive real-time hemodynamic monitoring feeds from multiple patients at any given time. This improves performance by decreasing the risk of inattentive omissions (failure of a bedside provider to see a dangerous rhythm). The stations also decrease the risk of knowledge-based errors. Typically, these stations are staffed with skilled technicians who are trained to monitor rhythms. This level of constant attentiveness by an expert trained in cardiovascular rhythms would be expensive to duplicate at every patient bedside.

Recently, wireless technology has facilitated unit-based information sharing. Not only are these devices useful for communication (via voice or text), but they are also being used to access patient data away from the point of care. Consider, for example, the use of smartphones. With an appropriate software interface, smartphones can communicate patient physiologic alarms to staff away from the point of care (Mosa, Yoo, & Sheets, 2012). These are gaining particular popularity due to their capability to propagate alarms generated at the bedside not only to the assigned nurse, but other members of the care team. The rules that govern the alert distribution can and often should be adjusted. The goal is to decrease the risk of omission errors caused when nurses are too busy or too far removed from the patient's physical location to audibly hear the bedside alarm. Typically, cascade alarms are configured so that if the original alarm is sent to the assigned nurse and is not acknowledged within a set time, the alarm will retrigger to other HCPs in the patient's care area.

When using technology that sends or receives patient-specific information, it is crucial that the intended associations are properly connected; medical devices need to be associated with the appropriate patient. Association in this context means electronically connecting the patient's chart to the appropriate component (e.g., connecting the bedside monitor to the patient's EHR in order to record the vital signs). This is rather easy to accomplish with wired connections, but less obvious when one seeks to "associate" bedside monitors with handheld devices. Two issues arise: (1) making the right association and (2) being aware of an interrupted association. Making the right association is important when propagating patient alarms or pulling patient-specific information into the EHR for documentation purposes. Often two levels of association are required—identifying the correct patient and identifying the correct episode of service within the patient record. Errors occur when the wrong patient is selected (a risk when more than one patient record is open at a time) or when the wrong episode is selected (observations entered on the wrong patient encounter within a record). Likewise, if a nurse believes that his or her smartphone is associated with a device alarm, but the association does not exist, alarms will be missed. In this case, the nurse will be following an implied rule ("all alerts will be forwarded to my smartphone") that is not applicable at that moment, which can result in an error of omission.

ELECTRONIC DOCUMENTATION

Data components are entered (or electronically imported) and stored, ideally with contextual information that can generate knowledge to improve care. The preceding section discusses data generated by medical devices. These data can be pulled into the EHR rather than manually entered with the use of device integration. A link must be made between the correct patient's physiologic monitor and the associated care event within the EHR. This information should be "validated" by staff prior to saving into the permanent record. Additionally, nurses or other healthcare staff may enter data manually into the permanent record. Connecting to a larger network allows for data storage beyond the level of a single medical device. With wired connections, transmission of data from the point of care to data storage is very reliable, so data loss is not generally a concern. Wireless connections, on the other hand, can experience variable connectivity, which in turn may impact data. If a wireless connection is interrupted, data may be dropped or delayed, which in turn could lead to lost or corrupted data.

Professionals enter much of the data generated at the point of care manually, and intermittently. A common example is the entry of the nurse's physical assessment into the EHR. Several issues become important when manual, intermittent processes are utilized. Humans routinely make mistakes when entering information manually into systems. Such errors may reduce the clarity of records but may also initiate an error that cascades and injures a patient. For example, if a nurse documents the wrong weight into the flowsheet for a dialysis patient, the prescriber may alter the therapy based on the erroneous weight. The relationship and/or the difference between the clinical event and the documentation of the event is more visible and receives more scrutiny in an EHR. For example, time stamps are ubiquitous in electronic records and are generated with great precision in computerized records. Small inconsistencies in time stamps become very noticeable and thus more problematic in the EHR. Decision rules that have algorithms based on time stamps may be negatively impacted by entry errors.

A more subtle problem is the loss of information when data or actions at the microsystem level are not "saved" in the central data repository, either because the appropriate save sequence was not followed or because an unexpected disruption of service interfered with saving the information. When information is entered in the EHR, it exists in a local temporary memory until the information is loaded into more permanent electronic storage. While the item may appear to have been saved at the point of care, it may not be recognized at the central data repository when connectivity problems occur or there was a lack of adherence to the proper save sequence.

In order to give data meaning, data elements must have definitions assigned to them. While this is a complex topic, and largely outside of the scope of this text, there is one important implication that all nurses should remember. Data entry, or documenting, in the EHR, must be done in standardized formats in order for data to have a format that allows for future use. Inevitably, achieving appropriate data context depends not just on computer systems, but also on nursing workflow and practice. For example, in pediatrics dose/weight calculations are essential to safe medication management. To make sure such calculations are performed appropriately, the organization must adopt a convention that defines the type of values that are permissible in the weight field. Entering pounds when kilograms are called for can be extremely hazardous.

INFORMED MEDICATION ADMINISTRATION

Data in a central data repository become available for more sophisticated interventions that have the potential to significantly improve the safety of care HCPs deliver. An example of how centralized data can be used to improve care is in the case of "smart" IV pumps—which haven't always been smart! For many years, nurses simply dialed in a rate for the medication to be administered and pushed "start." Unfortunately, this approach was not error proof. An estimated 1.5 million preventable adverse drug events (ADEs) are reported each year, of which 7,000 result in death (Agius, 2012). One-third occur at the point of order initiation, another third during the transcription and dispensing stage, and the remaining third during the actual administration of the medication (Agius, 2012). Ninety percent of patients receive an IV medication as a part of their treatment plan, and the delivery of IV medications is associated with more errors than other delivery routes (Husch et al., 2005).

The first step in the evolution of smart pumps is endowing them with a "brain." Smart pumps are IV devices that house a library of medications along with their corresponding concentrations and safe dose ranges. If the nurse mistakenly enters a dose that exceeds limits programmed into the pump, the pump will alert the nurse of the potentially dangerous dose. The alert can be programmed to be a soft-stop or hard-stop alert. A soft-stop alert only warns HCPs that something is out of the ordinary but does not keep them from executing the intended action. Hard-stop alerts, on the other hand, warn HCPs that their anticipated plan is not actionable and will keep them from moving forward in their current execution. The library of medications on the pump can be tailored to the specific location in which the pump will be utilized. For example, if a patient is admitted to an acute care unit, it is possible to prevent the nurse caring for the patient from accessing the library for vasoactive drips. Programming for medication administration of vasoactive drips can be limited to the intensive care unit setting; however, an override function can be created for floor nurses to utilize these medications in certain situations (e.g., during a code event).

Bedside smart IV pumps not only facilitate delivery of medications; they also provide data on the care process (the administration rate of a fluid over time) and also on the behavior of providers (data on nursing keystrokes during programming and the nurse response to alerts). Similar to the drug catalogue stored in the smart pump's memory, data on the care-delivery process are stored on the device for a period of time and then downloaded for examination if a negative event occurs.

Of course, smart pumps do not stay smart if their brains are not updated or if there are errors in the programming of the device. Updates generally occur on an intermittent basis, usually when the pump is not actively engaged in the delivery of patient care. Some institutions have moved to integration of the smart pumps with the eMAR. This requires continuous association of the pump with the patient record system. Such integration allows for the possibility of patient-specific information and related patient-specific clinical decision support to be available at the bedside. The goal is to close the medication-delivery loop. While the technology of smart pumps is appealing and can facilitate reducing the error rate of ADEs, it should not take the place of critical thinking skills or manual verification steps. Proper training is essential to ensure competency of programming the device. For pumps to be smart, they must be intelligently used. One of the dangers of a tightly coupled link between the pump and the electronic record is that vigilance may be diminished. Because infusion pumps address only IV medications, smart pumps do not close the medication loop for medications of other routes (e.g., oral medications, topical medications, and injections). To better close the gap with nonintravenous medications, barcoding technology may be leveraged.

The first goal of the 2013 National Patient Safety Goals published by The Joint Commission is to improve the accuracy of patient identification by using at least two patient identifiers when providing care, treatment, and services (The Joint Commission, 2013). In addition, while the numbers of "rights for medication administration" have increased over the years, the traditional five "rights" still remain: Ensuring the right patient, right medication, right dose, right route, and right time of the medication is one layer of protecting the patient against medication errors, but the use of Barcode Medication Administration (BCMA) can aid in compliance with and automation of verifying these rights. The U.S. Food and Drug Administration (FDA) has recognized how useful this technology can be to patient safety. In 2004, the FDA issued a rule requiring barcodes on thousands of human drugs and biological products. As a result, prescription drug manufacturers placed barcodes on most drugs used in hospitals (FDA, 2004).

Like smart pumps, barcode medication administration can be implemented from the bedside, allowing real-time integration with patient-specific information stored centrally. There are three levels of safety. Level 1 is the simplest layer and serves as the foundation to the automated double check of the prescribed order. This layer may also include nursing work lists, alerts for missed doses, and a reference to the hospital's formulary. Level 2 is more involved and incorporates educational tools such as medication reference libraries. These libraries can benefit the nursing staff and patients. Information on specific medications can be accessed and printed on demand for patient education. In addition, calculation tables are integrated within this phase that allow the nurse to reference dosing information. Level 3 is the most intricate layer, because it functions to present alerts and warnings specific to the medication regimen and patient condition to provide a proactive error-prevention structure (Yang, Brown, Trohimovich, Dana, & Kelly, 2002). Examples of warnings generated at this level include those that are triggered upon reaching a patient-specific maximum cumulative dose, medications that fall into the look-alike/sound-alike category or high-risk category, and medications that may require specific clinical actions. Additionally, this level can incorporate order reconciliation and near-miss reports (Yang et al., 2002).

While barcoding assists in timely documentation of medication administration and has the potential to decrease medication errors by as much as 86%, hospitals in the process of implementing this technology must take a serious look at the workflow and limitations of the technology when setting up the system (Patient Safety Authority, 2008). Most medications come barcoded from the manufacturer, which makes initiating the bacoding process even easier. A problem does arise, especially in the pediatric population, because barcoding of unit doses is not part of the FDA requirement. There is an opportunity for error when the pharmacist must print a barcoded label to place on the medication.

WHERE, OH WHERE, HAS MY PATIENT GONE? _____

The use of barcoding in health care extends beyond medication management. In fact, barcodes are one of several technologies used at the institutional level (Level 3 of Figure 10-1) to improve materials flow and also improve the safety of care delivery. Often operating room (OR) supplies are managed and documented in the EHR with the use of barcodes. The barcodes typically capture details about the particular supply, such as the name, lot number, and expiration date. Because specific information associated with surgical devices and supplies can be traced back to the surgical event, this information is extremely useful in the instance of an adverse event following a surgery. Expiration date tracking within the OR setting is not only useful for patient safety but also can help with inventory management. In addition, should an adverse event related to a device be discovered at a future date, the information captured and linked to the surgical procedure can be evaluated.

Barcoding is merely a "static" accounting for materials that is not conducive to tracking and monitoring flow of materials across the physical environment of an organization. RFID is used by healthcare organizations to give more detailed tracking information related to patient care, patient movement, and supply management. With RFID technology, an automated wireless data-collection process designed to capture location and movement of identified objects is possible ("Radio-Frequency Identification," 2005). This type of system is made up of four parts: a computer chip "sensor," antennas to transmit data, a computing device "reader," and software to analyze the data. As sensors move in and out of antenna range, nearby readers detect radio wave signals transmitted from tags. The radio wave signals are converted to digital or audio signals (i.e., alarms) for a user to interpret, or transmit to another device (such as a computer) for analysis (Roark & Miguel, 2006). The success of RFID depends on the reliability of the distributed network that registers the movement of tags through the environment.

In tracking information directly related to patient care, RFID can be used to prevent retention of foreign bodies within the OR. An example of this is RFID-enabled surgical sponges that are counted automatically when dropped into a "smart" bucket. If any sponges are missing at the end of the surgical case, a hand-held wand can alert the surgical team to the location of the misplaced sponge (Feldman, 2011).

In addition to tracking information on patient care, RFID is also used to better monitor the flow of patients throughout the hospital (Zone 3, Figure 10-2). One area

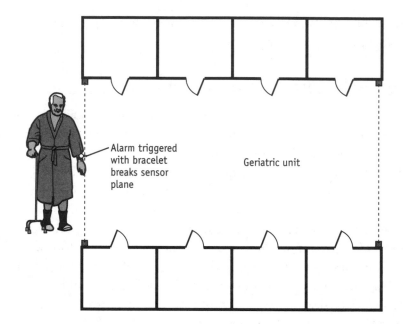

FIGURE 10-3   RFID in the geriatric unit.

of interest related to patient flow and RFID is infant abduction, which remains a major concern in nurseries and pediatric care environments. Affixing an RFID sensor to the infant's ID bracelet allows for the capability of an alarm to sound if the baby is moved out of the care area, adding an additional level of protection against abductions. Likewise, the same type of technology can be used in psychiatric and geriatric units where elopement and wandering are a high probability (Kamel, Boulos, & Berry, 2012; **Figure 10-3**).

Similarly, the management of supplies, equipment, and human resources can use RFID functionality. Expensive medical equipment can be tagged with an RFID sensor to prevent loss or theft. In the same respect, with an electronic map of the hospital, RFID-tagged wheelchairs and stretchers have the capability to be visible to staff, making patient transport between units and ancillary departments more streamlined. Because of this, hospitals can save time and resources by knowing exactly where equipment is at the precise time it is needed. In some organizations, RFID technology is used to track human resources. By affixing the RFID sensor to the employee name badge, senior management can better determine staff allocation in specific areas (Kamel, Boulos, & Berry, 2012). This same technology can help with employee hand hygiene compliance by putting the receiving sensors on the wall-mounted sanitizers within the patient room proximity. If the employee enters the room (RFID sensor can be attached to the employee badge) without stopping at the wall-mounted hand sanitizer, the lack of compliance can be accounted for and reported.

MEDICAL DEVICE SAFETY

As described earlier in this chapter, medical devices can be effective in reducing the risk of harm to patients. However, there are issues of safety that cannot be overlooked. The U.S. Food and Drug Administration (FDA, 2012) has the responsibility for regulating the approval and recall of medical devices. Because of this regulatory responsibility, the FDA has guidelines for medical device design, testing, and error reporting. Human factors are an important concern in the design and use of medical devices, and the outcomes of medical device use can be either safe and effective or unsafe and ineffective. First, medical devices should be designed for use by particular HCPs or by patients and their families. If people other than the intended user operate the device, the device may be unsafe. For example, ventilators are typically designed for use by physicians, respiratory therapists, and nurses. However, a patient who becomes ventilator-dependent may be sent home on a ventilator. The family becomes the user, and unintended, unsafe use errors can occur if the technology does not account for the different needs of this type of user. Second, medical devices should be tested in laboratory and clinical environments that are similar to the ones in which the device will ultimately be used. However, medical devices are often used in settings beyond the intended environment where varying conditions of lighting, noise, and chaos were not accounted for within the testing environment. These less-than-optimal environments can lead to use errors and unsafe patient outcomes. Finally, the medical device interface can be confusing to users. Lack of consistent interface design among a class of medical devices can complicate the problem. For example, if bladder ultrasound devices have different pathways to guide nurses through measurement of urine in the bladder and a hospital unit has three bladder ultrasound devices made by different manufacturers, use errors can occur.

The FDA regulates the use of medical devices through safety communications, post-market surveillance studies, recalls, and mandatory medical device error reporting through Medical Product Safety Network (MedSun). It is the responsibility of all HCPs to understand the risks of using medical devices and to report any device malfunction or involvement with patient harm to the FDA. The FDA issues email alerts to notify HCPs when a recall has been issued. These alerts are freely available to anyone who subscribes to the alert system on the FDA website (http://www.fda.gov).

Box 10-1   Case Study

Medical health technologies are designed to improve outcomes, particularly patient safety. While it may seem paradoxical that a technology designed to improve patient outcomes can actually facilitate errors, it is not so surprising when examined through the lens of human factors engineering. For instance, medication-dispensing systems do not exist in a vacuity of outside influence. Instead, these technologies are used by nurses, who are managing ever-changing patient needs with interruptions on busy hospital floors, with individual work cultures that are not always conducive to improving patient outcomes. The Systems Engineering Initiative for Patient Safety (SEIPS) model of work systems is a framework for examining how the work system elements affect clinical processes and, ultimately, patient outcomes. This case study uses the SEIPS model (Carayon, 2012) to analyze a specific aberrant outcome noted with the use of a medication-dispensing system.

According to the SEIPS model, "the work system in which care is provided affects both work and clinical processes, which . . . influence . . . outcomes of care" (Carayon, 2012, p. 71). The work system is comprised of the components that interact to help, or hinder, the ability of the person performing a task. These elements include *person, task, tools and technologies, physical environment*, and *organizational conditions* (Carayon, 2012, p. 67). The clinical process is the method, or means, of providing care, and the outcome is the assessment of the clinical results of the care provided. The SEIPS model asserts that "changes to any aspect of the work system will . . . either negatively or positively affect the work and clinical processes and the consequent patient, employee, and organizational outcomes" (Carayon et al., 2006). Thus, all elements of the work system need to be examined to understand the relationship between the work system, clinical processes, and patient outcomes.

Consider the following scenario: On a busy medical-surgical floor at a large hospital, a registered nurse (RN) entered her unit's clean utility room and used the hospital's medication-dispensing system to retrieve a dose of Lasix (furosemide). After verifying the name of the drug, the RN administered the drug to the correct patient at the correct time. However, a medication error occurred because the ordered route was IV, and the administered dose was oral. Despite using the dispensing system, a tool that purports to use "proven technology with actionable intelligence to prevent medication errors," the outcome was a medication error. The SEIPS model provides us with the framework to answer the question, "What happened?"

The center of this particular scenario's work system was a novice RN (*person*). She was working on a busy, noisy, well-lit hospital floor, inside of the clean utility room (*physical environment*). The medication-dispensing system (*tool/technology*) was located along a back wall in the clean utility room, and on this day there was a line to access the medication-dispensing system. While the RN's physical characteristics, including weight, height, and strength, did not directly affect the outcome—because the layout of the room and the design of the medication system were conducive to the physical task of removing medication from the medication system—other aspects of the environment did. The line of RNs waiting for their turn to use the medication system increased the level of noise in the room and provided a steady flow of conversational interruptions. These interruptions, according to Carayon (2012) are one of the leading reasons for errors in the healthcare environment.

The combination of environmental distractions, the hospital unit's "hurry up and finish" attitude, and a hospital-wide policy relating to administering medications within a prescribed amount of time (*organization*) provided sufficient motivation for the RN to rush her task. In her haste, the RN selected the correct patient from the medication system's drop-down menu, scrolled down the alphabetical list of medications until she found the name of the correct medication (Lasix 40 mg), and selected the drug. The drawer opened and the RN, who was simultaneously speaking to a coworker and removing the medication, withdrew a 40-mg Lasix pill from the same bin from which she had removed several doses of Lasix for other patients earlier that day. Despite having verified the medication name and dose, the RN neglected to verify the route (a slip error). The drug route was noted on the medication system's screen; however, it was not easily distinguished from the medication name, because both were presented in the same print and font on the screen. The outcome of this scenario was that the wrong route of the correct medication was administered to the correct patient, at the correct time. This medication error did not cause direct harm to the patient, but it did result in a suboptimal treatment outcome.

Numerous other factors in this scenario contributed to this error. The RN's previous experience with removing the oral Lasix led to a level of automaticity in the task, which set up favorable conditions for a slip error to occur (Carayon, 2012). Further, the design of the medication-dispensing system helped to facilitate the error, because the Lasix was stored in a drawer with other medications rather than in a bin that restricted access to only the medication selected (one of the many error-reducing features of the medication system). Rather, the drawer that opened was one of a few drawers in the machine that has open, numbered bins instead of bins with flip tops containing only one medication. The drawer had the oral Lasix located in the bin to the right of the IV Lasix. The proximity of two medications with the same name and dose created a design-induced error and further increased the risk of improper medication selection.

Analysis of this medication error with the SEIPS model clearly demonstrates that a poorly designed system facilitates mistakes. Using the SEIPS model, it is possible to recognize the flaws in a system and make adjustments to the system that will target the sources of poor patient outcomes. In this case, the nurse was executing a routine task, while working for an organization with policies that inadvertently encourage haste, in an environment that is filled with distractions, using a technology that does not always detract from errors. No one source of error was found. Rather, it was the interaction of all of these elements that produced a work system that adversely affected clinical outcomes.

SUMMARY

There is a constant desire in health care to improve quality without significantly impacting costs. Yet, how can nurses assist the healthcare team in making quality decisions, support their clinical workflow, and mandate an EHR while at the same time achieving safe care? While there is no single answer for this complex question,

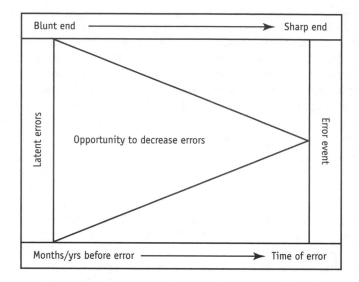

FIGURE 10-4   Human factors and medical device use.

Source: Reprinted from *The Journal of Pediatrics,* 142(4), Napper, C., Battles, J., & Fargason, C., Pediatrics and Patient Safety, pp. 359–360. Copyright 2003, with permission from Elsevier.

continuous advances in health IT can assist nurses and other HCPs in achieving these goals. This chapter has focused on care delivery and the potential benefits of adapting health IT to the various levels of care, but it has not addressed how HCPs and organizations must mobilize in order to ensure that the technologies put into place actually improve care delivery. As noted earlier, the point of care is the sharp end of care. Using time as the key variable, **Figure 10-4** shows the relationship between the sharp end of care and the blunt end. Decisions about technology adoption are made at the blunt end of the process. Such decisions must take into consideration the impact of new tools on the entire sociotechnologic system if adoption is to lead to better care. The complexity found in the present environment of health care requires everyone, including nurses, to ensure patients are well taken care of and protected against harm throughout their medical journey.

For a full suite of assignments and additional learning activities, use the access code located in the front of your book and visit www.jblearning.com. If you do not have an access code, you can obtain one at the site.

REFERENCES

Agius, C. R. (2012). Intelligent infusion technologies: Integration of a smart system to enhance patient care. *Journal of Infusion Nursing, 35*(6), 364–368. doi: 10.1097/NAN.0b013e3182706423

Boas, D. A., Gaudette, T., Strangman, G., Cheng, X., Marota, J. J., & Mandeville, J. B. (2001). The accuracy of near infrared spectroscopy and imaging during focal changes in cerebral hemodynamics. *Neuroimage, 13*(1), 76–90. doi: 10.1006/nimg.2000.0674

Carayon, P. (2012). Work system design in health care. In *Handbook of human factors and ergonomics in health care and patient safety* (2nd ed., pp. 65–79). Boca Raton, FL: CRC Press.

Carayon, P., Hundt, A., Karsh, B., Gurses, A., Alvarado, C., Smith, M., & Brennan, P. (2006). Work system design for patient safety: The SEIPS model. *Quality and Safety in Health Care, 15*(suppl. 1), i50–i58.

The Dartmouth Institute. (2013). *Clinical microsystems.* Retrieved from http://www.clinicalmicrosystem.org/about/background/

Feldman, D. L. (2011). Prevention of retained surgical items. *Mount Sinai Journal of Medicine, 78*(6), 865–871. doi: 10.1002/msj.20299

Healthcare Information and Management Systems Society. (2013). *HIMSS dictionary of healthcare information technology terms, acronyms and organizations* (3rd ed.). Chicago, IL: Author.

Husch, M., Sullivan, C., Rooney, D., Barnard, C., Fotis, M., Clarke, J., & Noskin, G. (2005). Insights from the sharp end of intravenous medication errors: Implications for infusion pump technology. *Quality and Safety in Health Care, 14*(2), 80–86. doi: 10.1136/qshc.2004.011957

Institute of Medicine. (1999). *To err is human: Building a safer health system.* Washington, DC: National Academies Press.

Institute of Medicine. (2011). *Health IT and patient safety: Building safer systems for better care.* Washington, DC: Committee on Patient Safety and Health Information Technology, Board on Health Care Services.

The Joint Commission. (2013). *Hospital: 2013 national patient safety goals.* Retrieved from http://www.jointcommission.org/hap_2013_npsg/

Kamel Boulos, M. N., & Berry, G. (2012). Real-time locating systems (RTLS) in healthcare: A condensed primer. *International Journal of Health Geographics, 11,* 25. doi: 10.1186/1476-072x-11-25

Lighter, D. E. (2013). *Basics of health care performance improvement: A lean six sigma approach.* Burlington, MA: Jones & Bartlett Learning.

Mosa, A. S., Yoo, I., & Sheets, L. (2012). A systematic review of healthcare applications for smartphones. *BMC Medical Informatics and Decision Making, 12,* 67. doi: 10.1186/1472-6947-12-67

O'Donnell, C. P. F., Kamlin, C. O. F., Davis, P. G., Carlin, J. B., & Morley, C. J. (2007). Clinical assessment of infant colour at delivery. *Archives of Disease in Childhood: Fetal and Neonatal Edition, 92*(6), F465–F467.

Patient Safety Authority. (2008). Medication errors occurring with the use of bar-code administration technology. *Pennsylvania Patient Safety Advisory, 5*(4), 122–126.

Radio-frequency identification: Its potential in healthcare. (2005). *Health Devices, 34*(5), 149–160.

Reason, J. (1990). *Human error.* New York, NY: Cambridge University Press.

Reason, J. (2000). Human error: Models and management. *The Western Journal of Medicine (0093–0415), 172*(6), 393.

Roark, D. C., & Miguel, K. (2006). RFID: Bar coding's replacement? *Nursing Management, 37*(2), 28–31.

Schmid, A., Hoffman, L., Happ, M. B., Wolf, F., & DeVita, M. (2007). Failure to rescue: A literature review. *Journal of Nursing Administration, 37*(4), 188–198.

U.S. Food and Drug Administration. (2004). Bar code label requirement for human drug products and biological products. Final rule. *Federal Register, 69*(38), 9119–9171.

U.S. Food and Drug Administration. (2012). *Overview of medical device regulations.* Retrieved from http://www.fda.gov/Training/CDRHLearn/ucm162015.htm#overview

Yang, M., Brown, M., Trohimovich, B., Dana, M., & Kelly, J. (2002). The effect of bar-code-enabled point-of-care technology on medication administration errors. In R. Lewis (Ed.), *The impact of information technology on patient safety* (pp. 37–56). Chicago, IL: Healthcare Information and Management Systems.

Use of Clinical Informatics Tools in Care Delivery Systems

CHAPTER 11

The Electronic Health Record

Susan Alexander, DNP, RN, ANP-BC, ADM-BC

Susan Alexander, DNP, RN, ANP-BC, ADM-BC

CHAPTER LEARNING OBJECTIVES

1. Define and describe the electronic health record (EHR) and its common features.
2. Review the benefits of EHR use in daily practice.
3. Describe the impact of the EHR upon tasks such as data management and the support of evidence-based practice.
4. Review the challenges of EHR use including interoperability, effects upon workflow patterns, system and system-related expenses, performance, and security concerns.
5. Examine the role of the nurse in use of EHR systems.

KEY TERMS

Access control tools
Clinical vocabulary
Computerized provider order entry
Decryption
Electronic health record (EHR)
Encryption
Health maintenance
Interface
Interoperability

Penetration testing
Point-of-care data entry
Recovery capabilities
Remote access
Security risk analysis
System downtime
Vendors
Virtual private network (VPN)

CHAPTER OVERVIEW

Any nurse who has spent valuable time in working with the traditional paper chart can appreciate the many features of the **electronic health record (EHR)**. The point-of-care data entry, rapid information retrieval, and decision support capabilities offered by EHR systems certainly seem to hold promise in streamlining the daily work of most nurses. However, there are other important potential benefits of EHR use, particularly in improving patient care, that have been recognized and supported by the federal government. The need for computerization of health records was addressed by President George W. Bush in his State of the Union Address in 2004 and quickly gained bipartisan support. The Health Information Technology for Economic and Clinical Health (HITECH) Act, which was designed to promote the adoption and meaningful use of health information technology (health IT) was signed into law on February 17, 2009. The HITECH Act provides the U.S. Department of Health and Human Services with the authority to establish programs to improve the quality, safety, and efficiency of health care by promoting health IT, including EHR systems and electronic health information exchange (HealthIT.gov, n.d.b). As a result of the HITECH Act, healthcare providers (HCPs) and facilities can receive incentive payments for the adoption and meaningful use of EHR systems. Current estimates suggest that EHR use in offices likely exceeds 34%, with $575 million in incentive payments having been distributed as of December 2011; similar results are seen in hospitals, with 35% having adopted EHRs, collectively receiving $2 billion in incentive payments (Emanuel, 2012).

As EHRs continue to proliferate, it is important for the nurse to become familiar with the features and capabilities of the systems. This chapter begins with a description of the benefits and features of EHRs, along with the problems that have been identified in using EHR systems. Issues of security, reliability, and accuracy are also reviewed. The chapter concludes with a description of the role of the nurse in preparing for and implementing the EHR, delivering care, and evaluating outcomes, and it discusses nurses' perceptions on interaction with EHR systems.

DEFINITIONS AND DESCRIPTIONS

Many students are experienced in the creation and management of electronic documents, but an EHR is more than a transposition of a paper chart into an electronic file. According to the Healthcare Information and Management Systems Society (HIMSS), an EHR is "a longitudinal electronic record of patient health information generated by one or more encounters in any care delivery setting" (HIMSS, 2012–2013). With optimum use, the EHR is a robust database with an almost endless capacity for customization that can be adapted to the needs of the patient, the HCP, and the healthcare organization. EHRs are designed to collect many types of data, ranging from patient demographics to radiology images, and contain features such as secure online messaging systems and order entry systems (**Table 11-1**). The

Table 11-1 Basic Features of Many Practice and Hospital-Based EHR Systems

EHR Feature	Example

Charting	• Note templates that are both predesigned and customizable
	• Patient "dashboards" containing multiple types of information such as:
	  • List of current medications
	  • Advance directives
	  • Past medical history
	  • Social history
	  • Growth charts
	  • Current vital signs

Medication Management	• Current and historical medication lists • Medication allergies and intolerances • Preferred pharmacies • E-prescribing capabilities • Computerized provider order entry
Scheduling	• Single and multiple provider appointments • Appointments for multiple locations and varieties (groups vs. individuals) • Automatic appointment reminders for patients and providers
Labs	• Most recent lab tests • History of all lab tests • Trends in lab results • Integration with in-house and reference labs for results via embedded interfaces
Referrals	• Immediate referrals to providers in the EHR system • Instant fax with confirmation to providers outside the EHR system • Secure messaging to providers outside the EHR system
Billing/Coding	• Creation of a superbill using elements from the note (ICD9 and CPT codes) • Streamlined billing using integrated vendors

Reporting/Surveillance Capabilities	• Customizable reports using various data elements such as:
	  • ICD9 codes
	  • CPT codes
	  • Medications

Health Maintenance	• Age-based templates for capturing recommended preventive health services (e.g., immunizations and colorectal cancer screenings) • Gender-based templates for capturing gender-specific health needs (e.g., mammograms and bone densitometries) • Disease-based templates for tracking clinical practice guidelines used in chronic disease management (e.g., eye and foot examinations for patients with diabetes mellitus)

data that are collected can then be made available to multiple providers across healthcare settings, however remote, through a system of shared networks. EHR system features can also be adapted to meet the needs of single-provider office practices or multi-user sites with remote locations. Systems that are designed for use in outpatient and inpatient care-delivery settings and that meet criteria for a minimum level of accuracy, reliability, security, and interoperability can obtain a designation for quality from the Certification Commission for Health Information Technology (CCHIT).

Under the HITECH Act, a hospital, HCP, or critical access hospital that adopts a certified EHR technology and uses it to achieve specified objectives can qualify for incentive payments from the Centers for Medicare and Medicaid Services (CMS). Referred to as "Meaningful Use Criteria," the sets are a group of core and menu objectives that are specific to the hospital or the HCP and must be met in order to receive incentive payments. Benefits of meaningful use of EHRs include the maintenance of complete and accurate information about patients, improved access to information for providers, and the empowerment of patients to take a more active role in their health (HealthIT.gov, n.d.b). Meaningful use criteria and objectives will evolve in stages over the next several years (**Figure 11-1**). Nurses will play an essential role in aiding healthcare facilities and other healthcare professionals to meet meaningful use criteria of EHR systems.

BENEFITS OF USING EHRs

When fully functional, an EHR has many prospective benefits for nurses that can make daily tasks easier, including the automation of manual repetitive tasks, streamlining of documentation, and enabling access to information, due to the features contained in the systems (Table 11-1). After the nurse enters a personalized username and password, **point-of-care data entry** allows the nurse to capture the activities of care as they occur, including the administration of medications, assessment of vital signs, physical exam, updating of medical histories, or other nursing duties (**Figures 11-2, 11-3, 11-4**). The data that are entered into the EHR are captured in a structured, coded format, and saved. These data can easily be retrieved for later quantitative analysis or use in decision support. For example, a nurse working at the bedside in a healthcare facility or practice could get access to a patient's chart from more than one location, for easier and more accurate charting. EHRs often include decision support tools, alerts, and reminders that can help to reduce medication errors and adverse events. Drug–drug interactions and intravenous drug incompatibility information are a common component of EHR systems. Another

Stage 1 2011–2012 Data capture and sharing	Stage 2 2014 Advance clinical processes	Stage 3 2016 Improved outcomes

Stage 1: Meaningful use criteria focus on:	Stage 2: Meaningful use criteria focus on:	Stage 3: Meaningful use criteria focus on:
Electronically capturing health information in a standardized format	More rigorous health information exchange (HIE)	Improving quality, safety, and efficiency, leading to improved health outcomes
Using that information to track key clinical conditions	Increased requirements for e-prescribing and incorporating lab results	Decision support for national high-priority conditions
Communicating that information for care coordination processes	Electronic transmission of patient care summaries across multiple settings	Patient access to self-management tools
Initiating the reporting of clinical quality measures and public health information	More patient-controlled data	Access to comprehensive patient data through patient-centered HIE
Using information to engage patients and their families in their care		Improving population health

FIGURE 11-1   Stages of meaningful use criteria.

Source: http://www.healthit.gov/policy-researchers-implementers/meaningful-use

good example is patient medication allergies and intolerances. Once this information is entered, it can populate many different fields, so that anyone who is prescribing or administering medications to the patient will automatically be given an alert if an incompatible drug is used. In an EHR, documentation of care that is provided is legible, so that time is not wasted in attempting to decipher the handwritten notes or orders of another HCP, and interfaces with labs ensure that results populate the chart automatically for review.

In addition to their benefits for direct nursing care, EHR systems can indirectly assist the work of the nurse by providing benefits to other staff in healthcare facilities. The rapid access to patient-related data that is possible when an EHR is used can simultaneously support many HCPs and ancillary staff, such as medical coding specialists, lab personnel, and billing departments. Information retrieval is almost immediate, and the record may be continuously updated as HCPs and other staff enter information related to patient care. In some care settings, the EHR may be

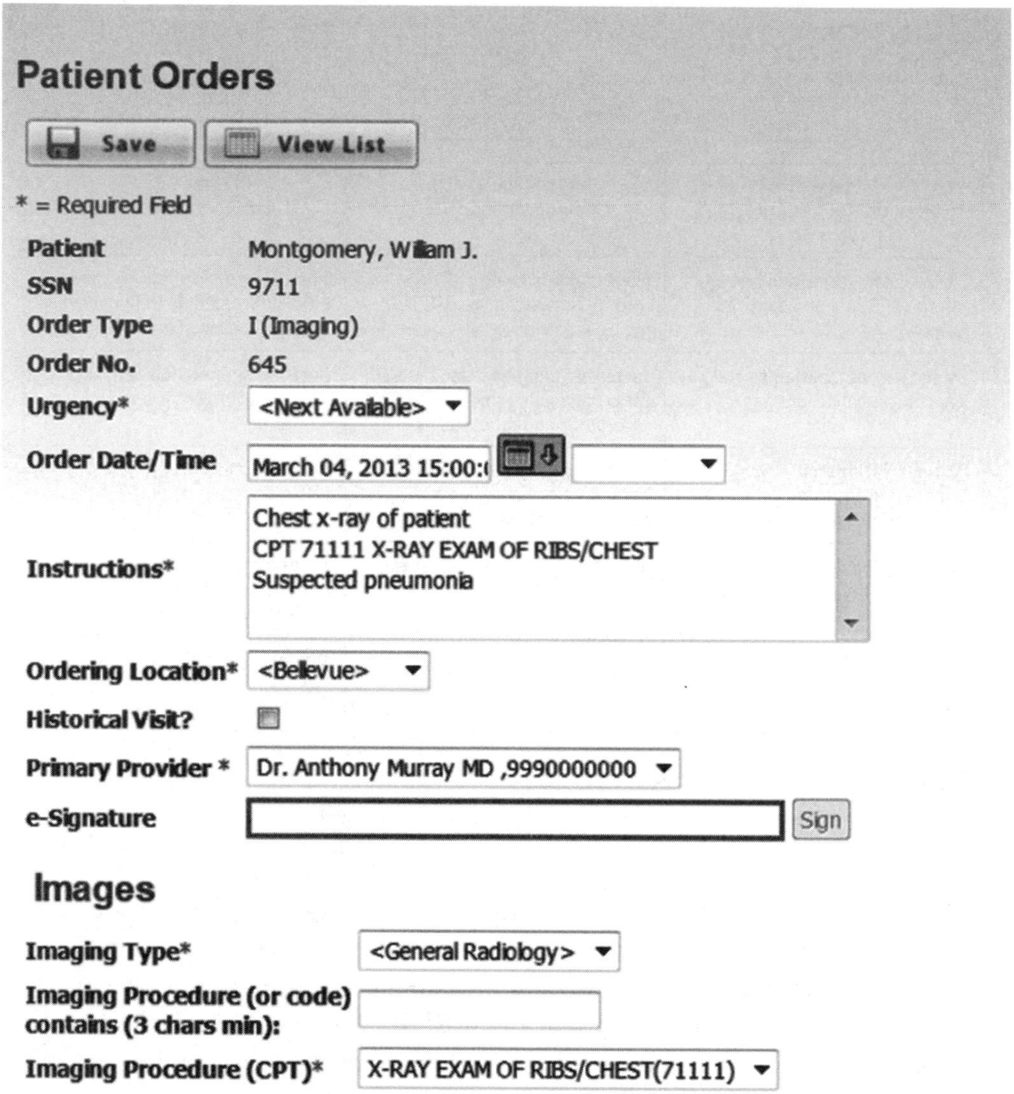

Patient Orders

[💾 Save]   [▦ View List]

* = Required Field

Patient	Montgomery, William J.
SSN	9711
Order Type	I (Imaging)
Order No.	645
Urgency*	\<Next Available\> ▼
Order Date/Time	March 04, 2013 15:00:0 [📅⬇] [▼]
Instructions*	Chest x-ray of patient CPT 71111 X-RAY EXAM OF RIBS/CHEST Suspected pneumonia
Ordering Location*	\<Bellevue\> ▼
Historical Visit?	☐
Primary Provider *	Dr. Anthony Murray MD ,9990000000 ▼
e-Signature	[ ] [Sign]

Images

Imaging Type*	\<General Radiology\> ▼
Imaging Procedure (or code) **contains (3 chars min):**	[ ]
Imaging Procedure (CPT)*	X-RAY EXAM OF RIBS/CHEST(71111) ▼

FIGURE 11-2 Computerized provider order entry screen.

Source: Courtesy of DataWeb Incorporated.

available using remote workstations, enabling access to patient data without having to be in the same physical location. This can be a great benefit for HCPs and staff who need access to patient charts for aspects of their jobs that do not necessarily need to be on site. Busy HCPs who are working in offices several miles away can access the EHR to get up-to-date information on hospitalized patients without leaving their office.

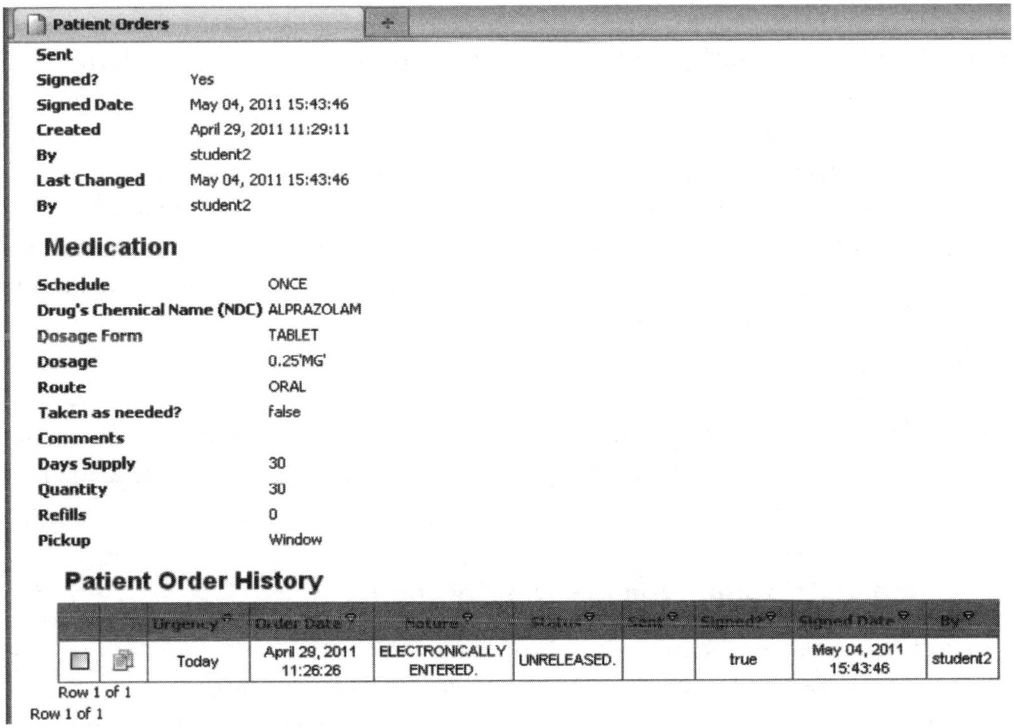

Patient Orders   +

Sent
Signed?   Yes
Signed Date   May 04, 2011 15:43:46
Created   April 29, 2011 11:29:11
By   student2
Last Changed   May 04, 2011 15:43:46
By   student2

Medication

Schedule   ONCE
Drug's Chemical Name (NDC) ALPRAZOLAM
Dosage Form   TABLET
Dosage   0.25'MG'
Route   ORAL
Taken as needed?   false
Comments
Days Supply   30
Quantity   30
Refills   0
Pickup   Window

Patient Order History

		Urgency	Order Date	Nature	Status	Sent	Signed?	Signed Date	By
☐	🗎	Today	April 29, 2011 11:26:26	ELECTRONICALLY ENTERED.	UNRELEASED.		true	May 04, 2011 15:43:46	student2

Row 1 of 1
Row 1 of 1

FIGURE 11-3 Medication order entry screen.

Source: Courtesy of DataWeb Incorporated.

Patient Information   **William Johnson**

Code   Prefix First MI Last Suffix DOB   Gender SSN   Primary Provider   Primary Care Team
DWVPT10012006   William Johnson   10/01/2003 Male 0061 Dr. Anthony Murray MD ,9990000000   Pediatrics 3

Patient Information

                                                        View List   + Add New Patient   **Age in photo**   6
                                                                                           Current Age   9
Patient Code Prefix First MI Last Suffix SSN (Last 4)   Rows 1-20 of 40
DWVPT10012006   William Johnson   0061   Previous 1 2 Next

Date Of Birth Age Gender Race   Ethnicity   Language Preference   **Patient Events**
10/01/2003

Default Providers

Primary Provider   Primary Care Team

Dr. Anthony Murray MD ,9990000000   Pediatrics 3

Contact Information

Address   Address 2 City   ST PostalCode
1001 Beech Street   Seattle WA   98101

Work #   Call #   Residence #
                         206-100-2006

Insurance Information

Insurance Type   Commercial

Group Name   DataWeb   Group Number   DW1965
Subscriber Name   James Johnson Subscriber Number DW1965-1
Member Number   DW1965-4   Payer Name   Blue Shield
Patient Name = Subscriber Name? false

Event	Description	Date
Patient	Johnson, William	03/18/2013
Order	C (Consultation)	11/26/2010
Order	M (Medication)	11/26/2010
Order	I (Images)	11/26/2010
Order	L (Lab)	11/26/2010
Appointment	Office visit	11/26/2010
Appointment	Office visit	11/19/2010
Appointment	Office visit	11/01/2010
Order	M (Medication)	10/01/2010
Appointment	Office visit	10/01/2010
Immunization	Polio	10/01/2010
Immunization	Chickenpox	10/01/2010
Appointment	Office visit	10/01/2010
Immunization	Influenza (Seasonal Flu)	10/01/2009
Appointment	Office visit	09/02/2008
Immunization	Hepatitis A	09/02/2008
Appointment	Office visit	01/02/2008
Immunization	Pneumococcal	01/02/2008

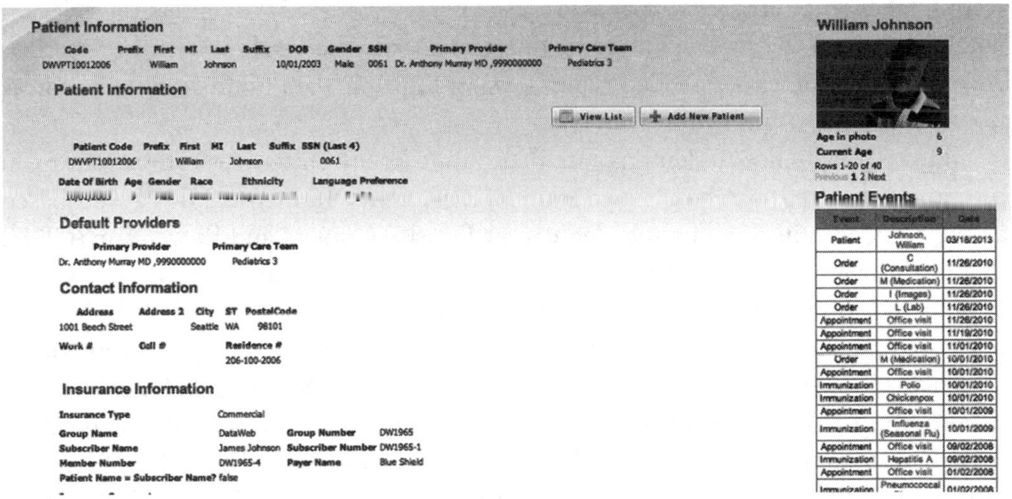

FIGURE 11-4 Patient demographics screen.

Source: Courtesy of DataWeb Incorporated; © Jaimie Duplass/ShutterStock, Inc. (photo)

Healthcare facilities are increasingly accountable for care that patients receive during their stays in such facilities. Hospital Compare (http://www.medicare.gov/hospitalcompare) is a consumer-oriented website created through the efforts of CMS and the Hospital Quality Alliance. Hospitals are required to report data on their performance in caring for patients with the most common conditions requiring admission to a hospital for treatment, including pneumonia, acute myocardial infarction, heart failure, and surgeries. Consumers can then select multiple hospitals and compare the performance of those hospitals using the performance data submitted to the website by each hospital. In reviewing a database of performance measures related to pneumonia, acute myocardial infarction, and heart failure from 2,021 hospitals, those facilities that maintained a basic EHR system (operational electronic patient record, clinical data repository, and decision support) realized a 2.6% improvement in quality of care scores for heart failure management (Jones, Adams, Schneider, Ringel, & McGlynn, 2010).

Collection, Aggregation, and Reporting of Data

In addition to caring for individual patients, nurses often work in positions that require the aggregation and review of data to guide policy or practice, such as infection and quality control. In the past, this could be a time-intensive process necessitating the collection of data from stacks of paper charts, entry of data into a statistical analysis software package, and generation of final reports for review. Fortunately, with the use of EHR systems, this process has become more simplified. The data collection takes place at the point of care, as the nurse or other HCP enters the relevant data points into the EHR. The reporting features of the EHR system can then be used to rapidly generate needed reports, using multiple data points such as medications, diagnoses, or procedures.

There is evidence to demonstrate that public health initiatives can benefit from the timely data that can be gleaned from EHR systems. BioSense 2.0 is a web-based application, administered by the Centers for Disease Control and Prevention (CDC) that can provide a real-time picture of any health condition, anywhere in the country. It pulls together information on emergency department visits and hospitalization from sources including the Department of Veterans Affairs and the Department of Defense. Civilian hospitals with EHR systems that meet Stages 1 and 2 criteria for meaningful use can also contribute data to the BioSense 2.0 program. Analyses of data that are contributed to the BioSense 2.0 tool can help public health officials to track health issues as they evolve, offer detailed insight into the health of communities, and support national, state, and local responses to health threats (CDC, 2012a).

Updates on evolving issues pertinent to national health, including the 2009–2010 H1N1 flu pandemic, the 2010 Gulf oil spill, and the 2011 U.S. heat wave, were transmitted to state and local health officials via the program website and social media tools such as Facebook and Twitter so that responsive protocols could be implemented (CDC, 2012b).

Decision Support and Potential for Evidence-Based Practice

With the capability to embed evidence such as clinical practice guidelines and best practice protocols, EHR systems can rapidly facilitate the translation of research into practice and influence decisions that nurses and other HCPs make at the actual point of care. Weaver, Warren, and Delaney (2005, pp. 991–995) describe three case studies in which EHR systems were used to generate evidence-based knowledge to guide nursing practice:

- Case Study 1: Querying practice to generate best practice evidence
  - Embedding of the Braden Pressure Sore risk assessment tool into the admission assessment for a hospital in Naples, Florida, resulted in a total pressure ulcer rate of 4.8%, half the national average.
- Case Study 2: Adoption of a clinical information system to teach evidence-based practice in an undergraduate nursing program
  - Faculty at the University of Kansas School of Nursing, in conjunction with Cerner Corporation, use the Simulated e-Health Delivery System (SEEDS) to combine education on pathophysiology, assessments, and plan of care development for virtual patients with evidence-based practice content.
- Case Study 3: Bench informatics—embedding evidence-based nursing protocols into front-line clinical workflows
  - The University of Iowa College of Nursing, in partnership with Cerner Corporation, is developing a method to translate evidence-based nursing protocols and guidelines into both the reference features and point-of-care decision support tools in EHR systems for nurses at the bedside.

Other mechanisms to support evidence-based decision making by nurses in multiple care settings may include the use of standing order sets. Such order sets can allow nurses to carry out specific protocols of patient care prior to examination or approval by an HCP. Order sets are frequently used for the management of common disorders found in hospital and ambulatory care settings, such as pneumonia, diabetes, and chest pain. A study of office-based practices across the United States reviewed the implementation of standing orders sets using the **health maintenance** reminder feature in an EHR for health screenings, immunizations, and diabetes care. Findings from the study revealed statistically significant improvements in osteoporosis screening, pneumococcal vaccination for adults older than 65 years and younger adults at high risk, tetanus/diphtheria and zoster vaccinations, and measurement of urinary microalbumin in patients with diabetes (Nemeth, Ornstein, Jenkins, Wessell, & Nietert, 2012).

CHALLENGES OF EHR USE

Despite the many benefits associated with use of EHR systems, challenges related to widespread implementation continue to permeate health care. The lack of **interoperability**, the economic aspects of system adoption and maintenance, and threats to performance and security may prevent installation or full utilization of an EHR and its features in many delivery settings. Practical, scalable solutions that address these challenges do exist. If possible, healthcare facilities and providers should craft plans to address anticipated challenges prior to installation or expansion of EHR systems.

Lack of Interoperability

In the manufacturing world, a silo is a structure that is capable of storing bulk materials for later use. Informatics science has modified the term, using it to designate an information storage system that is incapable of reciprocal operations with other, similar systems. Though an EHR typically has a substantial capacity for information storage, it should not serve only to accumulate data for later use. HIMSS (2010b) defines *interoperability* as "the ability of different information technology systems and software applications to communicate, exchange data, and use the information that has been exchanged" (p. 190). In an ideal setting, an EHR system acts a hub for the flow of information to improve care for the patient, from many different sources in a healthcare setting, including reference labs, specific areas within the facility (emergency departments, operating rooms, or critical care units), or outside HCP practices. The point at which the separate systems meet and communicate is called the **interface**. The phenomenon of communicating health-related information across multiple platforms and care-delivery settings is known as interoperability, and it has been notoriously difficult to achieve between various EHR systems and components. Many reasons for the failure to achieve interoperability in health care have been proposed.

A significant reason for the lack of interoperability among EHR systems is the need for a common **clinical vocabulary**, or a common terminology that can be used globally in all computerized health information systems. This need was addressed by the Institute of Medicine (2003) report, *Patient Safety: Achieving a New Standard for Care:*

> If health professionals are to be able to send and receive data in an understandable and usable manner, both the sender and the receiver must have common clinical terminologies for describing, classifying, and coding medical terms and concepts. Use of standardized clinical terminologies facilitates electronic data collection at the point of care; retrieval of relevant data, information, and knowledge; and reuse of data for multiple purposes (e.g., disease surveillance, clinical decision support, patient safety reporting). (pp. 37–38)

Encouraging the use of a common clinical vocabulary in EHR systems is one way to improve the interoperability of systems. SNOMED Clinical Terms (SNOMED CT) is a comprehensive, multilingual clinical healthcare terminology developed by the International Health Terminology Standards Development Organisation (IHTSDO). Already used in more than 50 countries around the world, SNOMED CT contains 311,000 active concepts organized into hierarchies, which can then be integrated into software applications to consistently represent the clinical activities of health care (IHTSDO, n.d.). As a member country of the IHTSDO, the United States is eligible to distribute the SNOMED CT language in multiple formats free of charge via the National Library of Medicine (http://www.nlm.nih.gov/research/umls/Snomed/snomed_main.html).

Other issues that prevent full interoperability of EHR systems include both the reluctance to share data among system developers, known as **vendors**, and the lack of unique identifiers for each patient. The highly competitive market for EHR systems and their proprietary software makes many companies reluctant to develop the interface tools necessary to share data between systems. However, recent recommendations from HIMSS support the development of standards and criteria that will encourage vendors to build robust interoperability into systems to facilitate the exchange of information across healthcare-delivery settings, disaster response, and public health initiatives (HIMSS, 2010a). The use of financial incentives to encourage vendors to produce EHR systems with greater inoperability has been suggested as an additional strategy (Hoffman & Podgurski, 2012).

The exchange of healthcare information across systems could also be assisted by the use of unique patient identifiers to prevent errors associated with mismatching of patient identities. Although HIMSS acknowledges that the need for correct linkage of patients to their data is key to achieving quality health care with EHRs, privacy and security concerns have prevented Congress from successfully passing legislation that will address the issue. At this time, the accurate pairing of patient identifiers and healthcare data is managed within an EHR system (Hillestad et al., 2008).

Change in Workflow Patterns

The adoption and implementation of an EHR system often poses a significant change to the daily workflow patterns of staff, which can be a source of stress for a facility and its HCPs—be it a small medical practice or a multi-site healthcare organization. Despite the promise of ongoing EHR use in improving patient care and reducing errors, the failure to consistently engage clinicians in decision making about usability aspects of systems can result in unintended consequences that lead to patient harm. The largest body of research to date has reviewed the impact of **computerized provider order entry** (CPOE) features on the number and character of patient care errors, finding that the use of CPOE can inadvertently increase the need for coordination of activities among clinicians and result in errors (Cheng, Goldstein, Geller, & Levitt, 2003; Harrington & Kennerly, 2011). The source of errors may be due to the assumptions inherent in the construction of CPOE features by designers. Cheng and colleagues (2003) found that the use of CPOE gave HCPs the freedom to place patient care orders at many locations within the facility, even at points far away from traditional patient care areas. While this change in workflow processes can reduce conversations at the bedside between staff and HCPs and can be more convenient for HCPs when entering patient care orders, it can also be a source of miscommunications or errors.

In reviewing the implementation of CPOE in multiple facilities, Campbell, Sittig, Ash, Guappone, and Dykstra (2006) identified new sources of potential causes of patient care mistakes: juxtaposition errors (selection of an item adjacent to an intended choice), desensitization to alerts, confusing presentation of order options, and system design issues (poor organization and display of data). Yet, there are strategies that EHR system users and developers can take to minimize sources of error. Clinician champions to maintain performance improvement (PI) processes should be appointed and a multidisciplinary PI group should be established to regularly review processes and errors as they occur and continuously communicate with facility leadership so that durable solutions can be designed. This approach was identified in studies of patient errors that occurred after implementation of emergency department information systems and could be extrapolated to facility areas

(Farley et al., 2013). Additionally, Farley and colleagues (2013) call attention to the need for EHR vendors to distribute the need for patient safety improvements to all installation sites.

In the past, entry of information into a chart was often the responsibility of a single person in an office or a ward. This clerk, or secretary, bore the full responsibility of familiarity with the system, along with transcription of medical and nursing orders. Responsibilities for data entry continue to disseminate, and the skillsets of HCPs in many care-delivery settings now include familiarity with the manipulation of an EHR system, in addition to their clinical knowledge. Systems with poor usability can serve as sources of frustration for busy HCPs and amplify the potential for error in the entry of documentation data. Examples of data-entry errors include the insertion of information into incorrect fields, transposition of numbers, and the copying and pasting of narratives from previous encounters that may no longer be accurate (Hoffman & Podgurski, 2012).

System and System-Related Expenses

The initial and ongoing fees for EHR systems represent a significant investment of capital. Evidence on the expenditures associated with the implementation and ongoing maintenance of systems is limited and often conflicting. While the direct expenses of an EHR system can vary according to its features and the way its data storage for the system is maintained (either on site with in-house servers or remotely via cloud-based applications), there are indirect costs that are associated with implementation that are often harder to quantify. In testimony delivered July 24, 2008 to the U.S. House of Representatives Ways and Means Committee, Subcommittee on Health, Peter R. Orszag, Director of the Congressional Budget Office (CBO), stated that the total costs for implementation of an EHR system (regardless of the care-delivery setting) included the following (CBO, 2008):

- Initial fixed costs of the hardware, software, and technical assistance necessary to install the system
- Licensing fees
- Expenses necessary to maintain the system
- "Opportunity cost"—the time that HCPs could have spent in seeing patients but instead used in learning the system and adjusting work practices

Later in his testimony, Orszag estimated that the cost of office-based EHR systems ranges from $25,000–$45,000 per provider for initial implementation, with annual licensing and maintenance fees to add $3,000–$9,000 per provider (CBO, 2008). According to Orszag, the cost of implementation of an EHR system in a hospital could average $4,500 per bed (CBO, 2008).

Preparing a budget for EHR adoption and implementation is a process that is specific to each organization and that requires much planning in order to be successful. Initially, it may be best for facilities to prioritize implementation in areas that stand to create the greatest impact on patient care and organizational revenues, such as a pharmacy information system. Incremental approaches can distribute the financial burden over a lengthier period of time (HealthIT.gov, n.d.a). Adoption of an EHR system is no guarantee of an increase in return on financial investment. In a survey analysis of 49 community practices in Massachusetts, 27% reported a positive return on investment by using strategies such as increasing the numbers of patients seen daily by providers and a reduction in the number of rejected claims for billing (Adler-Milstein, Green, & Bates, 2013).

HealthIT.gov provides a variety of resources to assist HCPs and practices in planning for implementation and meaningful use of EHR systems. Regional extension centers (RECs) are available in every part of the United States to offer education, outreach, and technical assistance. The RECs help providers in specific geographic areas to select, successfully adopt, and meaningfully use certified EHR systems (http://www. healthit.gov/providers-professionals/regional-extension-centers-recs#listing). The National Learning Consortium, an ongoing collection of resources contributed by field staff from the Office of the National Coordinator for Health IT (ONC) outreach programs, is also available for health IT professionals, HCPs, and other staff who are working to implement health IT (http://www.healthit.gov/providers-professionals/ about-national-learning-consortium).

There are other strategies that office-based practices and hospitals can employ to save on start-up and annual maintenance costs. For smaller facilities, web-based EHR systems can be economic alternatives to satisfy the need for information systems. In a web-based system, HCPs or hospitals pay a monthly subscription fee to vendors to access EHR systems in lieu of permanent purchase of the systems. Users can then access the EHR system from any computer, without having to purchase dedicated servers and the extra hardware and software needed to work with those servers. Known as application service provider (ASP) or software as a service (SaaS), the concept of providing cloud-based access to software records is becoming more widespread in healthcare-delivery systems. Though there are drawbacks to the use of the cloud- or web-based systems, such as slower response times to retrieve information, particularly if the healthcare facility has low bandwidth, they remain a viable alternative to reduce the expenses of installing and maintaining EHR systems.

Performance and Security Concerns

Issues of system performance and security maintenance are critical for healthcare facilities that use EHR systems. Frequent reports of stolen healthcare data can be found in the news media. While unprotected EHR systems can be vulnerable to hackers, laptops with both unencrypted and encrypted information have been taken from employees of healthcare organizations (Walker, 2013). In another case, a thumb drive that was used to back up one hard drive from another on the campus of the Oregon Health and Science University Hospital (2012) was inadvertently taken home by an employee in a briefcase, which was later removed from the employee's home during a burglary. Even more disturbing are accounts of the targeting of healthcare data by hackers for use in identity theft and commercial ventures (Hall, 2013). To protect electronic healthcare information, it is essential that employees, HCPs, and facility leaders understand their role in maintaining the privacy, security, and confidentiality of the information.

The Health Insurance Portability and Accountability Act (HIPAA) Security Rule requires that facilities take specific measures to safeguard electronic protected health information so that its confidentiality, integrity, and security are ensured (U.S. Department of Health and Human Services, 2013). Safety measures to protect information are often built into EHR systems, such as **access control tools** like user-specific passwords and personal identification numbers. Stored information frequently undergoes **encryption**, meaning that health information cannot be interpreted by anyone unless it is translated by an authorized person who has a specialized key for **decryption** of the information. To further comply with HIPAA Security Rules, organizations must have physical safeguards in place that limit access to their facilities, particularly workstations, and policies for the secure use of electronic media. Technical safeguards are requirements that limit access to electronic health information to authorized personnel; ensure that electronic health information is not improperly altered, destroyed, or transmitted; and require that the facility has the procedural mechanisms in place to generate audit trails of access to electronic health information, if needed. Facilities that use in-house servers to store data generated in their EHR system employ redundant forms of daily backup of data, so that data can be recovered in case of the failure of a system or loss of power. Remote storage of data, or transmission of data to be stored at a site away from the physical location of the EHR system, is another strategy that healthcare facilities use to keep healthcare data safe and retrievable.

Healthcare organizations should use regular tactics to assess the security of their EHR systems. A **security risk analysis** compares present security measures in the

EHR to those that are legally required to safeguard patient information, and the analysis can help in identifying high priority threats and vulnerabilities. The security risk analysis is the initial step in creating an effective action plan for addressing threats and vulnerabilities of the system. Guidance on conducting risk analysis in both small and large facilities can be found online from the U.S. Department of Health and Human Services (2010).

In addition to regular risk analyses, other approaches to assess the security of patient care information must be put into practice. **Penetration testing** is a method that has been used in other areas of electronic information management to assess the security of systems. It can be conducted by information technology personnel within the healthcare facility or by external providers. The results of penetration testing reveal gaps in the system's security that can make it vulnerable to attackers. Results can be used to further refine the action plan to prevent breaches and loss of patient information.

Clinicians who use their own computers to access EHR systems from their homes or offices, known as **remote access**, can pose special risks to the security of EHR systems. Data tampering and theft can occur by hackers' exploitation of weaknesses in the perimeter protection of the network and at the home or office locations. The use of a **virtual private network (VPN)** can reduce risks, because the remote user accesses the EHR network through the VPN, which also uses a tightly configured firewall. The process generates little activity on the Internet that could be detected and exploited by hackers. Use of a home computer, which is likely already compromised due to its use by multiple family members, to access EHR networks remotely should be discouraged. There are significant risks associated with the use of home computers that are not subject to organizational control, such as virus protection, that can inadvertently create security risks for the EHR system. A similar situation can occur if an HCP or other employee brings a home laptop into a healthcare facility and attempts to access the organization's network where the EHR is housed. In most instances, it is best to restrict remote access from unknown networks unless secure access methods have been previously established by organizational policies.

A further issue of concern for healthcare facilities in using EHR systems is unplanned **system downtime** and **recovery capabilities**. Downtime can occur for reasons as simple as short-term power outages, or can be prolonged if natural disasters, such as floods, affect healthcare facilities. Regardless of the size of the facility, mechanisms to retrieve necessary data during downtime to carry on normal operating procedures and to prevent the loss of data when downtime occurs suddenly must be in place. Battery-powered backups that plug directly into the server can be one option; facilities can also opt for automated remote backups at sites located geographical distances away from the healthcare facility. Recovery capabilities of EHR systems vary considerably, and it is important to remember that once power is restored to a system, a time period of several minutes or more may be necessary in order for it to return to full operation. Commonly, the reactivation of interfaces within the system may take several minutes. During this time, the system can be vulnerable to crashes if overwhelmed with an excessive number of users attempting to get back online. The appointment of a single person who can communicate to staff with instructions on system access can be valuable in rapid restoration of system use.

ROLE OF THE NURSE AND THE EHR

An emphasis on the roles and responsibilities of the nurse related to EHR systems should originate in prelicensure education. Conceptual understanding and practical experience, while increasing the prelicensure nurse's level of comfort in working with EHR systems, can also foster improvements in understanding how components of EHR features work together to create outcomes for patients and HCPs. Unfortunately, the literature suggests that academic programs do not sufficiently prepare students for using EHRs in the clinical setting. Students are unaware of the types of patient errors that can result from the use of EHR systems, and even those students with a greater degree of comfort with technology have been reported as experiencing difficulties in using EHRs (Borycki, Joe, Armstrong, Bellwood, & Campbell, 2011). Strategies to reduce barriers to EHR use in academic programs may include using faculty members who have prior experience with EHR systems to integrate their use into the curriculum of prelicensure programs (Borycki et al., 2011).

While nurses in professional practice can be expected to achieve a minimum level of competence with use of EHR systems, it is likely that nurses who seem to have a special flair for working with the system will also emerge. Often referred to as superusers, these nurses tend to display a positive attitude toward EHR use, are willing to take the time for extra training, and serve as a resource for others in use of the system (**Figure 11-5**). Superusers lead other staff and HCPs in the implementation and ongoing use of EHR systems and are crucial to the success of EHR systems in healthcare facilities. Superusers can facilitate the initial and ongoing training of employees in healthcare facilities regarding EHR use, which has been identified as an important factor in their successful implementation and continued use (Ash & Bates, 2005).

Nurses' Perceptions of EHR Systems

With more than 3 million registered nurses in the United States, some consideration of their opinions on the use of EHR systems must be given, if continued proliferation

Are you a superuser?
• Can you maintain a positive attitude during times of technological stress? • Do you have the patience to train others, answer questions, and take calls when you least expect them? • Are you committed to the successful use of an EHR at your healthcare organization?

FIGURE 11-5   Are you a superuser?

and success of the systems can be expected (U.S. Bureau of Labor Statistics, 2010). For the implementation of EHR systems to succeed, nurses need to be convinced that the benefits of electronic records will outweigh benefits of paper records. There is evidence that nurses' attitudes toward EHR implementation is changing. Positive attitudes on EHR use are more frequent, particularly in nurses who report more prior computer experience (Huryk, 2010). A positive attitude from administration creates a more positive attitude in staff, and this can be fostered by continued training opportunities with frequent facility-specific examples of how EHRs are used to improve patient care (Huryk, 2010). Adequate training time and sessions that are staggered according to technological ability are also mechanisms that can improve nurses' positive perceptions of EHR implementation (Huryk, 2010).

Care Surveillance and Delivery

The multiple features of EHR systems can make it simple for the nurse to identify and facilitate the delivery of care to patients. In one study (Feifer et al., 2007) of medical practices that used a common EHR tool, records revealed that an estimated 89.5% of female patients (above the age of 40 years) associated with one practice were found to have received annual mammograms. An examination of the strategies used to achieve this remarkable goal revealed that the project leader, a licensed vocational nurse within the practice, used the health maintenance feature of the EHR system to identify and contact females who needed to be scheduled for mammograms (**Table 11-2**).

Increased Time for Documentation

Nursing documentation often varies little from patient to patient in terms of the forms that are used. Standardized care plans, assessments, admission/registration

Table 11-2   Success Strategies for Projects Involving EHR Systems

Select the leader.	The leader is responsible for summarizing the baseline performance of the organization, and how the project can be implemented in order to improve patient care.
Find the vision.	With input from other staff, the leader clarifies the vision for the project implementation and sustainability.
Choose measurement criteria.	Select a realistic set of performance measurements that can be assessed regularly throughout the project implementation, and used to indicate successes and areas for improvement.
Support the vision.	Though transition can be difficult, remember the need to work together toward the common vision.
Empower the patients.	Use the features available in many EHR systems, such as patient education tools, to assist patients in taking an active role in their care.
Remember the ultimate goal.	Improving the quality of care for each patient is the purpose of the project.

forms, and medication lists may be used for each patient. Nurses will often access and review similar sets of documentation, in the same physical location, several times throughout the course of a day's work. For this reason, nurses can realize greater gains in efficiency with use of electronic documentation. Despite the existence of a Nursing Intervention Classification system for the time spent in documentation of patient care, many nurses do not regard documentation as a true patient-care activity. In a review of 11 studies examining the impact of EHR implementation on the amount of time nurses spent in documentation, six studies demonstrated a reduction in the average time spent in documentation, ranging from 2.1–45.1% (Poissant, Pereira, Tamblyn, & Kawasumi, 2005). However, further review of the studies suggested that location of the computer terminals could affect nurses' efficiency in documentation. Two of the studies found that the use of bedside terminals increased the amount of time needed for documentation (7.7% and 39.2%, respectively (Poissant et al., 2005). Specific strategies for integration of computer-assisted documentation into the daily workflow of nurses are listed in **Table 11-3**.

Table 11-3   Don't Let the Computer Be an Intruder! Five Strategies for Making the Computer Work for You When the Terminal Is in the Room

- **The patient comes first.** When you walk into the room, address the patient and the patient's family first. Introduce yourself and assess the patient's needs. After you finish your preliminary care, explain that you are going to move to the computer terminal, laptop, or other device to continue your care.

- **Positioning is everything.** The computer is a tool and not the focus of attention. The terminal should be placed in a position between you and the patient, so that you can change your focus between the screen and the patient with a slight turn of the head.

- **Focus, focus, focus.** Changing your attention from the patient to the computer screen, while maintaining rapport with the patient or family, may seem difficult at first. Don't worry; this is a skill that will improve with practice, as your comfort in using the EHR system and computer terminal increases.

- **The computer is never the patient.** Do not walk into a patient's room and begin to use the computer without addressing the patient. Always explain what you are about to do.

- **Use the power of the system for you and your patient.** EHR systems have a variety of features that can be used to enhance patient care at the bedside or in the exam room. Investigate graphing functions that can be used to display trends in lab results, vital signs, or other measures that could serve as teaching moments for patients. Many EHRs also have embedded patient education tools that can be downloaded and printed for on-demand use.

Source: Adapted from Communication Tips for Nurses when Electronic Health Records Enter the Exam Room. Accessed online at http://career-advice.monster.com/in-the-office/workplace-issues/nurse-communication-tips-ehr/article.aspx. Reprinted by permission of Monster.com.

SUMMARY

The proliferation of EHRs is expected to continue, and it is the nurse who can play a key role in optimizing use of systems to improve outcomes for patients and healthcare facilities. Preparing nurses for integral roles in the design, selection, and implementation of EHR systems begins with exposure to systems in prelicensure education and continued training in the occupational setting. Nurses can offer unique perspectives on the workflow of common tasks, such as provider order entry, that designers can integrate into EHR systems, improving function and reducing the risk for patient errors.

Not every nurse will become an EHR superuser, but all can achieve a level of competence with system use if facility administrators and peers provide adequate training and support. Demonstration of skill in EHR use is essential if nurses are to have a part in crafting policies and systems for future use.

Box 11-1   Case Study

Jill is a nurse who works in a busy office-based practice that uses an EHR system. The practice has set a project goal of administering influenza vaccinations to 85% of eligible patients in the upcoming season, and Jill is tasked with coordinating the project. Her responsibilities include the ordering of adequate supplies of influenza vaccine, publicizing the availability of vaccine to patients, and ensuring that each vaccination is properly documented in the chart, in such a way that a record of its administration can be retrieved upon audit.

After reviewing recommended guidelines for the administration of influenza vaccine to children and adults, Jill begins the project by using the reporting tool embedded in the EHR to determine the number of patients eligible for vaccination, using the parameters of age and diagnosis. The results of the report help Jill to determine supplies of influenza vaccine that will need to be ordered in preparation for the upcoming flu season. Jill returns to her report to construct a mailing list, and uses physical addresses and email addresses to send notices of the recommendations for influenza vaccines to the eligible patients. After Jill receives the shipment of vaccinations, she continues to prepare for the high volume of vaccinations that are expected to be administered by designing a short note template containing the manufacturer, lot number, and expiration date of the vaccination. The note template also contains a procedural code unique to the administration of the influenza vaccine, and a choice of anatomical sites for administration. As nurses open individual patient charts upon administering the vaccination, the note template will automatically import the date of administration. With two clicks on the mouse pad, the nurse's notation of vaccine administration is complete. As the season concludes, Jill again uses the reporting feature of the EHR to create a report of patient charts containing the unique procedural code for influenza vaccine administration during the specified date range. Jill compares this number to the number of eligible patients from her initial report, finding that 87.6% of eligible patients in the practice received influenza vaccinations during the season, and concludes that her project was successful.

For a full suite of assignments and additional learning activities, use the access code located in the front of your book and visit www.jblearning.com. If you do not have an access code, you can obtain one at the site.

REFERENCES

Adler-Milstein, J., Green, C. E., & Bates, D. W. (2013). A survey analysis suggests that electronic health records will yield revenue gains for some practices and losses for many. *Health Affairs*, *32*(3), 562–570.

Ash, J., & Bates, D. W. (2005). Factors and forces affecting EHR system adoption: Report of a 2004 ACMI discussion. *Journal of the American Medical Informatics Association*, *12*(1), 8–12.

Borycki, E., Joe, R. S., Armstrong, B., Bellwood, P., & Campbell, R. (2011). Educating health professionals about electronic health records (EHR): Removing the barriers to adoption. *Knowledge Management & E-Learning: An International Journal, 3*(1), 51–62.

Campbell, E. M., Sittig, D. F., Ash, J. S., Guappone, K. P., & Dykstra, R. H. (2006). Types of unintended consequences related to computerized provider order entry. *Journal of the American Medical Informatics Association, 13*(5), 547–556.

Centers for Disease Control and Prevention. (2012a). BioSense 2.0. Retrieved from http://www.cdc.gov/biosense/biosense20.html

Centers for Disease Control and Prevention. (2012b). BioSense data in action. Retrieved from http://www.cdc.gov/biosense/action.html

Cheng, C. H., Goldstein, M. K., Geller, E., & Levitt, R. E. (2003). The effects of CPOE on ICU workflow: An observational study. *AMIA Annual Symposium Proceedings,* 150–154.

Congressional Budget Office. (2008). *Testimony of Peter R. Orszag, Director: Evidence on Costs and Benefits of Health Information Technology.* Washington, DC: U.S. House of Representatives Ways and Means Committee, Subcommittee on Health. Retrieved from http://www.cbo.gov/sites/default/files/cbofiles/ftpdocs/95xx/doc9572/07-24-healthit.pdf

Emanuel, E. (2012). *Results of HITECH Act "nothing short of spectacular."* Retrieved from http://www.ihealthbeat.org/articles/2012/3/7/ezekiel-emanuel-results-of-hitech-act-nothing-short-of-spectacular.aspx

Farley, H. L., Baumlin, K. M., Hamedani, A. G., Cheung, D. S., Edwards, M. R., Fuller, D. L., . . . Pines, J. M. (2013). Quality and safety of implementation of emergency department information systems. *Annals of Emergency Medicine, 62*(4), 399–407.

Feifer, C., Nemeth, L., Nietert, P. J., Wessell, A. M., Jenkins, R. G., Roylance, L., & Ornstein, S. (2007). Different paths to high quality care: Three archetypes of top performing practice sites. *Annals of Family Medicine, 5*(3), 233–241. doi: 10.1370/afm.697

Hall, S. D. (2013). *Stolen health data increasingly sought after for commercial ventures.* Retrieved from http://www.fiercehealthit.com/story/stolen-health-data-increasingly-sought-after-commercial-ventures/2013-03-25

Harrington, L., & Kennerly, D. (2011). Safety issues related to electronic medical record (EMR): Synthesis of literature from the last decade, 2000–2009. *Journal of Healthcare Management, 56*(1), 31–43.

HealthIT.gov. (n.d.a). *Answer to your question: How much is this going to cost me?* Retrieved from http://www.healthit.gov/providers-professionals/faqs/how-much-going-cost-me

HealthIT.gov. (n.d.b). *What is meaningful use?* Retrieved from http://www.healthit.gov/policy-researchers-implementers/meaningful-use

Hillestad, R., Bigelow, J. H., Chaudhry, B., Dreyer, P., Greenberg, M. D., Meili, R. D., . . . Taylor, R. (2008). *Identity crisis: An examination of the costs and benefits of a unique patient identifier for the U.S. health care system.* Santa Monica, CA: Rand Corporation. Retrieved from http://www.rand.org/content/dam/rand/pubs/monographs/2008/RAND_MG753.sum.pdf

HIMSS. (2010a). *2011–2012 Public policy principles.* Retrieved from http://www.himss.org/files/HIMSSorg/policy/d/PolicyPrinciples2011.pdf

HIMSS. (2010b). *Dictionary of healthcare information technology terms, acronyms and organizations* (2nd ed.). Chicago, IL: Author.

HIMSS. (2012–2013). *Electronic health records.* Retrieved from http://www.himss.org/library/ehr/?navItemNumber=513261

Hoffman, S., & Podgurski, A. (2012). Big bad data: Law, public health, and biomedical databases. *Journal of Law, Medicine, and Ethics, 41*(Suppl. 1), 50–60.

Huryk, L. A. (2010). Factors influencing nurses' attitudes towards health information technology. *Journal of Nursing Management, 18,* 606–612.

Institute of Medicine. (2003). *Patient safety: Achieving a new standard for care.* Washington, DC: National Academies Press.

International Health Terminology Standards Development Organisation. (n.d.). *About SNOMED Ct.* Retrieved from http://www.ihtsdo.org/snomed-ct/snomed-ct0/

Jones, S. S., Adams, J. L., Schneider, E. C., Ringel, J. S., & McGlynn, E. A. (2010). Electronic health record adoption and quality improvement in U.S. hospitals. *American Journal of Managed Care, 16,* SP64–SP71.

Nemeth, L. S., Ornstein, S. M., Jenkins, R. G., Wessell, A. M., & Nietert, P. (2012). Implementing and evaluating electronic standing orders in primary care practice: A PPRNet study. *Journal of the American Board of Family Medicine, 25*(5), 594–604.

Oregon Health and Science University. (2012). *OHSU contacts patients about data stolen during burglary.* Retrieved from http://www.ohsu.edu/xd/about/news_events/news/2012/07-31-ohsu-contacts-patients-a.cfm

Poissant, L., Pereira, J., Tamblyn, R., & Kawasumi, Y. (2005). The impact of electronic health records on the time efficiency of physicians and nurses: A systematic review. *Journal of the American Medical Informatics Association, 12*(5), 505–516.

U.S. Bureau of Labor Statistics. (2010). *Occupational outlook handbook.* Retrieved from http://www.bls.gov/ooh/Healthcare/Registered-nurses.htm

U.S. Department of Health and Human Services. (2010). Guidance on Risk Analysis Requirements under the HIPAA Security Rule. Retrieved from http://www.hhs.gov/ocr/privacy/hipaa/administrative/securityrule/rafinalguidancepdf.pdf

U.S. Department of Health and Human Services. (2013). Modifications to the HIPAA Privacy, Security, Enforcement, and Breach Notification Rules Under the Health Information Technology for Economic and Clinical Health Act and the Genetic Information Nondiscrimination Act; Other Modifications to the HIPAA Rules (to be codified as CFR Pts. 160 & 164). *Federal Register 5567.* Retrieved from https://www.federalregister.gov/articles/2013/01/25/2013-01073/modifications-to-the-hipaa-privacy-security-enforcement-and-breach-notification-rules-under-the

Walker, D. (2013). *Laptop stolen from California health care provider exposing data of 1,500.* Retrieved from http://www.scmagazine.com/laptop-stolen-from-calif-health-care-provider-exposing-data-of-1500/article/298999/

Weaver, C. A., Warren, J. J., & Delaney, C. (2005). Bedside, classroom, & bench: Collaborative strategies to generate evidence-based knowledge for nursing practice. *International Journal of Medical Informatics, 74,* 989–999.

CHAPTER 12

Clinical Decision-Support Systems

Jane M. Carrington, PhD, RN

CHAPTER LEARNING OBJECTIVES

1. Identify the typical parts of a clinical decision-support system.
2. Understand how clinical decision-support systems can improve patient safety.
3. Discuss a nurse's responsibility when using clinical decision-support systems embedded in electronic health records and other health information technologies.

KEY TERMS

Algorithms

Artificial intelligence

Clinical decision rules

Data quality and validity

Knowledge base

Natural language processing

Reasoning engine

Standardized/controlled data

CHAPTER OVERVIEW

This chapter introduces clinical decision-support systems (CDSSs). First, it introduces the underpinnings of CDSSs. User-technology interface is then discussed. Finally, CDSSs and professional practice issues are presented.

INTRODUCTION

The American Recovery and Reinvestment Act of 2009 (ARRA) set a mandate for technology to increase patient safety and reduce healthcare costs. Implementation and adoption of the electronic health record (EHR) is included in the technology requirements, along with use of computerized provider order entry (CPOE), electronic prescribing, drug–drug and drug–allergy interaction checks, active medication lists, trending of patient vital signs, and **clinical decision rules** (Centers for Medicare & Medicaid Services [CMS], 2010). To meet the criteria for implementation of clinical decision rules, the EHR must have a functioning CDSS.

Nurses and other healthcare providers (HCPs) collect and manage vast amounts of patient information each shift (Kannampallil et al., 2013; Moore & Fisher, 2012). In addition, HCPs have to recall evidence-based practice standards for allergies, medications, laboratory data, and so forth. A quick scan of patient rooms, hospital units, intensive care units, and outpatient settings reveals many types of medical devices including cardiac monitors, pulse oximeters, syringe pumps, and intravenous (IV) fluid pumps; many of these devices have CDSSs embedded in their operating systems. These CDSSs function in efficient ways to alert HCPs when a patient's physiological parameters are outside the accepted normal ranges.

CDSSs contain reference information, order sets, reminders, alerts, and condition-specific or patient-specific information accessible to HCPs when this information is critical to decision making (Ash et al., 2012). A CDSS contained in an EHR uses principles of **artificial intelligence** and information science to provide active knowledge systems combined with patient data to generate clinical, patient-specific advice (Demner-Fushman, Chapman, & McDonald, 2009). This definition has several implications. First, a computer can be trained to provide clinical advice that is patient specific. Second, patient information can be organized in such a manner as to fit the data structure required for computer logic. Finally, CDSSs are capable of providing advice to guide patient-care decisions (Demner-Fushman et al., 2009).

This chapter provides a detailed description of CDSSs including data capture, quality and validity of the data, applications, clinical reasoning, and alert fatigue. Examples are provided to increase understanding.

CLINICAL DECISION-SUPPORT SYSTEMS

Imagine standing at the patient's bedside and gathering blood pressure, heart rate, respiratory rate, temperature, and performing a complete patient assessment, and then entering these values into an EHR. The morning laboratory values for complete blood count (CBC) and blood chemistries are available in the EHR. Throughout the shift, this patient information is available to clinicians who are also caring for him or her. At a deeper level, well within the computer and software coding for the EHR, these values are now data inputs and have been entered into **algorithms** and further organized by established rules. Later in the shift, an HCP reviews the vital signs and assessment data and prescribes digoxin for the patient. Using CPOE, the order is entered and immediately the CDSS triggers an alert. The HCP sees a pop-up alert: "K < 2.5." This alert informs the HCP that the patient's potassium level needs to be elevated prior to starting the patient on digoxin. Because of the alert, the HCP will order a potassium infusion, supplements, and/or check for the influence of diuretics.

Now imagine that when the HCP entered the digoxin order, there were call lights indicating that other patients needed assistance, phones were ringing, and nurses were caring for five other patients. The CDSS provided essential information, enhancing patient safety, in the complex and chaotic system. This safety feature is one reason CDSSs are included as part of the meaningful use criteria of ARRA.

DATA CAPTURE

One interesting point about CDSSs is that they are designed to take clinical information and provide advice for the HCP. Stated another way, CDSSs are a form of artificial intelligence (AI) whereby a computer has been "trained" to perform human behavior. There are three essential elements to most CDSSs: **knowledge base, reasoning engine**, and a mechanism to communicate with the end user (Wright et al., 2009). Data are entered to the CDSS as part of the routine documentation process. For example, data such as patient age, gender, symptoms, diagnosis, medications, vital signs, and assessment data are entered into the EHR, which seamlessly populates the CDSS in a standardized or controlled manner.

One of the keys to a CDSS is the standardized or controlled data recognized by the reasoning engine of the CDSS. **Standardized or controlled data** are accepted laboratory values, vital signs, and pre-accepted items from a drop-down menu. This implies that free text is not recognized by the CDSSs; therefore, it does not contribute to the decision making of the system or alert.

The reasoning engine functions as a series of logic schemes for eventual output (Wright et al., 2009). Using the Bayesian network, for example, the reasoning engine will work to determine the likelihood of an event occurrence (Sim et al., 2001). The system might use "if-then" logic, for example, "if the K level is < 2.5, then alert." The knowledge base informed the reasoning engine of the pre-adopted K value and uses evidence-based practice guides from the literature, expert opinion, and pre-adopted normal values to link with the reasoning engine (Sim et al., 2001). The reasoning engine and knowledge base are simultaneously interchanging information to pre-established rules. Finally, the output is possibilities provided by rank of probability based on results from the reasoning engine and knowledge base (Sim et al., 2001). **Figure 12-1** illustrates this using a clinical example.

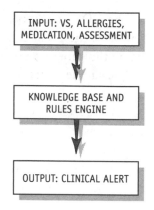

FIGURE 12-1   Architecture of clinical decision-support systems.
Data from Berner, ES and Ball, MJ, *Clinical Decision Support Systems: Theory and Practice,* Springer, 1998, p. 35.

DATA QUALITY AND VALIDITY

The familiar adage "garbage in-garbage out" is especially relevant with CDSSs. The CDSS can potentially threaten the safety of patients if the data entered as input and knowledge base lack **quality** and **validity**. Assuming the rules are written correctly, the threat to data quality and validity is data entry into the EHR. Berner, Kasiraman, Yu, Ray, & Houston (2005) examined 178 transcriptions of standardized patient visits to test the data quality and CDSS function. Focusing on the GI Risk Score, developed by Singh and licensed by Stanford University, data from the study suggest that missing data or incomplete documentation had an impact on the decision rule and CDSS potentially threatening patient safety (Singh, Ramey, Triadafilopoulus, Brown, & Balise, 1998).

A variety of clinical situations contribute to missing data. A chaotic and complex work environment and poor workflow contribute as HCPs rush through documentation. Another contributing factor could be the constraints put upon HCPs by the standardized response required by the system. For example, Carrington (2012) reported results from a study where nurses were interviewed to elicit their perceptions of the usefulness of standardized nursing languages to communicate a sudden change in patient condition. Researchers reported that nurses perceived standardized nursing languages as constraining, which fostered inaccurate patient information.

A possible solution is using natural language processing to include free text from the electronic documentation to inform the rules engine and trigger an alert. **Natural language processing (NLP)** is a method of taking free text from progress notes, nursing documentation, discharge summaries, or radiology reports, for example, and analyzing it for patterns and added meaning to create added rules and generate more individualized patient-specific alerts (Demner-Fushman et al., 2009). Natural language processing is considered a method that will increase alert sensitivity or ability to detect subtle data elements describing patient status. This is an exciting area of research in health care and CDSSs.

CDSS APPLICATIONS

CDSSs are often purchased from vendors of information systems such as EHR, CPOE, electronic medication-administration records, (eMAR), or Barcode Medication Administration (BCMA). Other CDSSs are designed for specific purposes by information analysts and HCPs such as physicians and nurses at the hospital or health system level. Refer to **Table 12-1** for a list of applications with a brief description.

CDSS Architecture

The strength of CDSSs lies within their architecture. CDSSs are very efficient in how they take patient information and generate an alert. This capability is due to the science of machine-learning or teaching the computer how to "think." Moreover, the reasoning engine requires two patient data points at minimum to construct a rule (Spooner, 2007). This requirement implies that elements included in routine patient

Table 12-1   Clinical Decision-Support Systems Applications

Application	Role	Example
Computerized Provider Order Entry (CPOE)	1. Medication incompatibilities, 2. Dosing and patient weight, 3. Medication and laboratory values 4. Medications and allergies	1. Patient is on a medication that is incompatible with another 2. For a patient weight, the dose or frequency is inappropriate 3. For a particular medication, a laboratory value is too high/low, or unknown 4. Known patient allergy and medication
Allergies	1. Allergies to medications 2. Allergies to intravenous nutrition	1. See above 2. Element in intravenous solution and patient allergy
Diagnostics	1. Patient diagnostics 2. Laboratory values 3. Vital signs	Link these patient information points for diagnosis support

care documentation are enough to create rules and generate alerts for safe care. Requiring only two data points to generate an alert further suggests that the alert could fire sooner than having the system wait for 3, 4, or 10 data points, which may not be entered at the same time or in the same area in the EHR.

USER ISSUES WITH CDSSs

Nurses and other HCPs collect, process, and filter vast amounts of data to assemble an accurate picture of the patient. The average human would not be able to accurately manage the quantity of data spread over multiple patients. The strengths of CDSSs, as previously mentioned are the ability to assist with the process of managing patient data and to provide alerts for decision making. By acknowledging CDSS alerts, the computer is told that the HCP has taken the information contained in the alert and made the appropriate decision for that case. Unfortunately, clinicians have demonstrated such dependence on the CDSS alerts that they have either become less confident in their own decision making or overly reliant on the CDSS alerts (Huryk, 2012; Weber, 2007).

Clinicians know that CDSSs lack the ability to reason beyond the programmed logic. For example, CDSSs recognize a low laboratory value or an issue with a medication, but CDSSs would not "know" to consider that the laboratory value was the result of dilution. Alerts are constructed from rules and knowledge, but some HCPs resist the alert, believing a machine could not "know" more than the HCP or that the HCP knows the whole patient situation required for decision making (Alexander, 2006).

Alert Fatigue

Despite the clinical assistance provided by CDSSs, alerts can also be disruptive. Imagine trying to enter orders for a patient and having three alerts trigger to remind you about allergies, laboratory values, medications, and/or diet and treatments or diagnostics. Then multiply the alerts by the number of patients in a shift. Eventually, alert fatigue sets in. Defined as simply disrupting clinical workflow, alert fatigue can result in dismissed alerts (quickly clicking to remove the alert) without taking the information into account (Kesselheim, Cresswell, Phansalkar, Bates, & Sheikh, 2011). Alert fatigue has contributed to clinicians' resistance to CDSSs when it interferes with their workflow (Huryk, 2012; Jaspers, Smeulers, Vermeulen, & Peute, 2011; Kleeberg, Levick, Osheroff, Reider, & Teich, 2011).

Slowly implementing rules in the CDSS in practice can minimize alert fatigue (Kuperman et al., 2007). For example, rules for medications with the highest frequency of errors or the highest risk for patient safety can be implemented first. Over time, the number of rules can be increased with appropriate alerts. The number of rules that can be supported by the knowledge base will be largely dependent on the vendor and the software supports. For any given EHR, the number of rules and alerts will vary.

Maintenance of the Knowledge Base

The knowledge bases in CDSSs are derived from research literature that is considered best evidence. The knowledge base must be updated and maintained when research evidence shows new findings important for patient care. Keeping up with the evidence can be challenging for an organization because of the fast pace of research and its dissemination across thousands of journals in health care. Moreover, healthcare organizations typically do not employ HCPs with expertise in evidence-based practice. The success of a CDSS depends on involving HCPs who can apply evidence to practice and informaticists who customize EHRs.

PROFESSIONAL PRACTICE

As part of professional practice, nurses must use CDSSs that are part of health information technology. Nurses can also participate in the development or customization of CDSSs, because the systems are composed of knowledge bases, algorithms, and clinical decision rules. Any of these parts must be refined to reflect the most effective care for patients possible. Nurses can work with information analysts on committees or on governing boards for CDSSs to bring about change in CDSSs. In fact, nurses may select an advanced role as an informaticist with more education and work with analysts in information system departments. Several principles for effective use of CDSSs are shown in **Box 12-1**.

Box 12-1 Effective Use of CDSS

- Recognize that alerts are presented in context to increase patient safety. This means that an alert should be taken seriously and not ignored without a sound rationale.
- Use the alerts to support patient care, but not to replace critical thinking and advanced human reasoning.
- Incorporate CDSSs into workflow. If an alert appears while entering patient information in the EHR, prepare for the added information and readily incorporate that information into decision-making.
- Recommend changes in practice (change to the CDSS logic) based on the research literature. Should a new practice standard be discovered in the literature, follow the appropriate procedures to communicate the suggestion to nursing leadership and eventually add it to the CDSSs knowledge base.

SUMMARY

CDSSs consist of input from the EHR, reasoning engine, knowledge base, and an output in the form of a clinical alert. CDSSs are designed to assist in managing clinical data to increase patient safety. Despite the impact on increasing patient safety, CDSSs also have had an impact on nursing practice. Issues with the user-technology interface consist of alert fatigue and dependence challenges. However, if used as designed and incorporated within workflow, CDSSs can have a positive influence in nursing practice and ultimately increase patient safety.

 For a full suite of assignments and additional learning activities, use the access code located in the front of your book and visit www.jblearning.com. If you do not have an access code, you can obtain one at the site.

REFERENCES

Alexander, G. L. (2006). Issues of trust and ethics in computerized clinical decision support systems. *Nursing Administration Quarterly, 30*(1), 21–29.

Ash, J. S., McCormack, J. L., Sittig, D. F., Wright, A., McMullen, C., & Bates, D. W. (2012). Standard practices for computerized clinical decision support in community hospitals: A national survey. *Journal of the American Medical Informatics Association, 19*(6), 980–987. doi: 10.1136/amiajnl-2011-000705

Berner, E. S., Kasiraman, R. K., Yu, F., Ray, M. N., & Houston, T. K. (2005). Data quality in the outpatient setting: Impact on clinical decision support systems. *American Medical Informatics Association Symposium Proceedings*, 41–45.

Carrington, J. M. (2012). The usefulness of nursing languages to communicate a clinical event. *CIN: Computers, Informatics, Nursing, 30*(2), 82–88.

Centers for Medicare & Medicaid Services. (2010). Medicare and Medicaid EHR incentive program. Retrieved from http://www.cms.gov/Regulations-and-Guidance/Legislation/EHRIncentive-Programs/Downloads/MU_Stage1_ReqOverview.pdf

Demner-Fushman, D., Chapman, W. W., & McDonald, C. J. (2009). What can natural language processing do for clinical decision support? *Journal of Biomedical Informatics, 42*, 760–772.

Ernesater, A., Holmstrom, I., & Engstrom, M. (2009). Telenurses' experiences of working with computerized decision support: Supporting, inhibiting and quality improving. *Journal of Advanced Nursing, 65*(5), 1074–1083.

Huryk, L. A. (2012). Information systems and decision support systems: What are they and how are they used in nursing? *American Journal of Nursing, 112*(1), 62–65.

Jaspers, M. W., Smeulers, M., Vermeulen, H., & Peute, L. (2011). Effects of clinical decision-support systems on practitioner performance and patient outcomes: A synthesis of high-quality systematic review findings. *Journal of the American Medical Informatics Association, 18,* 327–334.

Kannampallil, T. G., Franklin, A., Mishra, R., Almoosa, K. F., Cohen, T., & Patel, V. L. (2013). Understanding the nature of information seeking behavior in critical care: Implications for the design of health information technology. *Artificial Intelligence in Medicine, 57*(1), 21–29. doi: 10.1016/j.artmed.2012.10.002

Kesselheim, A. S., Cresswell, K., Phansalkar, S., Bates, D. W., & Sheikh, A. (2011). Clinical decision support systems could be modified to reduce 'alert fatigue' while still minimizing the risk of litigation. *Health Affairs, 30*(12), 2310–2317.

Kleeberg, P., Levick, D., Osheroff, J., Reider, J., & Teich, J. (2010). *HIMSS clinical decision support and meaningful use frequently asked questions.* Retrieved from http://www.himss.org/files/HIMSSorg/content/files/MU_CDS_FAQ_FINAL_April2010.pdf

Kuperman, G. J., Dobb, A., Payne, T. H., Avery, A. J., Gandhi, T. K., Burns, G., . . . Bates, D. W. (2007). Medication-related clinical decision support in computerized provider order entry systems: A review. *Journal of the American Medical Informatics Association, 14*(1), 29–40.

Moore, A. N., & Fisher, K. (2012). Healthcare information technology and medical-surgical nurses: The emergence of a new care partnership. *CIN: Computers, Informatics, Nursing, 30*(3), 157–163.

Sim, I., Gorman, P., Greenes, R. A., Haynes, R. B., Kaplan, B., Lehmann, H., & Tang, P. C. (2001). Clinical decision support systems for the practice of evidence-based medicine. *Journal of the American Medical Informatics Association, 8*(6), 527–534.

Singh, G., Ramey, D. R., Triadafilopoulus, G., Brown, B. W., & Balise, R. R. (1998). GI score: A simple self-assessment instrument to quantify the risk of serious NSAID-related GI complications in RA and OA. *Arthritis Rheumatology, 41*(suppl.), S75.

Spooner, S. A. (2007). Mathematical foundations of decision support systems. In E. S. Berner (Ed.), *Clinical decision support systems* (2nd ed., 23–43). New York, NY: Springer.

Weber, S. (2007). A qualitative analysis of how advanced practice nurses use clinical decision support systems. *Journal of American Academy of Nurse Practitioners, 19*(12), 652–667.

Wright, A., Sittig, D. F., Ash, J. S., Sharma, S., Pang, J. E., & Middleton, B. (2009). Clinical decision support capabilities of commercially-available clinical information systems. *Journal of the American Medical Informatics Association, 16*(5), 637–644. doi: 10.1197/jamia.M3111

CHAPTER 13

Telehealth

Kimberly D. Shea, PhD, RN

CHAPTER LEARNING OBJECTIVES

1. Define telehealth and understand its historical development.
2. Describe the many applications of telehealth.
3. Understand the relevant legal, policy, and ethical considerations associated with telehealth.
4. Assess the potential for the future development of telehealth.

KEY TERMS

Digital era

Internet era

Real-time applications

Store and forward applications

Telecommunications

Telecommunications era

Teleconsult

Telehealth

Telemonitoring

Telerehabilitation

Teletrauma

Televisit

CHAPTER OVERVIEW

In this chapter, the development of telehealth is briefly reviewed, and the nurse's role in field of telehealth is discussed. The chapter provides an overview of the health policy and ethical principles associated with the telehealth practice. Applications of telehealth technologies are also described.

INTRODUCTION

Telehealth, the process of using technological communication systems in the assessment and management of patients, is an evolving area of nursing practice. The goal of telehealth is to use the many communication technologies that are presently available to expand the provision of healthcare services to locations and populations who are in need of those services. A report issued by *Information Week* magazine estimates the telehealth sector was poised to grow by 55% in 2013 alone and could expand as much as six-fold by 2017 (Terry, 2013).

Advancements in technology and capacity for communication are allowing vast quantities of information to be sent and received quickly, closing gaps in access to health services created by disabilities and geography. Technology for information transmission has been evolving rapidly and consistently for more than a century and will continue to evolve as computer and information sciences provide more abilities and knowledge. It is and will continue to be important for healthcare providers (HCPs) to keep up to date with the technology and implement it appropriately in their workflow.

CORE CONCEPTS AND DEFINITIONS

Computers with electronic technologies and communication infrastructures enable the transfer of messages, in the form of data, from senders to receivers. When the data are given meaning, by interpretation or explanation, information has been created. The addition of knowledge, which is the recognition of patterns and insights within the data, to the interpretation of information aids the decision making of the HCP. Telehealth communication, in serving as the union of data, information, and knowledge, can use any or all parts of the union to promote desired outcomes.

The Health Resources and Services Administration (HRSA) defines telehealth as the "use of electronic information and telecommunications technologies to support long-distance clinical health care, patient and professional health-related education, public health and health administration" (HRSA, 2012). This definition provides the basis for this chapter and guides an examination of the components of telehealth. Although the American Telemedicine Association considers "telemedicine" and "telehealth" to be interchangeable terms, the use of telehealth encompasses all the health services (not only medical) that can be provided remotely.

As the definition indicates, telehealth can be used for many different communication purposes and serves as a general "umbrella" that contains many practices, many of which are designated by the prefix "tele" (e.g., telemonitoring, teleradiology, telenursing, telemedicine, televisits). Telehealth enables health expertise to be available regardless of the patient's ability to physically visit the provider of healthcare services. Applications for health promotion, treatment, and illness prevention are limited only by telecommunication abilities and imagination, and can be summarized into five groups (**Table 13-1**): referrals to healthcare specialists, patient consultations, remote patient monitoring, medical/nursing/allied health education, and consumer-oriented medical and health information.

The use of telehealth has great potential for improving health care in traditionally underserved populations, particularly those who are located in geographies isolated from HCPs and those in areas where HCPs and facilities are limited in number. Healthcare access for all is consistent with the missions of the World Health Organization (WHO) and the U.S. Department of Health and Human Services (HHS, 2013)—via its *Healthy People 2020* initiative. The HRSA works to increase and improve the use of telehealth through the creation of new telehealth projects, the administration and

Table 13-1 Summary of Current Telehealth Services	
1. Referrals to specialists	A specialist assists a general practitioner in arriving at a diagnosis. Many times, this involves the transmission of information such as diagnostic images, in addition to the patient interview, used to arrive at the diagnosis. Subspecialties of medicine including radiology, dermatology, cardiology, pathology, and mental health have used telehealth successfully in caring for patients.
2. Patient Consultations	Telecommunications technologies are used to connect a patient at a remote site and a healthcare provider for the purpose of interview, examination, and construction of a diagnosis and plan of treatment.
3. Remote patient monitoring	Devices are used to collect and send data to a site for interpretation. Examples include electrocardiogram, blood glucose monitoring, or ambulatory blood pressure.
4. Medical/nursing/allied health education	Continuing education for all specialties of healthcare providers can be offered at remote sites using telecommunications technologies.
5. Consumer medical and health information	Consumers use the Internet to access specific health-related information and connect to other consumers with similar care needs, such as disease-specific support groups.

evaluation of grant programs, and the promotion of a fluid exchange of knowledge about "best practices" in areas of telehealth.

Telecommunications, an essential component of telehealth, is defined as communication over a distance by cable, telegraph, telephone, or other broadcasting mechanism. Telecommunications networks include a transmitter that takes information and converts it to a signal. The signal is then carried by a medium to a receiver, where it is translated into usable information for the recipient. Telecommunications networks and the practice of telehealth were established well before the advent of the wireless networks that are present in today's society; however, the ability to move the signal from transmitter to receiver in a wireless fashion has enabled the field of telehealth to grow exponentially.

Televisit is a term used to describe an encounter involving a patient and an HCP that is enabled by telecommunications technologies. Determining the goal for the visit is the first step in deciding which type of televisit to use. Much has been written on the value of goal setting for healthcare encounters, and this is no less important in televisits (Davis, Kirby, & Curtis, 2007). Remote encounters with patients can often be quicker and may lack much of the casual interaction that is important in helping patients feel relaxed, so it is important for HCPs to adopt measures that prevent televisits from becoming impersonal (Shea & Effken, 2008). Just as a home health nurse would not just knock on the door to a home and immediately begin a physical assessment without a greeting, a televisit should start with "small talk." Nurses who connect electronically to a remote patient should ask about family, pets, or other things important to the patient. Five types of televisits have been described in the literature (Winters & Winters, 2007); **Table 13-2** identifies the categories of visits and the general goals associated with each type of visit.

Table 13-2 Categories and Goals of Televisits	
Type	**Goal**
Tele-assessment	Active and engaging remote assessment
Telemonitoring	Minimally intrusive detection using sensors and measurement devices
Telesupport	Encounter is to provide support for patients and/or providers (e.g., emotional support)
Telecoaching	Support and instruction for a prescribed therapy are conveyed
Teletherapy	Engage in interactive therapy (physical or mental)

One example of a televisit is a **teleconsult**. For example, dermatologists may be consulted using electronic information and photographic data about a patient's lesions. The dermatologist adds the missing knowledge needed to provide an expert decision that directs a patient's treatment. In telepathology, digitalized tissue and cell culture data can be given meaning in a detailed diagnostic report. The report is then sent electronically to an HCP, who could be thousands of miles away, who then adds his or her own knowledge about the specific patient situation. In the case of televisits, the general practitioner may already have data, information, and knowledge but is seeking confirmation from another expert. In **telemonitoring**, patient data such as blood pressure, weight, and pulse are delivered to HCPs so that they can keep track of the condition of a patient remotely.

A BRIEF HISTORY OF TELEHEALTH

HCPs, unless living with the sick or injured patient, have always had the obstacle of distance to surmount. While the proliferation of telehealth systems and technologies may be an emerging trend, the need to urgently assess patients is not a new problem. As recently as 40 years ago, hospitals began extending care to patients in remote geographical areas by exchanging medical information via electronic communication. Novel efforts at introducing and sustaining telehealth practice have occurred commonly over the last hundred years. In 1880, shortly after the invention of the telephone, attempts were made to transmit heart and lung sounds to an expert trained in auscultation of the organs. However, poor quality in the transmission of the sounds made the assessments virtually useless and the effort failed. Other more successful uses for phone lines were later identified. Einthoven, the father of electrocardiography, wrote an article about remote transmission of electrocardiogram (EKG) tracings using a string galvanometer to register the human electrocardiogram in 1906. Alternative telecommunications technologies, such as radio, were also utilized in the development of telehealth. In the 1920s, ships at sea were connected to public health physicians at shore stations via radio. In April 1924, *Radio News Magazine* published a futuristic story of children having their throats examined remotely by a physician. With the rapid spread of telecommunications networks that began in the 1960s came the development and proliferation of a number of different methods for the transmission of video telehealth.

Bashshur (2002) discusses three major eras that shaped the development of telehealth. Contributions from the telecommunications era (1970s–1980s), the digital era (late 1980s), and the Internet era (1990s–present) have built a complex, omnipresent, global communication environment. The **telecommunications era** was characterized by television and broadcast technologies. The **digital era** integrated computerized information that could transmit voice and video data at higher speeds. The **Internet era** has enabled telehealth services such as video-conferencing, remote access to patient data and information, and rapid communication between patients and providers. Most importantly, telehealth continues to enable the provision of healthcare services to areas that would otherwise be drastically underserved. Telehealth is the product of this continued technological development, and it is still being used to address the issues of rising healthcare costs, limited providers, and a lack of access to care in rural and underserved areas.

One example from the beginning of the telehealth movement comes from the Nebraska Psychiatric Institute, which installed closed-circuit television (CCTV) during its construction in 1955 for use as a teaching tool for medical residents and a monitoring tool for the nursing staff (Mallisee & von Rosenberg, 1965). By observing sessions between patients and physicians, residents in psychiatry were able to develop more advanced techniques of psychotherapy. Nurses used CCTV to assist in monitoring areas of maximum security within the hospital. Vocational counselors at the institute later used CCTV for long-distance patient interview sessions at remotely located state hospitals.

In 1967, collaboration between Logan International Airport and Massachusetts General Hospital (MGH) resulted in the establishment of the Logan International Airport Medical Aid Station. At the aid station, employees in the airport and airline travelers could receive medical care from MGH physicians via a two-way audiovisual microwave circuit. The aid station was staffed continuously by nurses, while physicians were present during the 4 hours of each day that were determined to be peak passenger-use times. Nurses triaged each patient who visited the station, identifying those who needed further medical care. The National Aeronautics and Space Administration (NASA) also played an important part in the development of telehealth in the 1960s with the initiation of space exploration. Physiological data from the astronauts were collected by space suits and spacecraft, and transmitted to medical staff on the ground for monitoring during missions.

In the 1970s, HCPs in remote Alaskan villages, often nurses and nurses' aides, used high-frequency radio and satellite systems to connect with physicians and obtain remote care for residents. Consisting of fixed blocks of time available 3 days per week, HCPs relied on two-way voice and video technologies that allowed the transmission of electrocardiogram, electronic stethoscope, and slow-scan video for x-rays. Though project participants were glad to have video capability, the image quality of color images was poor, and therefore limited to black and white photos, and the transmission of video images required expensive equipment. Due to limited bandwidth, video transmissions frequently failed. Lessons learned from the project were later used in larger projects created to serve the people of Alaska, including creation of the Alaska Telemedicine Project (ATP; Hudson & Ferguson, 2011). Remote transmission of complex images has experienced problems resulting from limited bandwidth, connection speed, bit rates, and complications with point-of-care technology. However, telehealth applications have continued to develop for almost every facet of healthcare, with a general understanding that increased transmission speed and capacity are always on the horizon.

CURRENT APPLICATIONS OF TELEHEALTH

Application Types

Technological communication provides the opportunity for the optimal delivery of services without complications related to the physical transportation of messages or people. Being able to work outside the realm of familiar face-to-face interactions provides greater efficiency and increased frequency of communication. In the modern-day use of telehealth, two types of applications are available: real-time applications and store and forward applications. The availability of telecommunications technologies and the type of information to be transmitted plus concerns about urgency and budget influence which type of telehealth application is most appropriate. **Real-time applications** are commonly transmitted in the form of live audio/video, telephone, or webcam with transmission occurring simultaneously with the capture of the information (**Figure 13-1**). Using Skype to visit with a colleague is an example of a real-time telehealth application. Video-chat platforms, such as Skype, were developed for marketing to the general consumer, and not for health care. The choice to use Skype would be optimal if the user has a computer with high-speed Internet access and anticipates a casual discussion without the need for strict privacy. **Store and forward applications** capture data and store the data to be forwarded to HCPs at a later time (**Figure 13-2**). An example of this would be recording a visit or treatment to be consulted at a later date. Laws and policies that pertain to the protection of patient healthcare information are important in the selection of telehealth applications (these are discussed later in the chapter).

There are a number of different means for telehealth implementation ranging in complexity and capacity. Some of the simplest systems consist of a basic system to video monitor the patient. The advent of networked computing enabled the communication of vital signs and other patient data to devices at remote locations. Today, many of these systems have developed smartphone applications that enable HCPs, patients, and even family members to monitor and track illnesses. Some telehealth applications are actual medical devices on the patient's person. One example of this

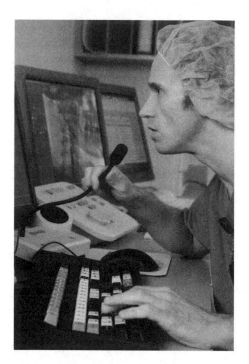

FIGURE 13-1   Remote home health using real-time transmission of video and heart sounds for a patient with heart failure.
Source: © Jupiterimages/Photos.com/Thinkstock.

type of telehealth is the advent of continuous glucose monitoring (CGM). CGM devices are minimally invasive devices that track interstitial glucose levels at intervals through the day independently of patient actions. This method of glucose observation provides a much clearer look at patients' glucose dynamics, alleviates the need for patients to actively monitor their glucose, and is capable of being communicated directly with HCPs (Klonoff, 2005).

The Need for Telehealth

Telehealth for Chronic Conditions

In 2005, 133 million Americans were living with at least one chronic illness, and that number is expected to grow to 157 million by 2020. Chronic illnesses account for 78% of the country's total health spending (Bodenheimer, Chen, & Bennett, 2009). These conditions, which include diabetes, heart disease, obstructive lung disease, and mental illness, require frequent if not constant monitoring to minimize the potential

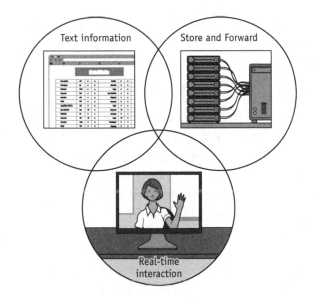

FIGURE 13-2 Types of telehealth applications: real time, regular text, and store and forward.

for exacerbation of acute disease. This makes them perfect for telehealth applications. The most common form of telehealth associated with chronic conditions is telemonitoring. Telemonitoring enables HCPs to monitor the relevant signs and symptoms of chronic diseases even when patients are out of the clinic. Telemonitoring systems not only provide HCPs with patients' vital signs, but they also give patients a way to update their HCPs on their subjective experiences of the illness.

From 2003 to 2007, the Veterans Health Administration (VHA) rolled out a national home telehealth program known as Care Coordination/Home Telehealth (CCHT). The goal of the program was defined as:

> The use of health informatics, disease management, and home telehealth technologies to enhance and extend care and case management to facilitate access to care and improve the health of designated individuals and populations with the specific intent of providing the right care in the right place at the right time. (Darkins et al., 2008)

The program focused on caring for patients with diabetes mellitus, congestive heart failure, hypertension, posttraumatic stress disorder (PTSD), chronic obstructive pulmonary disease (COPD), and depression. The tools available for use in the system included biometric devices that measured vital signs, messaging devices for patient input, videophones, and telemonitoring devices. In 2003 there were 2,000 patients enrolled in CCHT. By 2007 that number had grown to 31,570 (Darkins et al., 2008).

The most common conditions treated in CCHT were diabetes mellitus and hypertension, accounting for 48.4% and 40.3% of patients, respectively. This was followed by congestive heart failure and COPD, accounting for 24.8% and 11.6% of patients, respectively. Depression, PTSD, and other mental disorders accounted for 2.3%, 1.1%, and 1.2% of patients, respectively. The efficacy of CCHT was measured by the decrease in utilization of hospital services, as measured by both hospital admissions and bed days of care (BDOC). Each of the conditions treated saw utilization of hospital services fall by 20% or more. The largest decreases in hospital services were associated with conditions such as depression, PTSD, and other mental disorders, with declines of 56.4%, 45.1%, and 40.9%. Hypertension and chronic heart failure saw decreases of 30.3% and 25.9%; treatment for COPD and diabetes declined by 20.7% and 20.4%.

Patients and HCPs reported that the most beneficial aspect of home telehealth associated with the CCHT program was the messaging system. A direct line of communication from patient to provider greatly increased the efficacy of and capacity for self-management of chronic disease (Darkins et al., 2009). Increased communication between patients and HCPs also may have improved patient satisfaction. Quarterly patient satisfaction surveys assessed over the duration of the 4-year CCHT project revealed an average satisfaction rate of 86% (Darkins et al., 2008).

Telerehabilitation

Telerehabilitation, also known as telerehab, is defined by the American Telemedicine Association as the use of information and communication technology services to deliver rehabilitation services (Brennan et al., 2010) (**Figure 13-3**). Speech-language pathology services, with their attention to auditory and visual communication, are ideally suited for telerehabilitation services. However, many sources suggest that the routine practice of telerehabilitation in the United States has been limited due to regulatory issues relating to licensure and reimbursement, and variations in state-to-state requirements regarding the use of telerehab services (Cherney & van Vuuren, 2012). Despite these difficulties, a review of the literature suggests telerehabilitation technologies can be used to assist patients with motor speech disorders.

In a review of the international literature, Cherney and van Vuuren (2012) compared results of face-to-face assessments of dysarthria due to traumatic or hypoxic

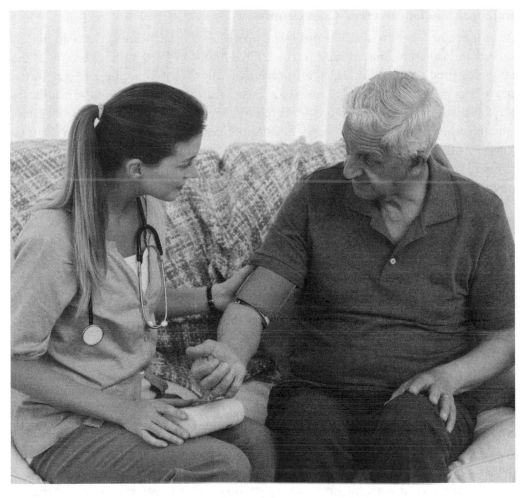

FIGURE 13-3   Providing education about oxygenation using home telemonitoring equipment in patient's home.

Source: © wavebreakmedia ltd/ShutterStock, Inc.

brain injury, Parkinson's disease, or stroke to those conducted in the telerehab environment. Though there were technical difficulties within the telerehab environment, for the majority of acoustic and perceptual parameters, clinical criteria for both face-to-face and video conferencing were similar. Cherney and van Vuuren further noted that the use of the small 128-kbit/second bandwidth hindered the detection of fine motor movements during video conferencing, and that these difficulties were more apparent for patients with severe dysarthria.

Telehealth in Underserved Communities

An important function of telehealth is the provision of healthcare services to underserved and isolated communities. In the United States in 2000, although 20% of the country's total population resided in rural areas, only 9% of U.S. physicians reported practicing in a rural area, and there was an even greater shortage of nurses, healthcare technicians, and nonphysician providers in those areas (Shea & Effken, 2008). Unfortunately, the lack of healthcare services and providers in rural areas can contribute to a self-reinforcing cycle. As the HCPs and facilities serving rural areas find themselves overworked and understaffed, rural opportunities may be less appealing to graduating medical students, and the cycle of underservice continues (Shea & Effken, 2008).

A primary purpose of the VHA's CCHT program was to address the geographical diversity of its patients (Darkins et al., 2008). Of the 31,570 total patients in the program, 31.2% lived in urban areas, 21% lived in rural areas, and 1% lived in highly rural areas. Patients who were located in highly rural areas saw the largest declines in hospital utilization, with an average reduction of 50.9%. Patients residing in urban areas utilized hospital services an average of 29.2% less, while patients living in rural areas utilized hospitals 17% less frequently over the course of the project. These declines are substantial and highlight the fact that telehealth may be most useful for those who are the most isolated.

The VHA CCHT program numbers also illustrate how telehealth programs may benefit urban communities as well as rural communities (Darkins et al., 2008). Though rural communities can suffer from a lack of HCPs in close proximity, the density of urban communities can make it more difficult to get timely appointments with HCPs despite increased numbers of HCPs in the communities. In addition, urban communities typically have more consistent access to Internet services. For these reasons, telehealth for underserved groups within urban communities should also be high priority.

Telehealth in Public Schools

Public schools in underserved areas have been identified as important opportunities for telehealth and in many cases may serve as the only exposure to assessment by HCPs that children receive (Whitten, Kingsley, Cook, Swirczynski, & Doolittle, 2001). School-based telehealth includes using telephones, teleconferences, or web cameras in the school to connect to a distant HCP. Pediatric equipment such as an otoscope or camera that transmits a static image or a stethoscope that transmits respiratory and heart sounds are valuable assets that enhance decision making for treatment when school nurses teleconsult with specialists. School nurses can use telehealth for managing common ailments encountered in the school setting, such as the examination of skin conditions (rashes, wheals, eruptions, blisters, and petechiae) and ear, nose, and throat disorders (infections of ears, tonsils, adenoids, and sinuses). Pediatric HCPs, nurses, and parents reported primary care school-based telehealth as an acceptable alternative to traditional healthcare delivery systems (Young & Ireson, 2003).

Connecting Patients with Specialists

A particularly difficult problem within health care is how to connect the most qualified HCPs with the patients who need their specific skill sets. Far too often patients have to travel hundreds or even thousands of miles to visit an appropriate specialist. Telehealth can give these patients a way to meet with the specialist they need, without having to endure the costly, troublesome process of long-distance travel. In many circumstances telehealth enables a patient's primary HCP to communicate directly with a specialist about the patient's illness and adapt treatment based on the specialist's recommendations.

Teletrauma, the remote treatment of trauma situations, is an example of a real-time application that can connect patients with specialists (**Figure 13-4**). In teletrauma, patients in rural areas or towns without access to a trauma center are able to receive the expertise of a trauma surgeon via telecommunications networks. Teletrauma services are initiated as soon as a trauma patient arrives at the rural hospital.

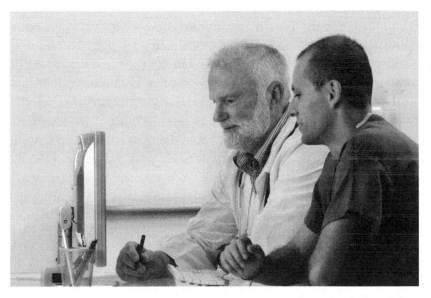

FIGURE 13-4   Teletrauma.
Source: © iStockphoto.com/YinYang.

Immediate consultation using real-time video allows the remote expert trauma surgeon to evaluate the patient's condition on arrival and work with the local emergency provider to stabilize and engage in a diagnostic workup. Early intervention from the Level I trauma expert can prevent painful, time-consuming, and unnecessary transfers. If air transfer to a Level I trauma center is required, the expert surgeon's familiarity with the case from the initiation of care can improve the quality of care that patients receive (Bjorn, 2012). One example of lifesaving teletrauma services was the case of an 18-month-old child who was the only surviving victim of an automobile accident in the remote desert near Douglas, Arizona. At the time of the accident, a trauma surgeon was able to provide direct supervision to an on-site physician via telecommunications networks. After endotracheal intubation, the delivery of blood products, and large amounts of intravenous fluids, the child was stabilized and transported to the University of Arizona Medical Center (Erps, 2008).

PRIVACY, ETHICS, AND LIMITATIONS IN TELEHEALTH

Patient Privacy

Privacy concerns are the some of the most important issues HCPs face. Patients have the right to keep their healthcare information private and protected, and it is the responsibility of HCPs to ensure this right is upheld and respected to the fullest. The use of telehealth services carries with it a host of specific privacy issues. HCPs must ensure that any means of communication that is used, be it video conferencing, direct messaging, or vital sign communication through biometric devices, is compliant with the Health Insurance Portability and Accountability Act (HIPAA). One of the most important caveats of HIPAA compliance relating to telehealth is the rule that HCPs use technology with the ability to produce audit trails, so that any potential security breaches can be tracked. HCPs are ethically driven to use telehealth to offer healthcare services to those who might otherwise not receive those services, but in doing so they should strive to adhere to best practices and a code of ethics. According to Fleming, Edison, and Pak (2009), the ethical code for telehealth pledges commitment to benevolent action, fairness, integrity, respect for others, avoiding harm, pursuing sound scholarship, and ensuring appropriate oversight. In order to ensure quality care without harm, a standardized code for telehealth practice would be valuable as an ongoing guide and reference.

Telehealth Ethics

The use of telehealth should not adversely affect the relationship between the patient and the HCP, which should be characterized by trust and respect. In addition, telehealth should not impair the ability of the HCP to engage in autonomous decision making for the best interests of the patient. Telehealth technology can be overwhelming for some older adults who are unfamiliar with communication using video and webcams; it is unethical to expect older adults to use a technology that creates stress. HCPs question the ethics of delivering a terminal diagnosis or other bad news to patients using telehealth technology (Fleming et al., 2009). Because privacy is always a concern in the use of Internet-based services, the use of telehealth is no exception. The use of any video or other recording of patients must be handled in a secure and safe manner, in such a way that it cannot be used for exploitation.

System Limitations and Downtime

As with all technological systems, the use of telehealth can have drawbacks. Computerized networks are subject to network errors and unscheduled episodes of downtime that, in the event of a health emergency, could prove devastating. HCPs who intend to implement telehealth services should make reasonable efforts to provide safeguards against the different threats to technological integrity, such as network downtime and hardware failure. In addition to the concerns associated with physical technology are the inherent limitations associated with telehealth services. Despite advances in technology, at times there is simply no acceptable substitute for a face-to-face examination by an HCP. Video and audio may not be clear enough to enable HCPs to gather all the information from a patient that is needed, and a personal visit may be warranted. It is the role of HCPs to be aware of the limitations of telehealth systems and be willing to admit those limitations, provide acceptable solutions, and, if necessary, assert the need for in-person examinations.

Licensure Issues in the United States

A regulatory aspect that has proven to be an obstacle to the delivery of telehealth services is medical and nursing licensure across state boundaries. In the United States, medical and nursing licenses are assigned at the level of the states; physicians, advanced practice nurses, and nurses may legally practice only within the boundaries of their respective state licenses. With the advent of telehealth services, there has been an increased movement to enhance licensure portability within the United States (see **Table 13-3**). However, at this time, the ability to practice telemedicine within a particular state resides within the jurisdiction of the medical board of that state. According to information from the Federation of State Medical Boards (2012), all states require that interested parties obtain a license to practice medicine within the state in which the patient is located. However, if the physician desires to practice

Table 13-3   Alternative Proposals for Licensure That Would Facilitate the Practice of Telehealth by Healthcare Providers

Model	Explanation
Consulting exceptions	With a consulting exception, a physician who is unlicensed in a particular state can practice medicine in that state at the request of and in consultation with a referring physician. The scope of these exceptions varies from state to state. Most consultation exceptions prohibit the out-of-state physician from opening an office or receiving calls in the state. In most states, these exceptions were enacted before the advent of telehealth and were not meant to apply to ongoing regular telehealth links. However, some states permit a specific number of consulting exceptions per year.
Endorsement	State boards can grant licenses to health professionals in other states with equivalent standards. Health professionals must apply for a license by endorsement from each state in which they seek to practice. States may require additional qualifications or documentation before endorsing a license issued by another state. Endorsement allows states to retain their traditional power to set and enforce standards that best meet the needs of the local population. However, complying with diverse state requirements and standards can be time consuming and expensive for a multistate practitioner.
Reciprocity	A licensure system based on reciprocity would require the authorities of each state to negotiate and enter agreements to recognize licenses issued by the other state without a further review of individual credentials. These negotiations could be bilateral or multilateral. A license valid in one state would give privileges to practice in all other states with which the home state has agreements.
Mutual recognition	Mutual recognition is a system in which the licensing authorities voluntarily enter into an agreement to legally accept the policies and processes (licensure) of a licensee's home state. Licensure based on mutual recognition is comprised of three components: a home state, a host state, and a harmonization of standards for licensure and professional conduct. The health professional secures a license in his or her own home state and is not required to obtain additional licenses to practice in other states. The nurse licensure compact is based on this model.

Table 13-3 (continued)	
Model	**Explanation**
Registration	Under a registration system, a health professional licensed in one state would inform the authorities of other states that he or she wished to practice part-time there. By registering, the health professional would agree to operate under the legal authority and jurisdiction of the other state. Health professionals would not be required to meet entrance requirements imposed upon those licensed in the host state but they would be held accountable for breaches in professional conduct in any state in which they are registered. California had the authority to draft this type of model but never did so.
Limited licensure	Under a limited licensure system, a health professional would have to obtain a license from each state in which he or she practiced but would have the option of obtaining a limited license for the delivery of specific health services under particular circumstances. Thus, the system would limit the scope rather than the time period of practice. The health professional would be required to maintain a full and unrestricted license in at least one state. The Federation of State Medical Boards has proposed a variation of this model. According to the Federation, 16 states have adopted a limited licensure model.
National licensure	A national licensure system could be adopted at the state or national level. A license would be issued based on a universal standard for the practice of health care in the United States. If administered at the national level, questions might be raised about state revenue loss, the legal authority of states, logistics about how data would be collected and processed, and how enforcement of licensure standards and discipline would be administered. If administered at the state level, these questions might be alleviated. States would have to agree on a common set of standards and criteria ranging from qualifications to discipline.
Federal licensure	Under a federal licensure system, health professionals would be issued one license, valid throughout the United States, by the federal government. Licensure would be based on federally established standards related to qualifications and discipline and would preempt state licensure laws. Federal agencies would administer the system. However, given the difficulties associated with central administration and enforcement, the states might play a role in implementation.

Source: Wakefield, M. K., Puskin, D. S., & Tipping, K. (2010). *Telehealth Licensure Report.* U.S. Department of Health and Human Services Health Resources and Services Administration. Retrieved from http://www.hrsa.gov/healthit/telehealth/licenserpt10.pdf

> **Box 13-1   Case Study**
>
> Mr. Kenneth Lister (65 years old) has multiple health problems including type 2 diabetes mellitus, severe congestive heart failure, and history of lung cancer. He was recently taken to the emergency department after he fell when trying to get out of bed. There, he was found to have a blood glucose level of 35 mg/dL and was diagnosed with uncontrolled type 2 diabetes mellitus and hypoglycemia, despite many years of well-maintained blood glucose levels. After further assessment, Mr. Lister was transferred to a medical room in the hospital. He has the following characteristics:
>
> - Medicare Parts A & B
> - Lives with wife in a remote area that is 180 miles from the closest HCP
> - Has a computer and Internet at home
>
> Mr. Lister's hospital roommate is Frank Barnes. Mr. Barnes is a 47-year-old truck driver who has been admitted for exacerbation of heart failure. Mr. Barnes is a long-haul truck driver, who is privately insured. Mr. Barnes' place of residence is his truck.
>
> Both Mr. Lister and Mr. Barnes are going home with telehealth, consisting of a telemonitoring device that transmits weight, blood pressure, blood glucose levels, and pulse oximetry to a remote telehealth nurse. Even though the use of telehealth does not often include hands-on interaction, the goal of keeping patients out of the hospital is consistent with quality nursing practice. Telehealth applications are designed to enhance the patient experience and improve clinical outcomes while providing care for patients in their home environment, rather than in institutional settings. Nurses can use telehealth in a manner that supports self-care by empowering patients, which is a central tenet of nursing practice.
>
> How will these patients benefit from telehealth services? What other applications might be necessary to reduce their risk of rehospitalization or injury? What types of telehealth applications could reduce or replace home telemonitoring?

only telemedicine, 10 states will allow for the provision of special purpose licenses that provide only for the practice of telemedicine. In addition, not every state requires that telemedicine services be reimbursed by insurers.

Licensure across state boundaries within the profession of nursing is slightly different. In 1994, the National Council of State Boards of Nursing (NCSBN) crafted a model of mutual recognition of licensure, entitled the Interstate Compact Agreement (Office of the Advancement of Telehealth, 2003). For nurses who were licensed in states that agreed to participate in the Interstate Compact Agreement, physical or electronic practice in the participating states was allowed, unless a nurse was under discipline or in a monitoring agreement that restricted practice to a home state. Currently, 24 state boards of nursing are members of the NCSBN Nurse Licensure Compact agreement. Because of the reciprocity agreements between the 24 state boards of nursing, nurses who hold unencumbered licenses within those 24 member states may practice, physically or electronically, without incurring additional applications or fees (NCSBN, n.d.).

SUMMARY

The future of telehealth is limited only by policy and the imagination, not by technology. Continued research is required to develop best practices for telehealth delivery. Telehealth should not be considered a replacement for face-to-face interventions, but another tool to be utilized alongside face-to-face interventions in the pursuit of the highest quality of care. As research and practice continue, the telehealth field will continue to grow and change. HCPs should embrace this change, work to stay abreast of technological changes, and constantly be reassessing their methods and standards of care. The ability to reach patients who otherwise would not have access to care is a tremendous opportunity for improving the quality of health in the United States. Whether in an urban or rural community, a busy hospital or a small private practice, patients and HCPs across all spectrums of health care can and will continue to benefit from telehealth services.

> (WWW) For a full suite of assignments and additional learning activities, use the access code located in the front of your book and visit www.jblearning.com. If you do not have an access code, you can obtain one at the site.

REFERENCES

Bashshur, R. L. (2002). Telemedicine and health care. *Telemedicine Journal and E-Health*, *8*(1), 5–9.

Bjorn, P. (2012). Rural teletrauma: Applications, opportunities, and challenges. *Advanced Emergency Nursing Journal*, *34*(3), 232–237.

Bodenheimer, T., Chen, E., & Bennett, H. D. (2009). Confronting the growing burden of chronic disease: Can the U.S. health care workforce do the job? *Health Affairs*, *28*(1), 64–74. doi: 10.1377/hlthaff.28.1.64

Brennan, D. M., Tindall, L., Theodoros, D., Brown, J., Campbell, M., Christiana, D., . . . Lee, A. (2010). A blueprint for telerehabilitation guidelines. *Telemedicine E-Health*, *17*, 662–665.

Cherney, L. R., & van Vuuren, S. (2012). Telerehabilitation, virtual therapists, and acquired neurologic speech and language disorders. *Seminars in Speech and Language*, *33*(3), 243–257. doi: 10.1055/s-0032-1320044

Darkins, A., Ryan, P., Kobb, R., Foster, L., Edmonson, E., Wakefield, B., & Lancaster, A. E. (2008). Care coordination/home telehealth: The systematic implementation of health informatics, home telehealth, and disease management to support the care of veteran patients with chronic conditions. *Telemedicine and e-Health*, *14*(10), 1118–1125. doi: 10.1089/tmj.2008.0021

Davis, M. A., Kirby, S. L., & Curtis, M. B. (2007). The influence of affect on goal choice and task performance. *Journal of Applied Social Psychology*, *37*(1), 14–42.

Erps, K. (2008). A life saved through new teletrauma service. The University of Arizona Telemedicine Program. Retrieved from http://www.telemedicine.arizona.edu/app/press-releases/A%20 Life%20Saved%20through%20New%20Teletrauma%20Service

Federation of State Medical Boards. (2012). Telemedicine overview: Board-by-board approach. Retrieved from http://www.fsmb.org/pdf/grpol_telemedicine_licensure.pdf

Fleming, D. A., Edison, K. E., & Pak, H. (2009). Telehealth ethics. *Journal of Telemedicine and eHealth*, *15*(8), 797–803. doi: 10.1089/tmj.2009.0035

Health Resources and Services Administration. (2012). Telehealth. Retrieved from http://www.hrsa.gov/ruralhealth/about/telehealth/

Hudson, H., & Ferguson, S. (2011). Telemedicine in Alaska: From ATS-1 to AFHCAN. Anchorage, AK: The University of Alaska at Anchorage's Institute of Social and Economic Research. Retrieved from http://www.iser.uaa.alaska.edu/Projects/akbroadbandproj/telecomsymposium/ HudsonATS1toAFHCAN.pdf

Klonoff, D. C. (2005). Continuous glucose monitoring. *Diabetes Care*, *28*(5), 1231–1239. doi: 10.2337//diacare.28.5.1231

Mallisee, M. E., & von Rosenberg, R. H. (1965). Closed circuit television in the rehabilitation of the mentally ill (unpublished manuscript). Retrieved from http://library.ncrtm.org/pdf/357.015.pdf

National Council of the State Boards of Nursing. (n.d.). *Nurse licensure compact*. Retrieved from https://www.ncsbn.org/nlc.htm

Office of the Advancement of Telehealth. (2003). *Telemedicine licensure report*. Retrieved from http://www.hrsa.gov/ruralhealth/about/telehealth/licenserpt03.pdf

Shea, K., & Effken, J. A. (2008). Enhancing patients' trust in the virtual home healthcare nurse. *CIN: Computers, Informatics & Nursing*, *26*(3), 135–141.

Terry, K. (2013, January 23). Telehealth to grow six-fold by 2017. *Information Week*. Retrieved from http://www.informationweek.com/healthcare/mobile-wireless/telehealth-to-grow-six-fold- by-2017/240146847

U.S. Department of Health and Human Services. (2013). *Healthy people 2020*. Retrieved from http://www.healthypeople.gov/2020/default.aspx

Whitten, P., Kingsley, C., Cook, D., Swirczynski, D., & Doolittle, G. (2001). School-based telehealth: An empirical analysis of teacher, nurse, and administrator perceptions. *Journal of School Health*, *71*(5), 173–179.

Winters, J. M., & Winters, J. M. P. (2007). Videoconferencing and telehealth technologies can provide a reliable approach to remote assessment and teaching without compromising quality. *Journal of Cardiovascular Nursing*, *22*(1), 51–57.

Young, L., & Ireson, C. (2003). Effectiveness of school-based telehealth care in urban and rural elementary schools. *Pediatrics*, *112*(5), 1088–1094.

CHAPTER 14

Mobile Health Applications

Mladen Milosevic, PhD
Emil Jovanov, PhD
Aleksandar Milenkovic, PhD

CHAPTER LEARNING OBJECTIVES

1. Define mobile health (mHealth) and mHealth applications.
2. Describe mHealth systems architecture.
3. Identify the potential of mobile applications in health care.
4. Describe challenges to the adoption of mHealth applications.

KEY TERMS

mHealth	Smartphones
Mobile apps	Wearable sensors
Mobile health monitoring	

CHAPTER OVERVIEW

This chapter discusses mobile health, or **mHealth**—an emerging practice of medicine, public health, and wellness enabled and supported by mobile communication devices such as **smartphones** and tablets. Continual advances and proliferation of mobile computing and communication devices, wearable health monitors, cellular networks, satellites, and cloud computing services will likely make mHealth a mainstream healthcare service in the future. The mHealth technologies can be used by healthcare providers (HCP) to improve healthcare delivery and by consumers to improve their own health. The use of mHealth has the potential to reduce healthcare costs and improve quality of life, but challenges with the technology exist.

INTRODUCTION

The National Institutes of Health (NIH) Consensus Group defined mHealth as "the use of mobile wireless communication devices to improve health outcomes, health care services, and health research" (Health Resources and Services Administration [HRSA], n.d.). mHealth holds the promise to radically modernize and change the way healthcare services are deployed and delivered. mHealth applications can enhance diagnosis, prevent disease, improve treatments, improve accessibility to health care, and advance health-related research. There is overlap of mHealth with telehealth, but mHealth tends to be more distributed and includes technology used by HCPs with patients and by consumers without the supervision of HCPs.

A typical mHealth system used by HCPs consists of devices used by patients such as weight scales, glucometers, or **wearable sensors** that transmit data by wireless technology to a patient's smartphone or other mobile communication device (Rajan, 2012). The communication device uses cellular technology to send data to a designated server, which in turn sends data to the HCP. In this way, patients use devices that allow monitoring of particular health parameters anywhere, called **mobile health monitoring**, and data from patients' medical devices populate HCPs' electronic health records (EHR). The transactions are transparent to patients and HCPs, but sophisticated networks make mHealth possible (Rajan, 2012).

mHEALTH BENEFITS

mHealth represents a new trend in healthcare management and delivery. Improved availability and immediate feedback facilitate a shift in care from reaction to symptoms to promotion of wellness and health. Mobile health monitoring and integrated information system support provide distinct benefits to each segment of the healthcare system. Benefits for patients include increased access to healthcare information, increased quality of life by focusing on prevention and early detection of disease, better diagnostics, affordability, instantaneous feedback, improved confidence, and promotion and encouragement of healthy lifestyles. Benefits for HCPs include better diagnostics and treatment facilitated by collection and processing of records collected at home and during daily living activities, monitoring of reaction (including adverse) to drugs and treatment, and instantaneous suggestions and advice to patients. Benefits for informal caregivers include remote monitoring and access to real-time and long-term trends of healthcare parameters. This is particularly important in the case of care for chronically ill family members. Researchers will benefit from significantly larger and more relevant databases of patient records. Physiological records collected at home will better represent the state of users and dynamics of daily and monthly changes of relevant physiological parameters. Data mining of large databases will provide assessment of patient-specific responses and treatments and discovery of new approaches.

DRIVING FORCES FOR mHEALTH

The anticipated change and emerging new services are well timed to help cope with the imminent crisis in healthcare systems caused by current economic, social, and demographic trends. The overall healthcare expenditures in the United States reached $2.5 trillion in 2009 (U.S. Census Bureau, 2012), though almost 49.9 million Americans do not have health insurance (DeNavas-Walt, Proctor, & Smith, 2011). On the other hand, many companies have already been plagued by high-rising costs of health care. With current trends in healthcare costs, it is projected that the total healthcare expenditures will reach $4.5 trillion by 2020 or almost 20% of the gross domestic product (GDP), threatening the wellbeing of the entire economy (Centers for Medicare & Medicaid Services [CMS], 2010). The Brookings Institute estimates that nearly $200 billion could be saved in healthcare expenditures with the use of mHealth (West, 2012).

The demographic trends are indicating two significant phenomena: an aging population due to increased life expectancy and the demographic peak of Baby Boomers in the over-65 age group. Life expectancy has significantly increased from 49 years in 1901 to 77.6 years in 2003, and it is projected to reach 82.6 years by 2040 (National Institute on Aging, 2013). According to the U.S. Census Bureau (2011), the number of elderly over age 65 is expected to double from 39.6 million in 2009 (or 13% of the total population) to nearly 70 million by 2025 when the youngest Baby Boomers retire, and reach 88.5 million by 2050 (or 20% of the total population). This trend is global, and the worldwide population over age 65 is expected to almost triple from 545 million in 2011 to 1.55 billion in 2050 (National Institute on Aging, 2013). These statistics underscore the need for more scalable and more affordable healthcare solutions.

At the same time, advances in technology are occurring at a rapid pace, and technology is being adopted by millions of people in the United States and across the world. The Pew Internet and American Life Project reported that as of May 2013, 91% of adult Americans own cell phones, and half of those cell phones are smartphones (Brenner, 2013). The ownership of all mobile technologies in the United States is on the rise, while stationary technology is losing favor (see **Figure 14-1**). New wearable technology—electrocardiography (ECG) sensors, electroencephalography (EEG)

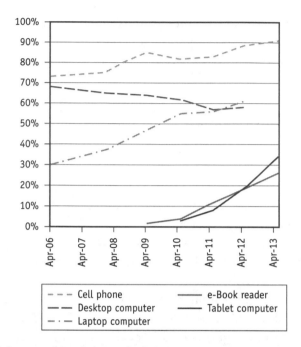

FIGURE 14-1   Adult ownership of electronic devices.

Source: Pew Internet surveys 2006–2013 at http://pewinternet.org/Commentary/2012/February/Pew-Internet-Mobile.aspx. Used by permission.

sensors, motion sensors, and many other types—is emerging rapidly (Wearable Technologies, 2013). Electronic sensors, power sources, and wearable materials are integrated in fabrics, polymers, and metals. The market for wearable technology is expected to exceed $6 billion by the year 2016 (Wearable Technologies, 2013). The company, Wearable Technologies, describes a new gadget each month on its website; however, not all technologies are for health and wellness (refer to the companion website of this text).

mHEALTH SYSTEMS FOR HCPs AND RESEARCHERS

Jovanov, Milenkovic, Otto, and De Groen (2005) developed an mHealth system incorporating a number of components, ranging from personal health monitors worn by patients to medical services running on computer servers accessed over the Internet. **Figure 14-2** shows a three-tiered mHealth architecture, which is described in detail in the sections that follow (Jovanov et al., 2005; Milenkovic, Otto, & Jovanov, 2006). Tier 1 consists of one or more wearable monitors (mHealth monitors), Tier 2 includes an mHealth application (mHealth app) running on a personal communication device, and Tier 3 includes mHealth services accessed via the Internet.

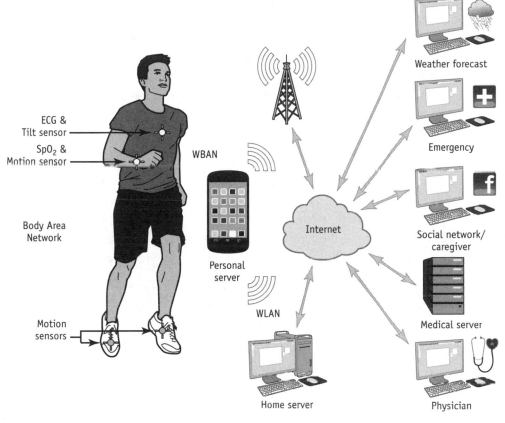

FIGURE 14-2 mHealth architecture.

Tier 1

A pivotal part of the mHealth system is Tier 1. It includes one or more wearable devices strategically placed on the human body that can monitor (a) physiological signals; (b) body posture, type, and level of physical activity; and (c) environmental conditions (Jovanov et al., 2005; Milenkovic et al., 2006). The exact number and type of physiological signals to be measured, processed, and reported depends on mHealth application. Tier 1 may include any subset of the following physiological sensors:

- ECG sensor for monitoring heart activity
- EEG sensor for monitoring brain electrical activity
- Electromyography (EMG) sensor for monitoring muscle activity

- Photoplethysmography (PPG) sensor for monitoring of pulse and blood oxygen saturation
- Cuff-based pressure sensor for monitoring blood pressure
- Resistive or piezoelectric chest belt sensor for monitoring respiration (breathing rate)
- Galvanic skin response (GSR) sensor for monitoring a subject's autonomous nervous system arousal
- Blood glucose level sensor
- Thermistor for monitoring of body temperature

In addition to the physiological signals, mHealth wearable monitors may include sensors that can help determine user's location, discriminate between user's states (e.g., lying, sitting, walking, or running), or estimate the type and level of the user's physical activity (e.g., low-, moderate-, or high-intensity aerobic activity; Jovanov et al., 2005; Milenkovic et al., 2006). These monitors typically include the following:

- Localization sensor (e.g., global positioning system [GPS])
- Tilt sensor for monitoring of trunk position
- Gyroscope-based sensor for gait-phase detection
- Accelerometer-based motion sensors on extremities and trunk to estimate type and level of the user's activity
- Smart sock or an insole sensor to count steps and/or delineate phases and distribution of forces during individual steps

Environmental conditions may often influence the user's physiological state (e.g., it has been shown that blood pressure may depend on the subject's ambient temperature) or accuracy of the sensors (e.g., background light may influence the readings from photoplethysmography sensors). Consequently, mHealth monitors may benefit from integrating the third group of sensors that provide information about environmental conditions, such as humidity, light, ambient temperature, atmospheric pressure, and noise (Jovanov et al., 2005; Milenkovic et al., 2006).

A number of commercial wearable monitors have been introduced recently. **Figure 14-3** shows a subset of commercially available wearable monitors used at Tier 1. For example, the Zephyr Technologies BioHarness device placed in a chest belt or shirt with a conductive textile can monitor a user's heart activity, including heart rate, R wave to R wave (RR) intervals, or even ECG signal; breathing rate; and body posture and level of activity by integrating inertial sensors (Zephyr BioHarness BT, n.d.). Several manufacturers introduced headphones with EEG sensors for monitoring brain electrical activity (Emotiv, 2013).

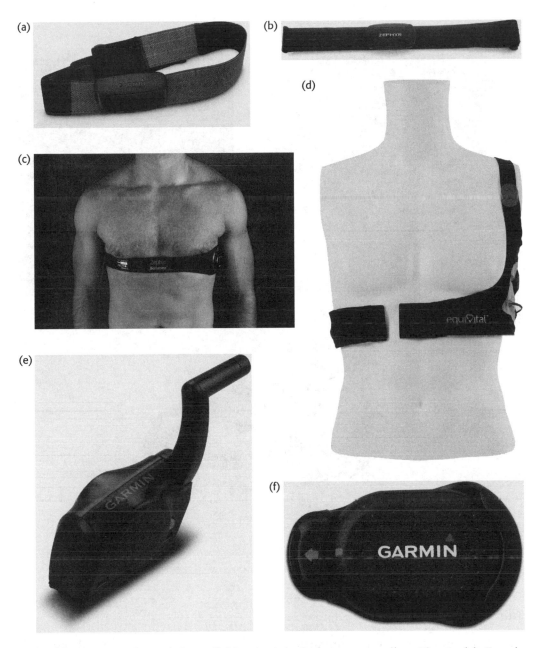

FIGURE 14-3 Commercially available physiological sensors used on Tier 1: (a) Garmin ANT+heart monitor, (b) Zephyr HxM heart rate monitor, (c) Zephyr BioHarness 3 physiological monitor, (d) Hidalgo Equivital 2 physiological monitor, (e) Garmin ANT+bike and cadence sensor, (f) Garmin ANT+foot pod, (g) Zeo sleep monitor, (h) NeuroSky MindSet EEG sensor, (i) Emotiv EEG neuroheadset.

(g)

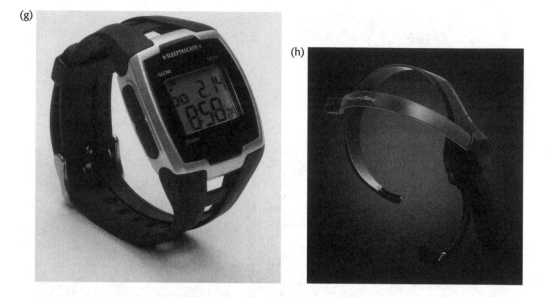

(h)

(i)

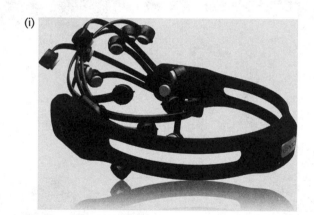

FIGURE 14-3   *(continued)*

Tier 2

Tier 2 encompasses a personal mHealth application that runs on a personal device. A typical mHealth app provides interfaces to (a) the mHealth monitors to configure them and retrieve data periodically from them; (b) the user to report the status, and provide feedback and guidance; and (c) the medical servers to upload the status information and receive feedback generated at the server (Jovanov et al., 2005; Milenkovic et al., 2006).

Proliferation of smartphones with standardized operating systems (OS) such as Apple's iOS or Google's Android makes smartphones an ideal platform for mHealth applications. User's health data collected from mHealth monitors can be sent to the medical servers and then integrated into the user's medical record. **Figure 14-4** shows several recent smartphones suitable for running mHealth applications.

Tier 3

Tier 3 includes mHealth servers accessed via the Internet. In addition to the medical server, the last tier may encompass other servers, such as informal caregivers, commercial healthcare services, and even emergency services (Jovanov et al., 2005; Milenkovic et al., 2006). The medical server keeps electronic medical records of

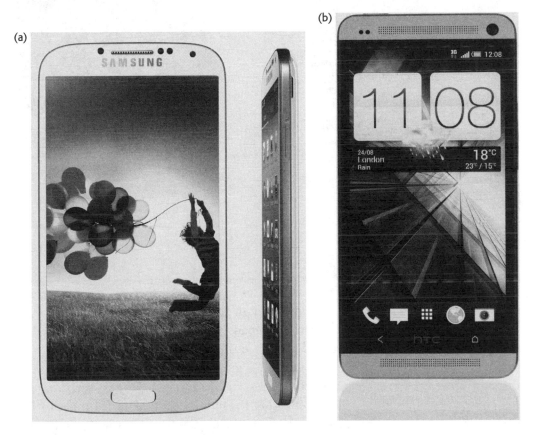

FIGURE 14-4   Smartphones: Samsung Galaxy S4, HTC One, Apple iPhone 5, and Blackberry 10.

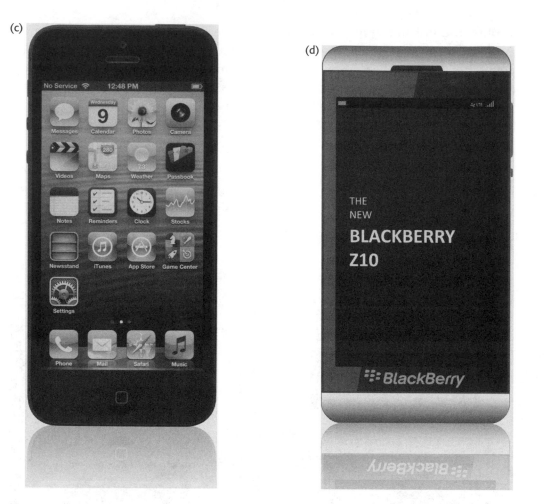

FIGURE 14-4   *(continued)*

registered users and provides various services to the users, medical personnel, and informal caregivers. It is the responsibility of the medical server to authenticate users, accept health-monitoring session uploads, format and insert the session data into corresponding medical records, analyze the data patterns, recognize serious health anomalies in order to contact emergency caregivers, and forward new instructions to the users, such as HCP-prescribed exercises (Jovanov et al., 2005; Milenkovic et al., 2006). The patient's HCP can access the data from his or her office via the Internet and examine them to ensure the patient is within expected health metrics (heart rate, blood pressure, activity), ensure that the patient is responding to a given treatment, or that a patient has been performing prescribed exercises. A server agent may inspect the uploaded data and create an alert in the case of a potential medical condition.

The large amount of data collected through these services can also be used for knowledge discovery through data mining. Integration of the collected data into research databases and quantitative analysis of conditions and patterns likely will prove invaluable to researchers trying to link symptoms and diagnoses with historical changes in health status, physiological data, or other parameters (e.g., gender, age, weight). In a similar way, mHealth systems could significantly contribute to monitoring and studying of drug therapy effects (Jovanov et al., 2005; Milenkovic et al., 2006).

mHEALTH SYSTEM IN ACTION: A CASE STUDY OF CARDIAC REHABILITATION

Peter is recovering from a heart attack. After his release from the hospital, Peter attended supervised cardiac rehabilitation for several weeks. His recovery process goes well, and Peter is to continue a prescribed exercise regimen at home. However, the unsupervised rehabilitation at home does not go well for Peter. He does not follow the exercise regimen as prescribed. He exercises but does not truthfully disclose to the treating HCP the minimal intensity and duration of his exercise. As a result, Peter's recovery is slower than expected, which raises concerns about his health status by his HCP. Is the damage to Peter's heart greater than initially suspected, or is he not adherent to the medical plan? The latter question is not answerable if his HCP has no way to verify his adherence to the exercise program.

An mHealth monitoring system offers a solution for Peter and all persons undergoing cardiac rehabilitation at home. Peter is equipped with an mHealth monitor that captures his heart activity and his physical activity. The time and duration of his normal and exercise activity are recorded, and the level of intensity of the exercise can be determined by calculating an estimate of energy expenditure from the motion sensors. The information is available on Peter's smartphone, which runs an mHealth app for cardiac rehabilitation. This app may also assist Peter in his exercise efforts: It may alert him that he has not initiated or is not reaching his intended goals, or generate warnings in case of excess exercise (e.g., heart rate is above the maximum threshold for a person of his age, weight, and condition).

Through the Internet, his HCP can collect and review all data, verify that Peter is exercising regularly, issue new prescribed exercises, adjust data threshold values, and schedule office visits. Peter's description of his progress continues to be important, but his HCP no longer needs to rely on only subjective descriptions. Instead the HCP has an objective and quantitative data set of his level and duration of exercise. In addition, Peter's parameters of heart rate variability provide a direct measure of his physiological response to the exercise, serving as an in-home stress test. Substituting these remote stress tests and data collection for in-office tests, Peter's HCP reduces the number of office visits. This decreases healthcare costs and makes better use of the HCP's time.

mHEALTH APPLICATIONS (APPs) FOR HCPs

With the recent explosion of the number of smartphone applications and the increase in smartphone performance, a number of **mobile apps** for HCPs have become available. Mobile apps for HCPs are built primarily for Apple iOS and Android OS. The iTunes store contains a large number of apps for HCPs, as does the Google Play store. Both app stores include medical references, patient education, and healthcare workflow management.

Medical References

Medical reference applications help medical professionals and other users to find information related to a broad spectrum of medical topics, such as anesthesiology, cardiology, and dermatology. Medical reference applications, such as *Netter's Anatomy Atlas* (Elsevier, 2012; Skyscape, 2012), *Dorland's Illustrated Medical* (Mobile Systems, Inc., 2013a; Mobile Systems, Inc., 2013b), *Surgical Anatomy* (Archibald Industries, 2011), and *BioDigital Human* (BioDigital Systems, 2012), provide detailed information and graphical illustrations of the human anatomy. These applications can be used by students in many different health disciplines, HCPs, or other interested individuals. The *Epocrates* application (Epocrates, 2013) is designed to help HCPs, and it is particularly helpful to nurses. It allows reviewing of drug prescribing and safety information for thousands of drugs, checking for potentially harmful drug–drug interactions, provides national and regional healthcare insurance formularies for drug coverage information, and helps identify pills by imprint code and physical characteristics. *Epocrates* can also perform dozens of calculations, such as body mass index (BMI) and glomerular filtration rate (GFR). HCPs can access medical news and research information using *Epocrates*.

Mobile applications can significantly facilitate evidence-based practice (EBP) and allow easy integration of clinical expertise and external scientific evidence with high-quality services delivered to the patient. A widely used EBP app is *UpToDate* (2013). It provides synthesis of research evidence and recommendations for practice. Another application that facilitates EBP is the *Evidence Based Treatment of Behavioral Symptoms of Dementia* application (University of Illinois, 2013), which is used to assist HCPs to assess patients for dementia. Similarly, the *BrainAttack* application (PHI Consulting, 2012) facilitates determining tissue plasminogen activator (tPA) eligibility for acute stroke victims. *Heart Failure Trials* by Clinical AppStracts LLC (n.d.) is an app to help HCPs keep track of clinical trials for the treatment of heart failure.

Patient Education

Apps can be used to provide education for patients during interactions with HCPs. For example, the *Cardiac Catheterization* application (ArchieMD Inc, 2013) uses visual animations for patient education about heart procedures. *Assist Me with Inhalers* application (Saralsoft LLC, 2012) teaches patients how to use their inhalers. Another useful and highly rated patient education tool, *drawMD*, is available for iPads (drawMD, 2013). Using this app, HCPs in many different specialties can open anatomical images and draw directly on the image to explain procedures or surgery. The images can be saved to EHRs as documentation of patient education.

Healthcare Workflow Management

Healthcare workflow management applications assist HCPs in their everyday activities. HCPs can remotely access patients' historical health records, their current vitals, or use them for pharmaceutical calculations. Airstrip Technologies (2010) has developed a hospital workflow management mobile application, *AirStrip Patient Monitoring*, for real-time and historical access of patients' physiological data. Healthcare workflow management applications can also help patients to communicate with their HCP's office to see their appointment summary, lab results, and other personal health data.

mHEALTH APPLICATIONS (APPs) FOR CONSUMERS

Consumers like gadgets! The Pew Research Center's Internet & American Life Project reported smartphone users engage in many different activities including checking news and weather forecasts, getting navigation directions, using social media, checking bank balances, getting coupons, and getting health information (Brenner, 2013). Around 40% of adults responding to the Pew survey download apps, and 30% report using smartphones for health and wellness monitoring and management. Dolan (2012) reported that growth of health and wellness apps on iTunes increases every year; as of April 2012, there were more than 13,000 such apps available for download.

Most health-related smartphone applications are dedicated to health and wellness monitoring and management. Such applications include monitoring and management of cardio fitness, diet, medication adherence, stress, sleep, mental health, and chronic disease. In order to perform a specific task, the applications need some type of input information. This information can be manually entered by users or it can be automatically sensed by built-in sensors.

Calorie Counter by FatSecret (FatSecret, 2013) and *MyPlate* (LIVESTRONG. COM, 2011) are examples of applications that help users to keep track of their meals, exercise, and weight. These applications rely on user input as the source of the necessary information. Users can manually enter the name, type, and number of calories for each nutrient, or they can use a built-in barcode scanner through smartphone's camera. Similarly, *Fitness Buddy FREE* (Azumio Inc., 2013) is designed to help with training regimens. The application can help in learning new exercises, keeping track of all workouts, and potentially improving motivation and enforcing commitment to fitness goals.

Aforementioned applications rely solely on user input as their source of information. Although this approach can be cheaper and easier to use because it does not require additional devices to be purchased and connected to a smartphone, often user input is not accurate enough or in some cases it cannot be used. Tracking of physical activity is one example where manual user input through surveys can be used, but it is not accurate because it relies on user's subjective assessment. A better approach is using sensors for tracking physical activity. *Accupedo Pedometer* (Corusen LLC, 2013) is a smartphone applications that uses the smartphone's built-in sensors to assess the number of steps the user makes during his or her daily activities. Other applications such as *Endomondo Sports Tracker* (Endomondo Sports Tracker, n.d.) utilize external sensors such as external pedometers and bike speed and cadence sensors to assess user's physical activity. Furthermore, *Endomondo Sports Tracker* supports continuous tracking of cardio fitness using external heart rate monitors.

The effect of consumer mHealth apps on wellness or disease self-management is uncertain, and more research is needed (Vodopivec-Jamsek, de Jongh, Gurol-Urganci, Atun, & Car, 2012). However, studies of particular chronic conditions have shown some promise. Studies of smoking cessation with medications and text messaging to support behavior change and tips for quitting have been shown to be effective (Whittaker et al., 2012). For people seeking weight loss, one study showed that mobile technology that delivered messages enhanced adherence and improved weight loss (Burke et al., 2012). Other studies show that people who use mHealth applications have consistent exercise patterns and improved self-efficacy (West, 2012). **Box 14-1** provides a case study for consumer use of mHealth apps.

Box 14-1   Case Study

Julie and Rachel had been friends for several years and enjoyed spending time together. Both gained more than 20 pounds and realized they needed to change their eating and exercise habits to lose weight. Julie suggested that they become accountability partners for their weight loss journey. Because they both had smartphones, they decided to use apps to help themselves lose weight. Rachel found several apps to help them determine the number of calories in foods, plan low-calorie meals that were balanced among the food groups, and record food intake. Julie recommended they purchase a reliable mobile sensor that would send data to their smartphones with an mHealth app to track their energy expenditure. The app could be synchronized with a website. They could share the progress with friends using a social media plug-in. Julie also found apps that showed exercises for different muscle groups and a sensible running plan that moved them from no exercise to jogging for 1 mile. When one of the friends felt she was about to "stress eat," she would send an "SOS" text message to the other. A quick response provided the needed support to avoid food as a stress reducer. Although there were days when they ate foods higher in calories than planned or missed exercise, at the end of 3 months they reached their weight goals.

- Did Julie and Rachel need to be supervised by an HCP to use mHealth apps?
- Do Julie and Rachel need to be concerned about their health data on their smartphones or the website?
- Would the U.S. Food and Drug Administration (FDA) be interested in regulating the mHealth apps that Julie and Rachel used?

---

mHEALTH CHALLENGES

Health-monitoring systems have benefited from the fact that mHealth technologies are driven by consumer markets, particularly cell phone technology and portable communication platforms (e.g., smartphones, laptops, tablets). This is evident by significant improvement of power efficiency of processors and microcontrollers since the 1990s. This trend will continue as basic technologies continue to mature. However, the full potential of mHealth-based systems can be achieved only if all users are aware of the remaining technological challenges. As wearable monitoring technology progresses from academic prototypes to commercial products, it is important to understand current challenges and interaction of humans with technology. Acceptance of mHealth systems is and will continue to be determined primarily by ease of use and reliability, meaningful feedback to users, price, and privacy and security of data.

Human factors, such as wearability, reliability, and interface design are crucial for any personal technology, particularly if used by older adults. It is necessary to employ user-centered design and quantify users' satisfaction of wearable health monitoring systems for everyday use (McCurdie et al., 2012). Research and clinical studies are needed to further evaluate new systems to test the willingness of users to adopt mHealth technologies. Wearability is mostly determined by the size and weight of sensors, ease of mounting and application, and seamless integration of sensors in the system. Size and weight of sensors are mostly determined by the size and weight of batteries selected to support certain sensor functionality for a predefined period of time. Some of the widely accepted technologies, such as WiFi and Bluetooth, do not provide power efficiency necessary for the ambulatory health monitoring systems. Therefore, sensor design must take into account user factors from the beginning of sensor design. New technologies, such as smart textiles, allow for integration of sensors into clothing and commonly used objects, and this will likely improve acceptance of such systems (McCurdie et al., 2012).

Reliability issues span all components in mHealth systems. Individual sensors and their communication networks (short-range communication in the wireless body area networks and/or long-range communication over cellphone network) must provide continuous, high-quality service. Dropped data due to problems with sensors or communication technology remains an issue. Medical servers will need to have redundancy and backup. Servers will need to handle vast amounts of data generated from mobile health monitoring, and this means servers will need to be managed by network experts. The reliability and validity of feedback to HCPs and patients is particularly important if data analytical techniques are used. The techniques require advanced statistics and computer coding; data scientists who understand physiological data will be required.

Issues related to privacy, integrity, and confidentiality of protected health information were addressed by the Health Insurance Portability and Accountability Act of 1996 (HIPAA) and updated by the Health Information Technology for Economic and Clinical Health (HITECH) Act of 2009. mHealth systems must provide support for privacy and confidentiality on each level of the system. For covered entities (hospitals, medical practices, and other HCPs) and business associates of covered entities, administrative and technological practices to safeguard protected health information must be planned, implemented, and regularly evaluated. Failure to comply with regulations will result in fines (Rinehart-Thompson, 2013).

The FDA (2013) announced its regulation of a subset of mobile medical devices. The FDA regulations for mobile medical applications will:

> focus on a subset of mobile apps that either have traditionally been considered medical devices or affect the performance or functionality of a currently regulated medical device. The FDA believes that this subset of mobile apps poses the same or similar potential risk to the public health as currently regulated devices if they fail to function as intended. (FDA, 2013)

In its final report, *Mobile Medical Applications: Guidance for Industry and Food and Drug Administration Staff*, the FDA limited the regulatory reach based on the *intended use* for mobile medical apps. Apps available for use by the general public on iTunes or Google Play are specifically not regulated by the FDA. The definition of a medical device and intended use are provided below.

> Products that are built with or consist of computer and/or software components or applications are subject to regulation as devices when they meet the definition of a device in section 201(h) of the FD&C Act. That provision defines a device as ". . . an instrument, apparatus, implement, machine, contrivance, implant, in vitro reagent, or other similar or related article, including any component, part, or accessory", that is ". . . intended for use in the diagnosis of disease or other conditions, or in the cure, mitigation, treatment, or prevention of disease, in man . . ." or ". . . intended to affect the structure or any function of the body of man or other animals . . . ." Thus, software applications that run on a desktop computer, laptop computer, remotely on a website or "cloud," or on a handheld computer may be subject to device regulation if they are intended for use in the diagnosis or the cure, mitigation, treatment, or prevention of disease, or to affect the structure or any function of the body of man. The level of regulatory control necessary to assure safety and effectiveness varies based upon the risk the device presents to public health. (FDA, 2013, pp. 7)

Only a few mHealth apps have FDA approval at this time. **Table 14-1** provides two mHealth devices approved by the FDA. Other relevant mHealth resources and their Internet addresses are located in **Table 14-2** and at the companion website to this text.

Table 14-1 mHealth Apps Approved by the FDA	
mHealth App	**Available from**
AT&T mHealth DiabetesManager, FDA-approved mobile app designed to coach patients through positive behavior change and decision making	https://play.google.com/store/apps/details?id=com.welldoc.diabetesmanager&feature=search_result#?t=W251bGwsMSwxLDEsImNvbS53Wx-sZG9jLmRpYWJldGVzbWFuYWdlciJd
MedWatcher, created in collaboration with the FDA and Center for Devices and Radiologic Health (CDRH), provides news and alerts for medical devices, drugs, and vaccines.	https://play.google.com/store/apps/details?id=org.medwatcher&feature=search_result#?t=W251bGwsMSwyLDEsIm9yZy5tZWR3YXR-jaGVyIl0

Table 14-2 Internet Resources for mHealth	
Resource	**Website**
Health Resources and Services Administration: List of federal agencies involved in mHealth	http://www.hrsa.gov/healthit/mhealthfedpro.html#NIH
U.S. Department of Health and Human Services: Your Mobile Device and Health Information Privacy and Security	http://www.healthit.gov/providers-professionals/your-mobile-device-and-health-information-privacy-and-security
Wearable Technologies: Gadgets of the Month	http://www.wearable-technologies.com/gadgets-of-the-month/
Your Mobile Device and Health Information Privacy and Security: Videos and Education	http://www.healthit.gov/providers-professionals/your-mobile-device-and-health-information-privacy-and-security
Tips for HCPs using Mobile Devices Containing Protected Health Information	http://www.healthit.gov/providers-professionals/how-can-you-protect-and-secure-health-information-when-using-mobile-device
U.S. Food and Drug Administration: Draft Guidance for Industry and Food and Drug Administration Staff—Mobile Medical Applications	http://www.fda.gov/downloads/MedicalDevices/DeviceRegulationandGuidance/GuidanceDocuments/UCM263366.pdf

SUMMARY

The proliferation of mobile computing and communication devices designed to improve health and wellness will continue to influence the care provided by nurses and all HCPs in the future. As the life expectancy and healthcare needs of U.S. citizens increase, the capabilities of mHealth applications to collect physiological data and interface with smartphones and Internet-based medical servers will become critical in monitoring patients' responses and adherence to treatments. In addition, the aggregation of data generated from wearable physiologic sensors and their companion devices will continue to assist researchers and HCPs in answering clinical questions.

For a full suite of assignments and additional learning activities, use the access code located in the front of your book and visit www.jblearning.com. If you do not have an access code, you can obtain one at the site.

REFERENCES

AirStrip Technologies LLC. (2010). *AirStrip – Patient monitoring*. Retrieved from https://itunes.apple.com/us/app/airstrip-patient-monitoring/id399665195?mt=8

Archibald Industries. (2011). *Surgical anatomy - Premium edition*. Retrieved from https://itunes.apple.com/us/app/surgical-anatomy-premium-edition/id368728329?mt=8

ArchieMD Inc. (2013). *ICHealth: Cardiac catheterization*. Retrieved from https://itunes.apple.com/us/app/archiemd-ichealth-cardiac/id592468810?mt=8

Azumio Inc. (2013). *Fitness buddy Free*. (n.d.). Retrieved from https://itunes.apple.com/us/app/fitness-buddy-free-300+-exercise/id514780106?mt=8

BioDigital Systems. (2012). *BioDigital human*. Retrieved from https://itunes.apple.com/us/app/biodigital-human/id581713009?mt=8

Brenner, J. (2013). Internet & American Life Project. *Pew Internet: Mobile*. Retrieved from http://pewinternet.org/Commentary/2012/February/Pew-Internet-Mobile.aspx

Burke, L. E., Styn, M. A., Sereika, S. M., Conroy, M. B., Ye, L., Glanz, K., . . . Ewing, L. J. (2012). Using mHealth technology to enhance self-monitoring for weight loss: A randomized trial. *American Journal of Preventive Medicine, 43*(1), 20–26. doi: 10.1016/j.amepre.2012.03.016

Centers for Medicare & Medicaid Services. (2010). *National health expenditure projections 2010–2020*. Retrieved from https://www.cms.gov/Research-Statistics-Data-and-Systems/Statistics-Trends-and-Reports/NationalHealthExpendData/downloads/proj2010.pdf

Clinical AppStracts LLC. (n.d.). *Heart failure trials*. Retrieved from https://play.google.com/store/apps/developer?id=Clinical+AppStracts+LLC&hl=en

Corusen LLC. (2013). *Accupedo pedometer*. Retrieved from https://play.google.com/store/apps/details?id=com.corusen.accupedo.te&feature=search_result

DeNavas-Walt, C., Proctor, B., & Smith, J. (2011). *Income, poverty, and health insurance coverage in the United States: 2010*. Retrieved from http://www.census.gov/prod/2011pubs/p60-239.pdf

Dolan, B. (2012). *An analysis of consumer health apps for Apple's iPhone 2012*. Mobi Health News. Retrieved from http://mobihealthnews.com/17925/just-launched-our-2012-consumer-health-apps-report/

DrawMD. (2013). Retrieved from http://www.drawmd.com/

Elsevier Inc. (2012). *Netter's anatomy atlas*. Retrieved from https://itunes.apple.com/us/app/netters-anatomy-atlas/id461841381?mt=8

Emotiv. (2013). *EEG features*. Retrieved from http://www.emotiv.com/eeg/

Endomondo Sports Tracker. (n.d.). Retrieved from https://play.google.com/store/apps/details?id=com.endomondo.android&hl=en

Epocrates. (2013). *Epocrates*. Retrieved from https://itunes.apple.com/us/app/epocrates/id281935788?mt=8&ign-mpt=uo%3D6

FatSecret. (2013). *Calorie counter by FatSecret*. Retrieved from https://itunes.apple.com/us/app/calorie-counter-by-fatsecret/id347184248?mt=8

Health Resources and Services Administration (HRSA). (n.d.). mHealth. *Health Information Technology and Quality Improvement*. Retrieved from http://www.hrsa.gov/healthit/mhealth.html

Jovanov, E., Milenkovic, A., Otto, C., & De Groen, P. C. (2005). A wireless body area network of intelligent motion sensors for computer assisted physical rehabilitation. *Journal of Neuroengineering and Rehabilitation, 2*(1), 6. doi:10.1186/1743-0003-2-6

LIVESTRONG.COM. (2011). *MyPlate calorie tracker.* Retrieved from https://itunes.apple.com/us/app/calorie-tracker-livestrong.com/id295305241?mt=8

McCurdie, T., Taneva, S., Casselman, M., Yeung, M., McDaniel, C., Ho, W., & Cafazzo, J. (2012). mHealth consumer apps: The case for user-centered design. *Biomedical Instrumentation & Technology,* 49–56.

Milenkovic, A., Otto, C., & Jovanov, E. (2006). Wireless sensor networks for personal health monitoring: Issues and an implementation. *Computer Communications, 29*(13–14), 2521–2533. doi:10.1016/j.comcom.2006.02.011

Mobile Systems, Inc. (2013a). *Dorland's Illustrated Medical Dictionary.* Retrieved from https://play.google.com/store/apps/details?id=com.mobisystems.msdict.embedded.wireless.elsevier.dorlandsillustrated&feature=search_result#?t=W251bGwsMSwxLDEsImNvbS5tb2Jpc3lzdGVtcy5tc2RpY3QuZW1iZWRkZWQud2lyZWxlc3MuZWxzZXZpZXIuZG9ybGFuZHNpbGx1c3RyYXRlZCJd

Mobile Systems, Inc. (2013b). Dorland's Illustrated Medical Dictionary (32nd ed.). *App Store.* Retrieved from https://itunes.apple.com/us/app/dorlands-illustrated-medical/id447024921?mt=8

National Institute on Aging. (2013). *Unprecedented global aging examined in new Census Bureau report commissioned by the National Institute on Aging.* Retrieved from http://www.nia.nih.gov/newsroom/2009/07/unprecedented-global-aging-examined-new-census-bureau-report-commissioned-national

PHI Consulting. (2012). *BrainAttack.* Retrieved from https://itunes.apple.com/app/brainattack/id581546430?mt=83D2

Rajan, R. (2012). The promise of wireless: An overview of a device-to-cloud mHealth solution. *Biomedical Instrumentation & Technology,* 26–32.

Rinehart-Thompson, L. A. (2013). *Introduction to health information privacy and security.* Chicago, IL: American Health Information Management Association Press.

Saralsoft LLC. (2012). *Assist me with inhalers.* Retrieved from https://itunes.apple.com/us/app/assist-me-with-inhalers/id590417707?mt=8

Skyscape. (2012). *Netter's atlas: Human anatomy.* Retrieved from https://play.google.com/store/apps/details?id=com.skyscape.packagenetteranfivektwokgdata.android.voucher.ui&hl=en

U.S. Census Bureau. (2011). *Newsroom: Profile American facts for features: Older Americans.* Retrieved from http://www.census.gov/newsroom/releases/archives/facts_for_features_special_editions/cb11-ff08.html

U.S. Census Bureau. (2012). *National health expenditures—Summary: 1960 to 2009.* Retrieved from http://www.census.gov/compendia/statab/2012/tables/12s0134.pdf

U.S. Food and Drug Administration (FDA). (2013). *Mobile medical applications: Guidance for industry and Food and Drug Administration staff.* Retrieved from http://www.fda.gov/downloads/MedicalDevices/DeviceRegulationandGuidance/GuidanceDocuments/UCM263366.pdf

University of Illinois. *(2013). Evidence based treatment of behavioral symptoms of dementia.* App Store. Retrieved from https://itunes.apple.com/us/app/evidence-based-treatment-behavioral/id598716627?mt=8

UpToDate. (2013). *Product.* Retrieved from http://www.uptodate.com/home/product

Vodopivec-Jamsek, V., de Jongh, T., Gurol-Urganci, I., Atun, R., & Car, J. (2012). Mobile phone messaging for preventive health care. *Cochrane Database of Systematic Reviews, 12*(CD007457). doi: 10.1002/14651858.CD007457.pub2

Wearable Technologies. (2013). *Wearable technologies*. Retrieved from http://www.wearable-technologies.com/

West, D. (2012). How mobile devices are transforming healthcare. *Issues in Technology Innovation, 18*, 1–14.

Whittaker, R., McRobbie, H., Bullen, C., Borland, R., Rodgers, A., & Gu, Y. (2012). Mobile phone-based interventions for smoking cessation. *Cochrane Database of Systematic Reviews, 11*(CD006611). doi: 10.1002/14651858.CD006611.pub3

Zephyr BioHarness BT. (n.d.). Retrieved from http://www.zephyranywhere.com/products/bioharness-3

CHAPTER 15

Informatics and Public Health

Brenda Talley, PhD, RN, NEA-BC
Susan Alexander, DNP, RN, ANP-BC, ADM-BC
Ellise D. Adams, PhD, RN, CNM

CHAPTER LEARNING OBJECTIVES

1. Review concepts used in the study of public health.
2. Describe methods used to assess the health of populations and communities.
3. Examine informatics tools used in the surveillance and management of acute and chronic diseases.

KEY TERMS

Census Data Mapper
Community
Epidemiology
Population

Public health informatics
Reference maps
Thematic maps
Vital statistics

CHAPTER OVERVIEW

Innovative applications for health information technology (health IT) continue to emerge, including in the challenging field of public health where tools can be used in disaster planning, managing outbreaks of communicable disease, and addressing disparities in health among communities and populations. This chapter introduces the concepts needed to understand the study of public health, such as communities and populations. Tools that are widely used to assess the health of communities and populations are reviewed, along with innovative informatics approaches that can be applied to the study of public health. Finally, future directions in the study of **public health informatics** are reviewed.

CONCEPTS IN PUBLIC HEALTH

There are many ways in which communities and populations are examined, and there are many informatics tools that are used to assess various aspects of health and disease in communities and populations. To grasp the potential benefits of the tools, an understanding of concepts that are commonly used in the field of public health is necessary.

Population

The term **population** has a specific meaning to healthcare professionals in the field of public health. The American Nurses Association (2007) defines population as "those living in a specific geographic area or those in a particular group who experience a disproportionate burden of poor health outcomes" (p. 5). Analysis of health data demonstrates that some population subtypes may have a greater propensity toward disease and accidents. Targeted information about the health risks of populations can assist public health professionals in drafting programs to address these risks. For example, *Healthy People* is an ongoing project containing goals and objectives designed to improve the health of citizens of the United States (U.S. Department of Health and Human Services [HHS], 2013; **Table 15-1**). An updated version of *Healthy People* is released every 10 years, and *Healthy People 2020* is the fourth generation of the document. Although the entire *Healthy People 2020* document may be downloaded, it is quite lengthy. Specific topics are easier to access and review online. Searches can be conducted by topics, which include health conditions or specific populations, or by objectives that are contained in the document. *Healthy People 2020* can

Table 15-1   Mission of *Healthy People 2020*
• Identify nationwide health improvement priorities.
• Increase public awareness and understanding of the determinants of health, disease, and disability, and the opportunities for progress.
• Provide measurable objectives and goals that are applicable at the national, state, and local levels.
• Engage multiple sectors to take actions to strengthen policies and improve practices that are driven by the best available evidence and knowledge.
• Identify critical research, evaluation, and data-collection needs.

Source: U.S. Department of Health and Human Services. Office of Disease Prevention and Health promotion. *Healthy People 2020.* Washington, DC. Retrieved from http://healthypeople.gov/2020/about/default.aspx

be used as a foundation for health and wellness activities and as a guide for measurement of activities by local groups.

Community

Groups of people may be designated a **community** on the basis of many parameters. Each community has its own unique characteristics and dynamics. Those who reside in the community have similarities because they share a common greater environment and experience similar social interactions. Community residents may have shared histories, values, and concerns. However, some communities are more homogeneous than others. Understanding the similarities and differences among those who live in a given community is critical in defining and prioritizing the health risks specific to that community and in assessing the resources and motivations required to reduce risks. Priorities may differ within the community; the priorities of the community may well differ from those on the "outside" who find themselves engaged in trying to work with the community to improve health outcomes and the wellbeing (however that is defined!) of the community.

A community may be defined broadly as "a collection of people who interact with one another and whose common interest or characteristics is the basis of unity" (Allender, Rector, & Warner, 2009, p. 6), or slightly more specific as "a group of people who share something in common and interact with one another, who may exhibit commitment with one another and may share a geographic boundary" (Lundy & Janes, 2009, p. 16).

As with communities, tools are available for the systematic assessment of defined populations. Some, such as the Population Health Assessment and Surveillance, (PHAS), offer a general framework to gather and analyze information and provide guidance to implement and evaluate strategies (Government of Nova Scotia, 2011). The Vulnerable Populations Assessment Tool for assessing the risk to vulnerable populations especially during special conditions such as evacuation due to extreme weather conditions or disease outbreaks (which can occur in rapid succession) is used by the Florida Department of Health (n.d.) and is accessible online.

Epidemiology

Epidemiology is a field of science that studies health and disease in defined populations or communities. The statistical analysis of data that are collected in epidemiological research studies can assist public health professionals with tasks such as creating and revising public health programs or identifying risk factors for disease

(Porta, 2008). Principles of epidemiological research can be used in many ways. Field epidemiologists are often called upon to review the outbreaks of epidemics; hospital epidemiologists use similar techniques to identify patterns of disease occurrence, such as nosocomial infections, in hospitals (Porta, 2008). The techniques of epidemiological research can be applied to any community or population of interest and used to assess relationships between characteristics or behaviors of the community and health. In a sample of 173 nurses employed in North Carolina and West Virginia, Bae (2013) identified a significant association between mandatory overtime and verbal abuse, after controlling for other variables such as work setting, workload, and the educational level of the nurse.

Public Health Informatics

As public health professionals address issues within their field, knowledge of informatics tools and applications, in addition to training in concepts and practices specific to public health, is necessary for all disciplines within the specialty. In a recent survey of 56 public health workers, Hsu and colleagues (2012) identified the most important competencies as leadership and system thinking skills. Respondents identified the need to integrate health IT tools into the systems-level thinking as necessary for constructing and executing public health policy decisions. There is a global need for workforce development in the field of public health informatics to train a workforce familiar with concepts inherent in public health, health promotion, health services research, and information and communications technologies (Gebbie, Rosenstock, & Hernandez, 2003). When reviewing educational programs in the field of public health informatics, Joshi and Perin (2012) identified only 15 programs across 13 institutions, mainly in the United States. None of the programs offered a doctoral degree in public health informatics, and only seven could be taken in an online format.

Informatics and communications technology tools to support the work of the nurse in public health are widely available, particularly in the field of chronic disease management. However, barriers to the adoption of these technologies have been reported, including themes such as capacity building, confidence and trust in the technology, and competence (Courtney-Pratt et al., 2012). Without question, the adoption of tools, even as they are intended to reduce workload, can initially increase it. Strategies to increase ease of adoption, such as consideration of physical office setup, adequate resources, and initial and ongoing training, are needed (Courtney-Pratt et al., 2012). It is important to involve public health nurses in the design of informatics tools that can increase efficiency in daily work activities but also support them during times of public health crises.

METHODS OF DESCRIBING THE HEALTH OF COMMUNITIES AND POPULATIONS

Similar to the manner in which an individual is assessed, a community or population can be assessed in a manner using selected criteria. Statistics that describe the health of a population or a community cannot be fully understood without demographic information. For example, understanding the impact and significance of 100 cases of a disease may differ if the occurrence is in a city with a population of 1 million, rather than a smaller city with a population of 1,000. Making connections to demographic factors, such as socioeconomic status, age, gender, occupation, geographic location, and other parameters, provides context for the interpretation of the effects of a disease or disorder. By utilizing this approach to the analysis of information, a better estimate of the burden of disease, the vulnerabilities, and the disparities in health outcomes for a specific population can be acquired. Several models based in nursing and public health offer a framework for appraisal of communities and populations and are available in an online format.

An example of a resource that local communities can use to improve the health of their members is the Mobilizing for Action through Planning and Partnerships (MAPP) framework. The framework offers resources and tools to enhance community involvement in decision making, setting priorities, appraising needed resources, and community engagement in effecting change. Targeted assessments, such as the Community Themes and Strengths Assessment, Local Public Health Systems Assessment, Forces of Change Assessment, and the Community Health Status Assessment are available in the MAPP Clearinghouse. Specifically, the Community Health Status Assessment is used to analyze "data about health status, quality of life, and risk factors in the community" (National Association of County and City Health Officials, 2013). MAPP also gives annual Model Practices Awards to those partnerships that best demonstrate ways in which health departments and local communities work together to address local health issues.

Facilitating change in a community or a population can be a difficult and overwhelming task. The initial step in facilitating change is often the assessment of readiness to change. Other online tools are available for communities and populations who wish to begin the change process. The Community Health and Group Evaluation (CHANGE) Tool provides resources for building community teams, gathering and analyzing information, and developing plans to improve a community's health (Centers for Disease Control and Prevention [CDC], 2013b). The CHANGE tool can be used by community planners for focused assessments and to target change efforts in five sectors: the community at large, community institutions/organizations, health care, schools, and work sites. Successful change efforts include the substitution of healthy food items in school vending machines, the establishment of community gardens and farmers' markets in low-income areas to increase access to fresh fruits and vegetables, and enhancing the ability of pedestrians and bicyclists to use public streets (CDC, 2013b).

Populations and communities are multidimensional. Thorough assessment of these entities often includes collection of many different data points, such as personal income, gender, ethnicity, age, and home ownership, requiring the collection of data from discrete members. Historically, data have been collected telephonically, through in-person examinations or interviews, or by mailouts, all of which require entry into a database by someone other than the person who obtained the data point. Health-related data are frequently included in these assessments, typically by self-reports from patients. The proliferation of electronic records has allowed for healthcare facilities to export health-related data to larger, federally maintained databases, removing the step of indirect entry that is required with some surveys.

Assessments with Indirect Entry to Databases

The most inclusive and comprehensive source of demographic data is maintained by the U.S. Department of Commerce in the Census Bureau. According to Constitutional law, a census of the population of the United States is conducted every 10 years, and census records date back to 1790. According to the U.S. Census Bureau (2010), the largest city in the United States is New York, with a population of 8.1 million, and the population of the United States experienced a 9.7% increase from 2000 figures. Many data visualization tools, including mapping tools and other statistical analysis tools, are available on the Census Bureau's website. Census data are collected through mail canvass of state government offices that are involved with the administration of state-level taxes. If necessary, phone calls, repeat mailings, and emails can be used until a sufficient sample of the population is achieved. Data that are collected are aggregated and are accessible by the public on the Census Bureau website.

Census Bureau Maps

A variety of interactive maps enable the retrieval of census data in graphic form, which can be used for illustration and education. For example, **reference maps** are designed to show geographic locations and show features such as rivers but do not contain demographic data. **Thematic maps** display socioeconomic, demographic, or business-related data about an area and may build on reference maps. The **Census Data Mapper** is an application that allows users to create custom maps containing county-level demographic data (**Figure 15-1**).

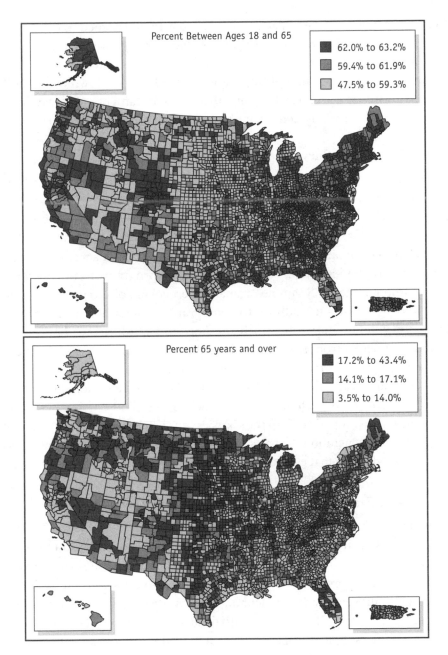

FIGURE 15-1   Percent of U.S. population aged 65 years and older.

Source: http://www.census.gov/geo/maps-data/maps/datamapper.html

To expedite real-time use of data, a mobile application designed to deliver updates on 19 key economic indicators is now available. Sponsored jointly by the U.S. Census Bureau, the U.S. Bureau of Labor Statistics, and the U.S. Bureau of Economic Analysis, the America's Economy mobile application is available for download on iOS and Android platforms (U.S. Census Bureau, 2013b). Users can get up-to-date information on topics such as employment, manufacturing, and retail sales (**Figure 15-2**).

American Community Survey

The American Community Survey (ACS) is an ongoing statistical survey used by the U.S. Census Bureau that samples a small percentage of the population every year to gather information needed by communities to plan investments and services (U.S. Census Bureau, 2013a). Data from the ACS help to determine priorities in allocating more than $400 billion in federal and state funds annually, and data analysis is used to make decisions on topics ranging from school lunch programs to the need for new hospitals. Although the ACS samples a smaller percentage of the population, it contains questions on topics in addition to demographics, such as family information, employment, veteran status, health insurance, and disabilities. The results are obtained by estimating from fewer individuals than the 10-year census, but the report provides a deeper set of information than the census.

One-, 3-, and 5-year estimates of data from the ACS can be retrieved from the website using interactive searches based on topics such as age, gender, geography, ethnicity, employment, and housing. Results of the searches can then be displayed visually by using embedded tools for generation of charts and maps. The website also contains a selection of pre-constructed charts that can be edited according to user preference (**Table 15-2**).

Behavioral Risk Factor Surveillance System (BRFSS)

The CDC initiated the Behavioral Risk Factor Surveillance System (BRFSS) in 1984 in an effort to systematically collect data on the health behaviors of Americans. Data collection expanded to all 50 states in 1993. The BRFSS is a phone-based survey tool designed to collect a person's self-reported responses to questions on health behaviors, covering items such as use of alcohol, tobacco, seat belts, or history of medical conditions. Responses are then entered into databases, and interested users can query the databases with a simple web-based tool (CDC, n.d.). Because survey items remain largely consistent from year to year, users can construct queries to compare responses between states and regions of the country by year of survey.

The BRFSS databases are maintained by the CDC and are available for use by investigators in assessing the health of specific populations and communities and

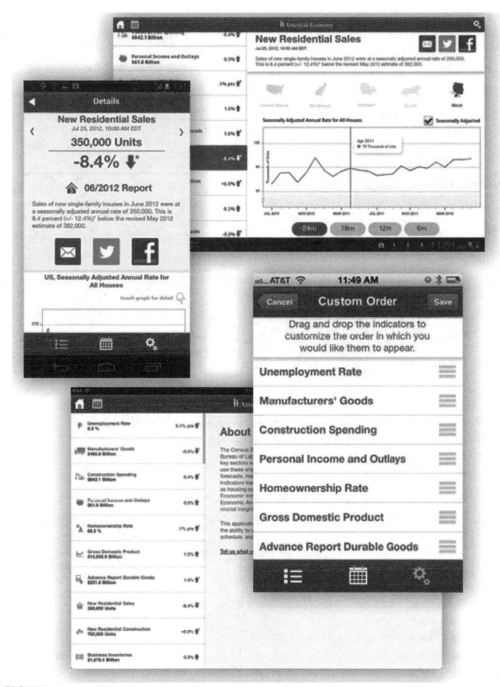

FIGURE 15-2   Screen capture of America's Economy App.

Source: http://www.census.gov/mobile/

Table 15-2   U.S. Department of Commerce, U.S. Census Bureau: 2009–2011 American Community Survey 3-Year Estimates

Disability Status of the Civilian Noninstitutionalized Population	Estimate	Margin of Error	Percent
Total Civilian Noninstitutionalized Population	304,085,860	+/−8,917	304,085,860
With a disability	36,499,048	+/−58,831	12.0%
Under 18 years	73,901,825	+/−11,968	73,901,825
With a disability	2,942,519	+/−16,660	4.0%
18 to 64 years	190,999,705	+/−12,599	190,999,705
With a disability	19,141,182	+/−44,271	10.0%
65 years and over	39,184,330	+/−8,251	39,184,330
With a disability	14,415,347	+/−26,918	36.8%

Source: U.S. Department of Commerce, Census Bureau, American Community Survey. (2010). *About the American Community Survey*. Retrieved from http://www.census.gov/acs/www/about_the_survey/american_community_survey/

health-related trends. Interested users must make an application to the CDC in order to obtain needed datasets. Information is available in datasets that can be queried by state, year, and category.

National Health and Nutrition Examination Survey (NHANES)

Using the National Health and Nutrition Examination Survey (NHANES), information is collected both from physical examinations and by interview (CDC, 2013c). NHANES collects and analyzes health and nutritional information on adults and children. NHANES is a major program of the CDC's National Center for Health Statistics (NCHS). Additional information gathered includes dental and eye health, information related to diabetes, kidney and heart disease, osteoarthritis, and other topics. NHANES is one of the earliest collections available, beginning in the 1960s. Numerous surveys and physical examinations have created searchable datasets on multiple populations and in many locations. Due to the complexity of the resources available, it is recommended that the brief, easily accessed tutorials be used before seeking information. Though the NHANES is intended to be representative of all Americans, intentional oversampling of some population subgroups allows for more reliable statistics. However, the health condition of older Americans is a stated objective.

Youth Behavioral Risk Surveillance System

While the CDC's BRFSS focuses on assessing the health-related behaviors of adults, the Youth Behavioral Risk Surveillance System (YBRSS) collects data on six categories of health-risk behaviors that are leading causes of death and disability in America's youth (CDC, 2013a). The YBRSS is administered annually in paper form to selected populations of middle- and high-school students across the United States. Survey items include questions about alcohol, drug, and tobacco use; sexual health; diet and physical activity; violence; and unintentional injuries. The prevalence of medical conditions such as obesity and asthma are also assessed. Much of this information is available in report form, with numerous publications available; responses are entered into databases that can be searched by data points such as sites of participation and survey topics. Searches may be further refined, with the selection of gender, age, race, and grade in school as additional data points. Results from the YBRSS are used by investigators to create projects designed to address high-risk health behaviors in adolescents.

Assessments with Direct Entry into Databases

Vital Statistics

Local and state departments of public health are charged with the responsibility of collecting **vital statistics**, including data points such as births, deaths, marriages, divorces, and fetal deaths. Although these data may be retrieved electronically from individual departments, they are aggregated by the National Vital Statistics System (NVSS). Users can get direct access to individual state and territory information, such as copies of birth or marriage certificates or aggregated national mortality data for a specified year. The site also contains pre-specified datasets on items such as multiple births, maternal and infant health, and family growth (**Table 15-3**). The NVSS site is maintained by the CDC, the Division of Vital Statistics, and the NCHS.

Though a vast array of data is collected by departments of health in each state, its use in research can be limited by difficulties in access. Not every state has the tools necessary to access the data so that they can be used for research purposes. Investigators at the University of Utah have developed an alternative method of querying the Utah Population Database (UPDB; Hurdle et al., 2013). The query tool, called Utah Population Database Limited, rapidly determines the availability of specified cohorts for researchers. Users can select a cohort from UPDB datasets, gain access to limited

Table 15-3   Programs Related to National Vital Statistics System

Programs	Internet Address
Linked Birth and Infant Death Data	http://www.cdc.gov/nchs/linked.htm
National Survey of Family Growth	http://www.cdc.gov/nchs/nsfg.htm
Matched Multiple Birth Data Set	http://www.cdc.gov/nchs/nvss/mmb.htm
National Death Index	http://www.cdc.gov/nchs/ndi.htm
National Maternal and Infant Health Survey	http://www.cdc.gov/nchs/nvss/nmihs.htm
National Mortality Followback Survey	http://www.cdc.gov/nchs/nvss/nmfs.htm
Vital Statistics of the United States	http://www.cdc.gov/nchs/products/vsus.htm
National Vital Statistics Reports	http://www.cdc.gov/nchs/products/nvsr.htm
Other selected reports	http://www.cdc.gov/nchs/products.htm

Source: Centers for Disease Control and Prevention. (2013). *National Vital Statistics System.* Retrieved from http://www.cdc.gov/nchs/nvss.htm

family or pedigree information, and gather preliminary results that are used to refine a query tool used to generate data for research (Hurdle et al., 2013). To date, the tool has been used to create cohorts for studying conditions such as spondyloarthritis, breast cancer, and pregnancy complications co-occurring with cardiovascular disease (CVD) (**Figure 15-3**).

Healthcare Cost and Utilization Project

Many states collect health-related information on hospital admissions, discharges, ambulatory surgeries, and emergency department visits. The Healthcare Cost and Utilization Project (HCUP) is a collection of databases maintained by the Agency for Healthcare Research and Quality (AHRQ). States may choose to participate in submitting de-identified data to the HCUP databases. Databases may then be queried to identify, track, or analyze national trends in healthcare utilization, access, charges, quality, and outcomes (AHRQ, 2013). Use of state-level data can yield similar information for a specific state or group of states. Investigators who are interested in using the data for research purposes can submit an application to obtain copies of necessary files, with fees ranging from $20–$800 (AHRQ, 2013).

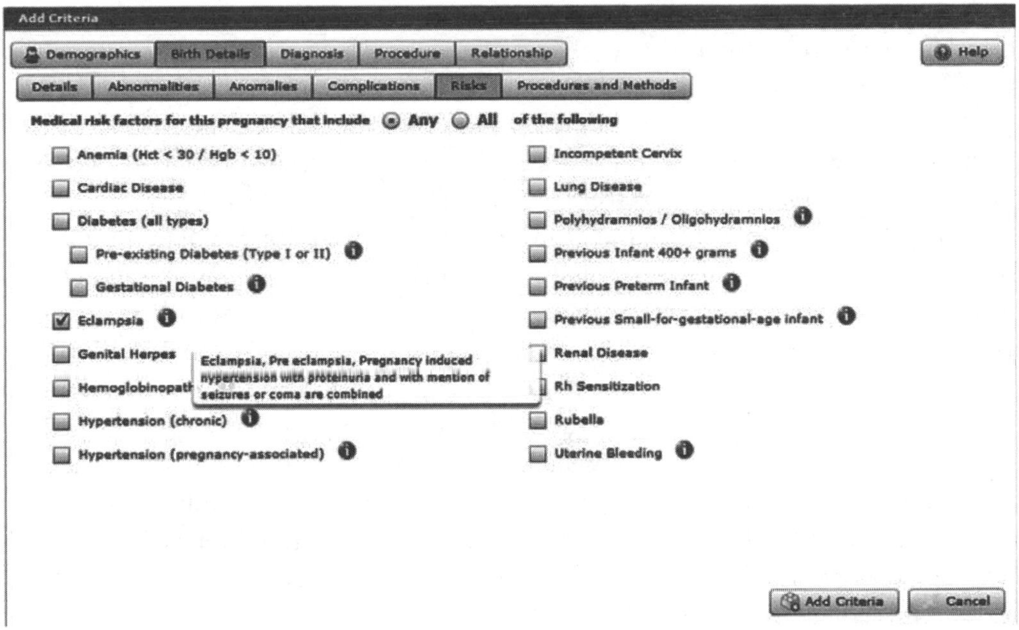

FIGURE 15-3 A sample screen shot showing the selection of birth details, specifically eclampsia, pre-eclampsia, and pregnancy-induced hypertension with proteinuria and with a mention of seizures or coma, which are all combined under 'eclampsia' as shown to the user in the pop-up help balloon.

Source: Reproduced from *Journal of the American Medical Informatics Association*, Hurdle, J. F., Haroldsen, S. C., Hammer, A., Spigle, C., Fraser, A. M., Mineau, G. P., & Courdy, S. J., *20*(1), 164–171, 2013 with permission from BMJ Publishing Group Ltd.

APPLYING INFORMATICS TOOLS TO IMPROVE PUBLIC HEALTH

Prevention and Surveillance of Communicable Disease

Some communities experience exceptional conditions that can have an adverse effect on the wellbeing of their citizens. Two of these conditions are disasters—natural and manmade—and occurrences of communicable disease outbreaks. Online resources can be helpful in assessing the state of the community. In addition to examining real-time information, examination of the experiences of other communities in similar experiences may aid a community in preparing or responding to adverse events.

Prevention of Disease Outbreaks

According to the World Health Organization (2012), more than 900 million international journeys are undertaken annually. Global travel exposes people to many varieties of health risks. Providing immunizations for diseases such as yellow fever or typhoid fever and empowering patients for self-treatment of conditions such as traveler's diarrhea are often necessary when people travel to less-developed areas of the world. A surveillance network known as Global TravEpiNet was created by the CDC, in conjunction with Massachusetts General Hospital, in 2009. It consists of member organizations scattered across the United States that contribute data on the demographic characteristics, travel patterns, and pre-travel health care of people traveling internationally from the United States. Analyses of the data on traveler population subtypes is ongoing, including pediatrics, immunocompromised individuals, frequent business travelers, those who travel to zones where yellow fever is endemic, and use of vaccines for rabies and Japanese encephalitis (Global TravEpiNet, 2012). In an analysis of data contributed to the Global TravEpiNet database by member sites, LaRocque and colleagues (2012) found that more than 90% of travelers to areas of West Africa, where malaria is endemic, were prescribed malaria chemoprophylaxis. These results are important, because they may reduce the risk of importing cases of malaria to the United States. Further analysis of data from Global TravEpiNet revealed reasons for missed vaccinations in international travelers, such as patient refusal, time constraints, or lack of vaccine availability (**Figure 15-4**; LaRocque et al., 2012). Targeting identification of the causes for missed vaccinations is the initial step in crafting strategies to improve vaccination rates and eventually reduce the risk of communicable diseases.

Surveillance of Communicable Diseases

In the United States, the responsibility for surveillance of disease and wellness lies with the CDC. The CDC is the collector of information, functions as its repository, and prepares the information for consumption on several levels. Originally called the Communicable Disease Center, the CDC was established in 1946 in Atlanta, Georgia to deal with the serious issue of malaria in the Southern United States. Probably the most traditional of the responsibilities expected of the CDC is surveillance of communicable diseases. The surveillance of reportable diseases actually involves many systems that report to the CDC. The CDC has the responsibility of aggregating, compiling, and communicating the information. The list of reportable conditions is revised as new trends emerge (CDC, 2010b).

Disease-specific data   Also accessible through the CDC data and statistics portal are links to collections of disease-specific resources. The CDC produces numerous collections of data and statistics on health and disease conditions. Especially useful in the assessment of community needs is information on incidence, prevalence, risk factors, and disparities in outcomes including differences in racial and ethnic groups. Factors such as cost and level of disability aid in describing the impact of the condition on the

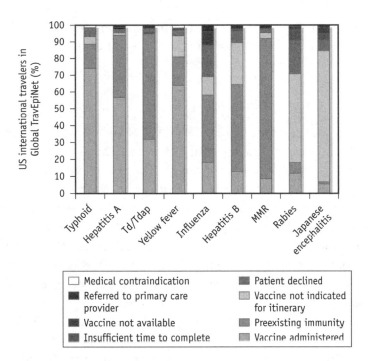

FIGURE 15-4   Selected immunization status and vaccine use among U.S. international travelers in Global TravEpiNet.

Source: Regina C. LaRocque, Sowmya R. Rao, Jennifer Lee, Vernon Ansdell et al, Global TravEpiNet: A National Consortium of Clinics Providing Care to International Travelers—Analysis of Demographic Characteristics, Travel Destinations, and Pretravel Healthcare of High-Risk US International Travelers, 2009–2011, Clinical Infectious Diseases 2011, p. 7 (Figure 2). Reprinted by permission of Oxford University Press.

community, and on the individual. Full-text articles relating current information are also available. Information specific and unique to the disease or condition is included with each topic. Relevant webinars and podcasts are included as resources on the site (http://www.cdc.gov/).

CDC Epi Info 7

Epi Info 7 is a resource of software and rapid assessment tools that can be deployed by public health professionals, including nurses, physicians, and field epidemiologists, in areas lacking in technological resources and/or by those who do not have extensive background in the use of technology (CDC, 2010a). It can be used when there are disease outbreaks or to develop small surveillance systems in rural areas. It is an Internet-based software package, available in the public domain that can be used to quickly construct questionnaires and databases, perform rapid data entry, and perform analysis with epidemiologic statistics. Analytical visualization, by use of graphs and maps, is also included. At this time, the application is limited to Windows-based operating systems. The website contains a variety of training resources and free downloads (http://wwwn.cdc.gov/epiinfo/).

Management of Chronic Diseases

According to estimates from the CDC (n.d.), CVD is the most common cause of death in the United States, occurring at a rate of 193.6 per 100,000 of the population. Myocardial infarction, commonly called a "heart attack," is one example of an acute manifestation of CVD that can result in sudden death. The insertion of a stent through an occluded coronary artery, and the restoration of perfusion to the cardiac muscle, may reduce the morbidity and mortality associated with CVD. Once inserted, the stent is left in place, and the risk of reocclusion of the stent is a great concern for the cardiologist and the patient. Efforts to reduce the risk of stent reocclusion led to the development of drug-eluting stents (DES). These types of stents are designed to slowly release drugs that block the proliferation of cells leading to restenosis. When a patient's CVD warrants the use of a stent to restore myocardial circulation, cardiologists can choose between use of the DES or a traditional bare-metal stent (BMS).

In 2006, the results of a randomized clinical trial on outcomes for patients who used DES were released, suggesting that patients who received this type of stent were at increased risk for restenosis within the first 6 months post-stent deployment, and further recommending that this group of patients use dual antiplatelet therapy for longer periods of time than originally recommended (Pfisterer et al., 2006). This incident is an example of the need for rapid translation of research findings into practice. Major medical societies in the United States jointly issued a Clinical Alert and Science Advisory to stress the importance of compliance with dual antiplatelet therapy. Staff members at Duke University Heart Center supplemented this education campaign by sending letters to each of their patients who had a history of DES insertion, using records from their in-house registry, instructing the patients to speak with their healthcare providers (HCPs) about the need for continued dual antiplatelet therapy to prevent restenosis of the stents. Results of their targeted patient campaign revealed increased patient self-reports of clopidogrel (an antiplatelet therapy recommended to be used along with aspirin) at 6 and 12 months following initiation of the campaign (Eisenstein et al., 2012). There was no reported increase in the use of clopidogrel for patients who received bare-metal stents (Eisenstein et al., 2012).

When combined with geospatial data mapping, clinical information mined from electronic health record (EHR) systems can offer rich insight into the strategies communities can use to help patients with chronic disease. Califf, Sanderson, and Miranda (2012) combined clinical data from Duke Medical Center with geospatial mapping data on points such as housing, social stressors, neighborhoods, and culture, hoping to gain more detail about the environmental factors that influence the lives and health of patients. A second project, focusing on adults with type 2 diabetes mellitus, extends the dual approach to other counties in North Carolina, Mississippi, and West Virginia. The projects are ongoing, and results are expected to better demonstrate the effects of community-based interventions on patients with chronic diseases. Studies such as these using geospatial mapping are expected to add to the knowledge base about long-term clinical outcomes for patients with chronic diseases, such as diabetes (Califf et al., 2012).

Disaster Planning—National and International

Planning for disasters requires the collaboration of multiple disciplines to achieve preparedness goals. In training exercises, staff can practice using technological devices, such as hand-held global positioning system (GPS) devices to produce specific coordinates that can be used for search and rescue efforts. Outbreaks of disease that can quickly become global health threats can occur in any country. In 2005, the World Health Organization (WHO) issued revised International Health Regulations (IHR). The revised IHR addressed the need for strengthening global alerting and response systems, and it required participating countries to "develop and strengthen field systems, tools, methodologies, and capacity for risk assessment, communication and information management, outbreak logistics, and field deployment" (WHO, 2007, p. 24).

In developed countries such as the United States, computerized disease biosurveillance systems are based on data reported from EHRs, such as claims data from office or hospital visits, prescription drug sales, or nurse hotline data, and reported to local and regional public health departments (Campbell et al., 2012). In countries without stable Internet access, extensive use of EHR systems, and other electronic resources, disease surveillance is more difficult, and outbreaks can be more difficult to detect until the disease has become widespread.

Two low-cost biosurveillance systems designed for use in areas with unreliable access to the Internet and data feeds from electronic records have been developed by the U.S. Department of Defense, the Veterans Administration, and the Johns Hopkins University Applied Physics Laboratory: the Electronic Surveillance System for the Early Notification of Community-Based Epidemics (ESSENCE) Desktop Edition (EDE) and an open source version of ESSENCE (OE). Both of the systems utilize freely available open source software and are low in cost. EDE can run on a stand-alone desktop computer, with data entered by personnel or by simple short message service (SMS) text messages via smartphones. OE can be used as a stand-alone system or connected to the Internet, with data being entered directly into the OE server or via the Internet. A pilot study of EDE use began in 2009 in the Philippines, where healthcare personnel used SMS messaging to send daily patient data to a receiver phone connected to a computer at a city health office. Prior to implementation of the SMS messaging system, a 2-week delay between case presentation of diseases and reporting to the city office was common. After implementation of the messaging system and the EDE surveillance, 90% of local health clinics were using SMS messaging to send daily reports of fever to local health offices (Campbell et al., 2012).

Federal Agencies Charged with Public Health Efforts

U.S. Department of Labor, Occupational Safety and Health Administration (OSHA)   OSHA (n.d.) offers educational programs for emergency workers and community leaders and planners. Modules range from natural disasters, chemical and biological hazards, radiation release, and oil spills to acts of terrorism. The guidelines are provided for communities. In conducting a community assessment, evaluation of the community's disaster plan is a critical component. These resources could be used as a benchmark for local communities in developing disaster planning.

U.S. Department of Homeland Security, Federal Emergency Management Agency (FEMA)
FEMA is probably the best known resource for community planning. In addition to the vast resources and support for disaster preparedness, FEMA also provides a framework for the establishment of a community's emergency preparedness plan. FEMA's *Comprehensive Preparedness Guide, Version 2.0* is available online as a tool for evaluation (http://www.fema.gov/plan). Two versions of the *Comprehensive Preparedness Guides* are available. Version 2.0 expands upon the fundamentals of planning and decision making regarding risk planning originally presented in Version 1.0 of the *Guide*. It emphasizes the need to engage the entire community and family, including children, service animals, and even household pets in emergency planning and preparedness.

FUTURE DIRECTIONS

This chapter contains numerous examples of the many ways data can be used to inform models of public health care and research, along with tools that are in development and present use. However, the need to further adapt and transform present surveillance systems to more fully meet the needs of public health practice is ongoing and has been identified by the CDC as an important future direction to meet the healthcare needs of the 21st century (Savel & Foldy, 2012). At present, the most pressing need is the further development of health IT tools in order to link to data that have not traditionally been available to public health professionals, such as data contained in the EHRs of medical practices and hospitals (**Figure 15-5**). Regularly sharing these data

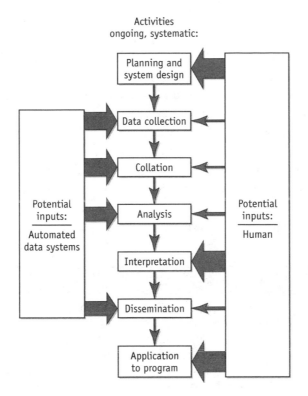

* The size of the arrow indicates the relative human and automated inputs into each activity

FIGURE 15-5 Optimal balance of humans and automated inputs into ongoing systematic public health surveillance system activities.

Source: Savel, T. G., Foldy, S., Centers for Disease Control and Prevention. (2012). The role of public health informatics in enhancing public health surveillance. *MMWR: Surveillance Summaries, 61* Suppl., 20–24.

would improve the timeliness of public health surveillance, but doing so is a source of controversy due to concerns of confidentiality violations and data ownership (Savel & Foldy, 2012). Strategies to improve data sharing include the following:

- De-identification of data
- Use of a subset of restricted data that complies with regulations concerning release
- Development of agreements in which data can be released only for public health surveillance purposes (Savel & Foldy, 2012, p. 32)

Savel & Foldy (2012) further suggest that the offer of feedback or incentives to the agency that owns the data may also be successful in promoting the sharing of data for public health purposes.

The personally controlled health record (PCHR) has been investigated as a mechanism for increasing the sharing of personal health data for public health surveillance efforts. In a PCHR, participants have control over a web-based, digital collection of their personal medical history, including elements such as medical illnesses and medications, age, weight, vital signs, immunization history, and other elements. Participants have the option to decide if they would like data from the PCHR released, and to whom the information would be released. In this model, patients could consent to sharing of their PCHRs to a public health agency, without the intervention or consultation of their HCP. Weitzman, Kelemen, Kaci, and Mandl (2012) conducted a web-based survey of 261 users on their willingness to share data maintained in a PCHR via a hospital patient portal system. In the survey, respondents reported greater willingness to share all categories of health information with a state or local public health

Box 15-1   Case Study

Andrea is an area coordinator for a public health office in a southeastern state. As Andrea visits the county health departments in her area, she is confronted with a seeming increase in sexually transmitted infections (STIs) in 15- to 19-year-old females. By consulting two resources, Andrea is able to determine whether the state and county statistics for STIs substantiate the clinical findings.

First, Andrea consults the National Center for HIV/AIDS, Viral Hepatitis, STD, and TB Prevention Atlas (http://www.cdc.gov/nchhstp/Default.htm) to determine state rates of the STIs (per 100,000). By choosing the parameters of disease, year, race, sex, and age, this tool provides rates for diseases, which can then be compared with other states. Many state health departments provide these same rates by county or region. For example, the Georgia Health Department uses a system called the Online Analytical Statistical Information System (OASIS) to provide information about STIs (https://apps.itos.uga.edu/DPHGIS/DPHGISQueryMap.aspx?infotype=S).

Once Andrea frames the scope of the problem, she prepares to address the clinical issue. Using the Community Health Assessment and Group Evaluation (CHANGE) method to address issues of health care, Andrea begins to assemble a team of leaders. Key partners, such as the city councils of all affected areas, school boards, providers of health insurance, girls' and boys' clubs, city sports leagues and YMCAs, and area hospitals and clinics, can combine efforts to make a stronger impact on this issue by developing common objectives. The CHANGE method advocates for a thorough community assessment to reflect the needs, wants, and desires of the people most directly affected by a rising STI rate among teenage girls. After the team is assembled and the community assessment is complete, the key partners can begin to design changes in policy, systems, and environments to address this healthcare need.

- How would the team assess the impact of their intervention?
- What tools could be used to assess the impact of the team's efforts?
- What other public health informatics resources are available to use in describing the at-risk behaviors for young adults?

authority than with an outside health provider (63.3% vs. 54.1%; Weitzman et al., 2012). Weitzman and colleagues suggest that further efforts are needed in order to increase public knowledge of the need to share comprehensive information, to support better understanding of the health of populations and communities.

SUMMARY

Health information and tools are rich in variety, but vary in reliability and quality. This chapter explores selected online, easily accessible resources for information and tools needed to assess communities and populations. Included are datasets, interactive tools, and frameworks useful to communities, though this is not an exhaustive presentation. The volume of resources could be overwhelming; individuals will find that employing an assessment framework will help focus the selection of resources. At the same time, new and updated resources are constantly being made accessible.

For a full suite of assignments and additional learning activities, use the access code located in the front of your book and visit www.jblearning.com. If you do not have an access code, you can obtain one at the site.

REFERENCES

Agency for Healthcare Research and Quality. (2013). *HCUP databases: Healthcare cost and utilization project*. Retrieved from www.hcup-us.ahrq.gov/databases.jsp

Allender, I. J., Rector, C., & Warner, K. (2009). *Community health nursing: Promoting and protecting the public's health* (7th ed.). Philadelphia, PA: Lippincott Williams & Wilkins.

American Nurses Association. (2007). *Public health nursing: Scope and standards of practice*. Silver Springs, MD: Author.

Bae, S. H. (2013). Presence of nurse mandatory overtime regulations and nurse and patient outcomes. *Nursing Economic$, 31*(2), 59–89.

Califf, R. M., Sanderson, I., & Miranda, M. L. (2012). The future of cardiovascular clinical research: Informatics, clinical investigators, and community engagement. *Journal of the American Medical Association, 308*(17), 1747–1748.

Campbell, T. C., Hodanics, C. J., Babin, S. M., Poku, A. M., Wojcik, R. A., Skora, J. F., . . . Lewis, S. H. (2012). Developing open source, self-contained disease surveillance software applications for use in resource-limited settings. *BMC Medical Informatics and Decision Making, 12*, 99. doi: 10.1186/1472-6947-12-99

Centers for Disease Control and Prevention. (2010a). *Epi info.* Retrieved from http://wwwn.cdc.gov/epiinfo/

Centers for Disease Control and Prevention. (2010b). Summary of notifiable diseases—United States, 2010. *Morbidity and Mortality Weekly Report, 59*(53), 1–111. Retrieved from http://www.cdc.gov/mmwr/preview/mmwrhtml/mm5953a1.htm

Centers for Disease Control and Prevention. (2013a). *Adolescent and school health: Youth Risk Behavior Surveillance System.* Retrieved from http://www.cdc.gov/healthyyouth/yrbs/index.htm

Centers for Disease Control and Prevention. (2013b). *Community Health Assessment and Group Evaluation (CHANGE) Action Guide: Building a foundation of knowledge to prioritize community needs.* Retrieved from http://www.cdc.gov/healthycommunitiesprogram/tools/change.htm

Centers for Disease Control and Prevention. (2013c). *National Health and Nutrition Examination Survey.* Retrieved from http://www.cdc.gov/nchs/nhanes.htm

Centers for Disease Control and Prevention. (n.d.). *BRFSS: Prevalence and trends data.* Retrieved from http://apps.nccd.cdc.gov/brfss/

Centers for Disease Control and Prevention. (n.d.). *Heart disease fact sheet, 2007–2009.* Retrieved from http://www.cdc.gov/dhdsp/data_statistics/fact_sheets/fs_heart_disease.htm

Courtney-Pratt, H., Cummings, E., Turner, P., Cameron-Tucker, H., Wood-Baker, R., Walters, E. H., & Robinson, A. L. (2012). Entering a world of uncertainty: Community nurses' engagement with information and communication technology. *CIN: Computers, Informatics, Nursing, 30*(11), 612–619. doi: 10.1097/NXN.0b013e318266caab

Eisenstein, E. L., Wojdyla, D., Anstrom, K. J., Brennan, J. M., Califf, R. M., Peterson, E. D., & Douglas, P. S. (2012). Evaluating the impact of public health notification: Duke clopidogrel experience. *Circulation: Cardiovascular Quality and Outcomes, 5*(6), 767–774. doi: 10.1161/CIRCOUTCOMES.111.963330

Florida Department of Health. (n.d.). *Vulnerable populations assessment tool.* Retrieved from http://www.floridahealth.gov/preparedness-and-response/healthcare-system-preparedness/vulnerable-populations/vp-resources.html

Gebbie, K., Rosenstock, L., & Hernandez, L. M. (Eds.). (2003). *Who will keep the public healthy? Educating public health professionals for the 21st century.* Washington, DC: National Academies Press.

Global TravEpiNet. (2012). *Materials, updates, and postings.* Retrieved from http://www2.massgeneral.org/id/globaltravepinet/materials/

Government of Nova Scotia. (2011). *Population health assessment and surveillance.* Retrieved from http://www.gov.ns.ca/hpp/populationhealth/

Hsu, C. E., Dunn, K., Juo, H. H., Danko, R., Johnson, D., Mas, F. S., & Sheu, J. J. (2012). Understanding public health informatics competencies for mid-tier public health practitioners: A web-based survey. *Health Informatics Journal, 18*(1), 66–76. doi: 10.1177/1460458211424000

Hurdle, J. F., Haroldsen, S. C., Hammer, A., Spigle, C., Fraser, A. M., Mineau, G. P., & Courdy, S. J. (2013). Identifying clinical/translational research cohorts: Ascertainment via querying an integrated multi-source database. *Journal of the American Medical Informatics Association, 20*(1), 164–171. doi: 10.1136/amiajnl-2012-001050

Joshi, A., & Perin, D. M. (2012). Gaps in the existing public health informatics training programs: A challenge to the development of a skilled global workforce. *Perspectives in Health Information Management, 9,* 1–13.

LaRocque, R. C., Rao, S. R., Lee, J., Ansdell, V., Yates, J. A., Schwartz, B. S., . . . Ryan, E. T. (2012). Global TravEpiNet: A national consortium of clinics providing care to international travelers—analysis of demographic characteristics, travel destinations, and pretravel healthcare of high-risk US international travelers, 2009–2011. *Clinical Infectious Diseases, 54*(4), 455–462. doi: 10.1093/cid/cir839

Lundy, K. S., & Janes, S. (2009). *Community health nursing: Caring for the public's health* (2nd ed.). Sudbury, MA: Jones and Bartlett.

National Association of County and City Health Officials. (2013). *Mobilizing for Action through Planning and Partnerships (MAPP)*. Retrieved from http://www.naccho.org/topics/infrastructure/mapp/

Occupational Safety and Health Administration. (n.d.). *Emergency preparedness and response*. Retrieved from http://www.osha.gov/SLTC/emergencypreparedness/index.html

Porta, M. (2008). *A dictionary of epidemiology* (5th ed.). New York, NY: Oxford University Press.

Pfisterer, M., Brunner-La Rocca, H. P., Buster, P. T., Rickenbacher, P., Hunziker, P., Mueller, C., . . . Kaiser, C. (2006). Late clinical events after clopidogrel discontinuation may limit the benefit of drug-eluting stents. *Journal of the American College of Cardiology, 48*(12), 2584–2591.

Savel, T. G., & Foldy, S. (2012). The role of public health informatics in enhancing public health surveillance. *MMWR: Surveillance Summaries, 61*(Suppl.), 20–24.

U.S. Census Bureau. (2010). *Interactive population map*. Retrieved from http://www.census.gov/2010census/popmap/

U.S. Census Bureau. (2013a). *American community survey*. Retrieved from http://www.census.gov/acs/www/about_the_survey/american_community_survey/

U.S. Census Bureau. (2013b). *Mobile apps*. Retrieved from http://www.census.gov/mobile/

U.S. Department of Health and Human Services. (2013). *Healthy People 2020*. Retrieved from http://healthypeople.gov/2020/default.aspx

Weitzman, E. R., Kelemen, S., Kaci, L., & Mandl, K. D. (2012, May 22). Willingness to share personal health record data for care improvement and public health: A survey of experienced personal health record cases. *BMC Medical Informatics and Decision Making*. 12:39. doi: 10.1186/1472-6947-12-39

World Health Organization. (2007). *International health regulations (2005): Areas of work for implementation*. Retrieved from http://www.who.int/ihr/finalversion9Nov07.pdf

World Health Organization. (2012). *International travel and health*. Retrieved from http://www.who.int/ith/en/

CHAPTER 16

Genetics/Genomics

Kelly M. East, MS, CGC
Neil E. Lamb, PhD

CHAPTER LEARNING OBJECTIVES

1. Describe basic concepts associated with genetics and genomics as they relate to health and disease.
2. Characterize the current landscape of genetic testing with respect to technology and clinical applications.
3. Identify the informatics components associated with generating, using, and storing patient genetic data.
4. Differentiate the current and future influence of genetic and genomic information in the healthcare decision-making process.
5. Recognize the role of nurses in understanding and administering genomic medicine.

KEY TERMS

Analytic validity
Bioinformatics
Clinical validity
DNA
Exome
Genetic risk assessment
Genetics
Genomic medicine

Genomic variation
Genomics
Nursing competencies
Privacy and confidentiality
Secondary findings
Sequencing
Testing technologies
Variants

CHAPTER OVERVIEW

This chapter focuses on the current and future applications of genetics and genomics to clinical practice and the associated informatics challenges. Informatics is more aptly termed **bioinformatics** because of the storage, organization, and retrieval of large sets of genetic data and the computing power and programming needed to analyze genetic data. Basic genetics and genomics concepts are described and resources for additional learning are provided. Current genomic **testing technologies** can produce massive amounts of data quickly and relatively inexpensively. This, coupled with an increased understanding of the impact of deoxyribonucleic acid (DNA) variation on disease, increases the likelihood that genomic information will become part of clinical care. A case study involving whole exome sequencing further highlights the potential benefits, limitations, and challenges associated with using genome data to make genetic diagnoses and influence patient care. Registered nurses and other healthcare professionals will play a critical role in the implementation of **genomic medicine**, which is the application of genetics in clinical care of patients.

INTRODUCTION

Scientific advances in genetics are reshaping our understanding of health and illness. Historically viewed as the domain of obstetric and prenatal specialists, today genetic risk factors are known to influence many common health conditions across the human lifespan. Multiple lines of evidence suggest these disorders are the collective result of lifestyle and environmental factors interacting against a susceptible backdrop of multiple genetic risks (Guttmacher, Collins, & Drazen, 2004). Research since 2000 has proven especially insightful, highlighting the relationship between genetic variation, disease risk, and responsiveness to treatment (Feero, Guttmacher, & Collins, 2010). **Genetics**, the study of individual genes, has expanded into **genomics**, which encompasses the study of all the genes in the human genome, including the interactions between genes and with the environment, and the influence of cultural and psychosocial factors (Consensus Panel on Genetic/Genomic Nursing Competencies, 2009). Genetic and genomic testing continue to move into mainstream health practice, necessitating a familiarity with DNA-based information and the ability to access, interpret, and act upon these findings. This has led to a focus on genomic nursing, that is, incorporating genetic and genomic findings into nursing practices beyond the traditional realm of genetic specialties (Calzone et al., 2010; Consensus Panel on Genetic/Genomic Nursing Competencies, 2009; Kirk, McDonald, Longley, & Anstey, 2003; McInerney, 2008). In this chapter, we explore ways genetic information is being applied for diagnosis, treatment, and prevention at the point of care. The intersection of genomics with informatics is highlighted at each stage of the clinical journey, from initial intake and data gathering to results reporting and integration into the medical record.

HISTORICAL PERSPECTIVES ON GENETIC TESTING AND DIAGNOSTIC TECHNOLOGIES

Karyotypes

Developed in the 1970s, the G-banded karyotype was the first DNA-based diagnostic test. A DNA stain visualizes condensed chromosomes present in cells just before they divide (**Figure 16-1**). Until recently, various versions of this technique were the gold standard for detecting anomalies involving entire chromosomes, as well as partial chromosome rearrangements of roughly 3 million bases or larger (Shaffer, Ledbetter, & Lupski, 2006). It was the original genome-wide analysis, albeit at very low resolution. In the 1990s, fluorescent in situ hybridization (FISH) was introduced, employing dye-tagged probes that would bind specific regions of patient DNA (Speicher & Carter, 2005). FISH probes could detect chromosome anomalies involving as few as 1 million bases of DNA.

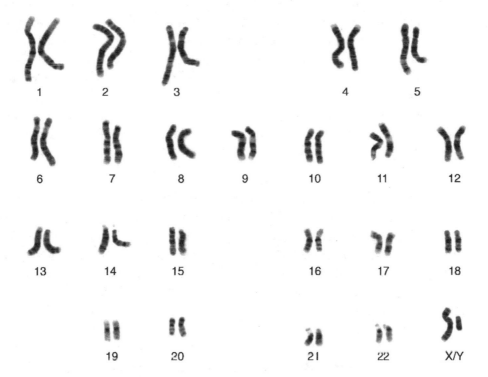

FIGURE 16-1   A human cell typically contains 46 chromosomes, organized into 23 pairs. A picture of human chromosomes is called a karyotype.

Source: NHGRI, Darryl Leja, www.genome.gov. http://www.genome.gov/dmd/img.cfm?node=Photos/Graphics&id=85192.

Microarray

More recent technologies have improved on the resolution and scale of FISH approaches, assembling a collection of up to a million probes on a single microscope slide. Known as chromosomal microarray, this method allows the genome to be quickly screened for imbalances in dosages as small as 50,000 DNA bases (Baldwin et al., 2008), and it has been shown to identify a significantly greater proportion of disease-causing chromosomal imbalances than detected by G-banded karyotype. It has become the first-tier genetic test for individuals with multiple congenital anomalies or developmental delays of unknown origin and for those with autism spectrum disorders (Manning & Hudgins, 2010).

Targeted Assays

For smaller scale DNA changes (involving a single nucleotide up to a few thousand), several detection methods are available. Many technologies confirm the presence or absence of known disease-causing mutations—for example, the beta-globin mutation associated with sickle cell anemia. These targeted assays focus on the mutation site, which is often a single-nucleotide change. If a number of potential mutation sites span one or several genes, an array of possible **variants** may be simultaneously interrogated. Using microarray technology, a single experiment can obtain the genetic results for over a million single nucleotide polymorphisms. This type of genome-wide analysis can be obtained for $100 or less (e.g., via http://www.23andMe.com).

Direct Sequencing

Directly **sequencing** the **DNA** is the current method of choice when searching for rare variants that are not likely to be detected by array-based approaches. This technology identifies single nucleotide changes, plus small insertions and deletions that can impact the function of the encoded protein. The gene of interest, or a panel of candidate genes, is divided into small overlapping fragments and analyzed using a method called capillary-based Sanger sequencing. This is the gold standard for sequence-based testing and can be ordered from clinical diagnostic testing laboratories for hundreds of individual genes.

CURRENT CLINICAL APPLICATIONS OF GENETIC INFORMATION _____

Today, genetics and genomics information and technologies are being applied in a wide variety of healthcare settings and specialties (Feero et al., 2010). The following are a few case examples of these applications.

Oncology

Steven, a 57-year-old male, was recently diagnosed with metastatic colon cancer. Tumors have been detected in his colon and in his liver. As Steven's oncologist works up a plan for chemotherapy, he orders genetic testing on Steven's tumor. Testing reveals a mutation in the KRAS gene (found in 40% of metastatic colon cancers) indicating anti-EGFR chemotherapies would not be an effective form of treatment (Allegra et al., 2009).

Sarah is a 25-year-old female with a family history of cancer. Her paternal grandmother died of ovarian cancer at 53, and her paternal aunt was diagnosed with breast cancer at 41. Her aunt recently tested positive for an inherited mutation in the BRCA1 gene associated with hereditary breast and ovarian cancer syndrome. Sarah has a 25% chance of having this same mutation, which would result in a significantly increased cancer risk (Lux, Fasching, & Beckmann, 2006). She undergoes testing to determine whether she has inherited the familial BRCA1 mutation and whether she needs to consider screening and surgical options to lower her cancer risks.

Obstetrics

Nicole is 37 years old and expecting her third baby. Because she is over 35 and classified as "advanced maternal age," she decides to pursue screening for chromosome imbalances such as trisomy 21 (Down syndrome). Nicole's nurse tells her about a new test available called noninvasive prenatal testing (NIPT) that is able to analyze fetal DNA present in maternal blood. With a simple blood draw from Nicole, the test is able to determine whether it is likely the fetus has trisomy 21 or other common chromosome conditions (Chitty, Hill, White, Wright, & Morris, 2012; Chiu et al., 2011).

Surgery

Prior to Don's coronary bypass for clogged arteries, Don's nurse asks about his family history of surgical complications. Don remembers that his mother had a near-fatal reaction to anesthesia during a routine hysterectomy that included rapid heart rate and rigid muscles. Don's healthcare team recognizes the symptoms of malignant hyperthermia—a severe adverse reaction to commonly used anesthesia gases. Don is tested and found to have an RYR1 gene mutation associated with malignant hyperthermia. Because he is at risk, alternative anesthesia medications are selected (Larach, Gronert, Allen, Brandom, & Lehman, 2010).

Pharmacology

Michael is being prescribed the blood thinner, warfarin, because of a recent blood clot in his left leg. Before determining the starting dose, his healthcare provider consults his genomic information, specifically two genetic variants in the CYP2C9 and VKORC1 genes that play a role in the metabolism of warfarin. His particular versions of these genes indicate that he is a "poor metabolizer." The drug will likely be processed more slowly and remain in Michael's blood longer, requiring a lower dose (Cavallari & Limdi, 2009).

Infectious Disease

Nigel visits his physician because he has a wound on his leg that has become increasingly painful. Upon evaluation, the healthcare team sees that the wound has become infected. Instead of prescribing a round of antibiotics that treat the most common pathogen suspects, they swab the wound and order a genetic test to determine the specific bacteria causing the infection. Within a day they determine that Nigel has methicillin-resistant *Staphylococcus aureus* (MRSA). This diagnosis drastically changes the treatment course for Nigel, because MRSA does not respond to first-line antibiotic therapy. Early diagnosis and genomic testing technologies help save Nigel, and his leg, from serious complications (Eiland et al., 2010).

The current state of genetic testing is very much in transition. Since the early 2000s, the cost of DNA sequencing has plummeted, thanks in part to so-called "next generation" technologies and associated analysis software (Mardis, 2011; Wetterstrand, 2013). Today, the entire **exome** (the approximately 1% of the genome that primarily encodes proteins) can be sequenced faster and more cheaply than a single gene using older methodology. The generation of the raw sequence data from an entire human genome can be completed in around 1 week. While analyzing the data to identify and validate clinically relevant sequence variants takes several additional weeks, this overall time frame is astonishing.

LARGE-SCALE SEQUENCING IN A CLINICAL SETTING _____

The following hypothetical case illustrates the informatics issues associated with this type of large-scale analysis. We describe each step in the process and return to the case study to illustrate the genomic concepts, the rationales behind the clinical decision-making process, and the bioinformatics concepts.

EVALUATING AND SELECTING GENOMIC TESTS _____

An ever-growing number of genetic and genomic tests is available to the clinician to aid in patient care. While most of these directly examine DNA at a sequence level, others analyze RNA or protein or even assess so-called epigenetic modifications—where

---

Box 16-1   Case Study

Sean is a 6-month-old baby boy. During a routine prenatal ultrasound, Sean was found to have tetralogy of fallot, a type of heart anomaly. No other anomalies were observed on ultrasound and no prenatal genetic testing was performed. After Sean was born, his pediatrician noticed some mild facial differences (a broad forehead and deep-set eyes) and a high bilirubin level indicating jaundice. There is no known family history of similar medical problems. Based on these findings, the physician ordered several baseline genetic tests, including karyotype, microarray, and 22q deletion testing, to try to determine a cause for Sean's symptoms. Although all results are negative, the healthcare team believes that Sean's symptoms are likely due to an undiagnosed genetic condition. Instead of continuing to order individual tests for a multitude of possible conditions (searching for a needle in a very large haystack), the physician decides to order whole exome sequencing.

---

small molecules bind DNA and impact overall gene expression. Regardless of the specific assay chosen, there are several characteristics to look for when evaluating the usefulness of a test for a particular patient. The clinician should select tests that are accurate and correctly detect and report genetic information (**analytic validity**). Healthcare providers should make sure that tests and testing laboratories have proper approval (i.e., from the U.S. Food and Drug Administration [FDA]) and certifications. All tests used for patient care should take place in a Clinical Laboratory Improvement Amendments (CLIA)–certified laboratory. The genetic information examined should also be strongly associated with the disease or trait of interest (**clinical validity**). The ideal test would detect 100% of disease-causing genetic mutations (no false negatives) while avoiding genetic changes that do not cause disease (no/few false positives). Even the best tests have some chance for error, but these risks should be minimized as much as possible.

Just because a test is valid does not mean it has a place in clinical practice and should be ordered for all patients. The clinical utility of a test—whether it will improve patient care—should also be considered. For example, a genetic test result may confirm a diagnosis that is not possible by physical exam alone. A test may also help direct treatment decisions or allow for disease prevention before symptom onset. Clinical utility should be determined each time a test is ordered, as the same genetic test may be meaningful in one situation, but not in others.

There are also practical issues to consider, such as the likelihood that the patient has a genetic change the test is capable of capturing and the financial burden of the test. It is a daunting task for the clinician to evaluate validity and utility of tests in a continually changing market. To make this job more manageable, several groups have begun creating tools and resources to help organize and evaluate genetic and genomic tests. The Genetic Test Registry, maintained by the National Institutes of Health

(NIH), contains a catalog of information (including validity and utility data) submitted by testing laboratories about genetic and genomic tests that are clinically available. The Evaluation of Genomic Applications in Practice and Prevention (EGAPP) working group is a multidisciplinary team that reviews genomic tests and publishes reports guiding clinicians on their validity, utility, and appropriate use.

USING PATIENT INFORMATION TO ASSESS RISK

A family health history can provide some important insight into a patient's future risk of disease and is the first step in a **genetic risk assessment** (Claassen et al., 2010). For single-gene diseases, such as Marfan syndrome and cystic fibrosis, the clinician can use family history and the knowledge of Mendelian patterns of inheritance (i.e., dominant, recessive, X-linked) to determine whether an individual is at risk for disease. For example, the proband (indicated by the arrow) in **Figure 16-2** has a 50% chance of having Marfan syndrome, a disorder characterized by an autosomal dominant inheritance pattern.

Risks are much less concrete when assessing complex diseases like lung cancer, heart disease, and diabetes for which there are a number of genetic and environmental risk factors, some known and many unknown. Family members share some

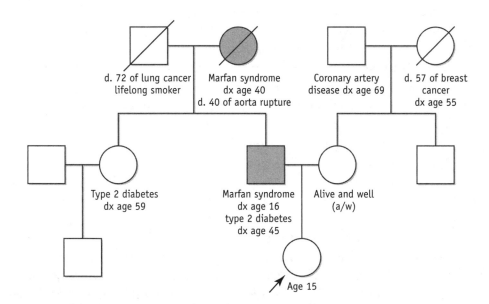

FIGURE 16-2 Example of an annotated pedigree for a family affected with Marfan syndrome.

percentage of genetic information with one another; therefore, they may share genetic variation that increases and/or decreases disease risk for complex diseases. In addition, family members often share an environment and environmental risk factors for disease.

Generally, a person's disease risk is influenced by the number of close relatives affected with that disease. For example, having a first-degree relative (parent, sibling, etc.) with a common complex disease is commonly thought to increase a person's risk approximately two- to three-fold above the general population (Scheuner, Wang, Raffel, Larabell, & Rotter, 1997). Other red flags include early onset of disease, having a disease present even in the absence of environmental factors known to raise the risk of that disease, being a race or ethnic background in which a disease is more prevalent, and having parents who are closely related by blood relationships. These red flags indicate a general increased risk for a disease with a genetic basis. However, it is important to remember that empiric risk estimates are based on population averages and that the actual risk in an individual family may be higher or lower than these estimates. Family health histories are currently an underused tool in clinical medicine (Acheson, Wiesner, Zyzanski, Goodwin, & Stange, 2000; Doerr & Teng, 2012).

Healthcare providers can collect family health history information in a variety of formats (pedigree chart, bulleted list, checklist, etc.). In particular, Brock, Allen, Keiser, and Langlois (2010) provide an excellent guide to creating three-generation patient pedigrees. Alternately, online tools have been developed to help patients and the public record family history information to share with relatives and healthcare providers (Giovanni & Murray, 2010). Computerized software such as Progeny is available to clinics to electronically input and store pedigree information. Regardless of format, it is important that the information be collected in a way that is meaningful, stored in the patient's medical record, and analyzed and updated regularly by the healthcare provider.

Environmental and genomic disease risk factors interact with one another in a very complex way, but healthcare providers can provide patients information as to whether their risk may be increased based on their environment and family history and actions they may be able to take to reduce risk for a particular disease (Claassen et al., 2010). For some conditions, computerized risk models are available that use information taken from a patient's family history and medical record to estimate a patient's risk. For example, a female's breast cancer risk can be estimated using risk models such as the Gail, Claus, and Tyrer-Cuzick models (Amir et al., 2003; Domcheck et al., 2003). For other conditions, the clinician currently has to use his or her best clinical judgment to estimate risk.

A small percentage of patients have red flags in their personal or family health history that point to hereditary disease and may benefit from referral for more specialized genetic services. For more information about making genetics referrals and a list of common referral indications, consult the 2007 *Genetics in Medicine* article written by Pletcher and colleagues entitled "Indications for Genetic Referral: A Guide for Healthcare Providers." Directories of certified genetics professionals can be found at http://www.acmg.net and http://www.nsgc.org.

GENERATING AND INTERPRETING LARGE-SCALE SEQUENCING DATA

Historically, DNA fragments were sequenced and analyzed individually, one stretch at a time. Today's next-generation systems simultaneously sequence billions of overlapping DNA fragments, making whole genome analysis possible. This results in an enormous text file containing billions of As, Ts, Cs, and Gs along with some quality measure that represents the accuracy of each base identified. Several sequentially applied analyses (reviewed in Moorthie, Hall, & Wright, 2013) provide meaning to this string of nucleotides, identifying clinically relevant variants (**Figure 16-3**). In a nutshell, the sequence of each DNA fragment is first aligned to its corresponding location on a reference sequence. Multiple alignment programs are available and each must be tolerant enough to allow mismatches that represent genetic variation yet exclude fragments that belong elsewhere in the genome or are of low accuracy. Ideally, multiple fragments will be aligned to each region—a concept known as "coverage." Increased coverage translates into greater confidence in the accuracy of the sequence, which is especially important for regions found to contain DNA variation. Current variant-detection software is quite good at identifying single-nucleotide changes but struggles with small insertions and deletions, and larger segmental gains, losses, or rearrangements. As the software matures, detection should improve.

Roughly 25,000 variants will be identified in each human exome, the vast majority of which will be benign, with no clinical implications. Further computational

---

Box 16-2   Case Study

A sample of blood is taken from Sean and sent to a laboratory for whole exome sequencing. The gene regions of Sean's genome are isolated and sequenced. Then a team of laboratory scientists culls through the data to determine whether any genomic variants identified in Sean might explain his symptoms or have other medical implications for Sean and his family.

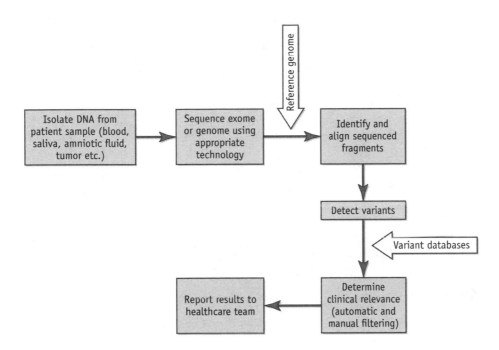

FIGURE 16-3 The pipeline for clinical genomic sequencing.

analysis and filtering software interprets the source, predicted functional impact, and relative frequency of each variant to identify a set of candidate clinically relevant DNA changes (**Figure 16-4**). As the algorithms, analytical tools, and databases linking DNA change to physiological symptoms are still evolving, this step is the bottleneck for the current clinical application of large-scale sequencing.

Existing protocols usually begin by excluding variants commonly found in the general population and those associated with benign conditions or traits. This filter often removes up to 90% of the identified variants (Bainbridge et al., 2011). Additional filters may be used, such as identifying changes that likely alter protein function, variants from genes that function in clinically relevant tissues, DNA changes in evolutionarily conserved regions, and an assessment of the protein's role in various biochemical pathways. Such analyses require access to databases of both normal and pathogenic **genomic variation**. A sampling of such databases is provided in **Table 16-1**. When the list of potential candidates has been shortened, software algorithms are replaced by manual interpretation, usually by a clinician or clinical scientist. Each variant must be evaluated in light of the patient profile. If a candidate causal variant is not identified at this point, the process is begun again with a less stringent set of conditions. If a putative

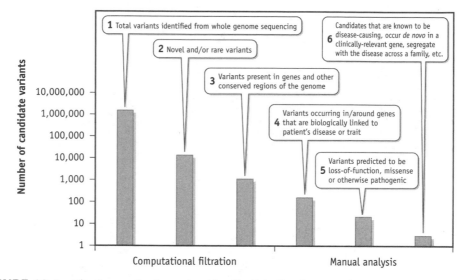

FIGURE 16-4   Filtration methods used to identify clinically relevant variants.

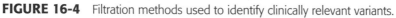

Table 16-1 Databases of Normal and Pathogenic Genomic Variation	
Genomic Category	**Databases**
Normal genomic variation	1,000 Genomes HapMap
Databases with variant-disease associations across genome	OMIM (Online Mendelian Inheritance in Man) HGMD (Human Gene Mutation Database) HGVbaseG2P (Human Genome Variation Genotype-to-Phenotype database)
Locus-specific databases	Cystic Fibrosis Mutation database LDLR Familial Hypercholesterlemia database
Disease-specific databases	AlzGene (Alzheimer disease) PDGene (Parkinson disease) T1Dbase (Type 1 diabetes)
Database of somatic cancer genome variation	TCGA (The Cancer Genome Atlas) HCMD (Human Gene Mutation Database)

Data from Moorthie S, Hall A and Wright CF (2013). Informatics and clinical genome sequencing: opening the black box. *Genet Med, 15*(3), 165–171.

(presumed) variant is found, its existence is ideally confirmed using an alternate method of detection. Unfortunately this is not always feasible, especially when confirming large numbers of variants.

In practice, genetic variants can be classified into one of four major categories: (1) those that have clear clinical implications in terms of disease causation or therapeutic intervention; (2) those with a plausible connection to disease, but which lack conclusive evidence; (3) those with no known disease association; or (4) variants of unknown significance. This last category presents a particularly thorny challenge, because changes with unknown significance may in fact truly be associated with disease, but simply lack current external validation. The evidence base that underlies variant classification is continually growing and evolving, and variants will transition from one category to another following further scientific discovery. The existence of actively curated and frequently updated variant databases is critical to tracking this movement and revising patient findings accordingly.

REPORTING AND STORING GENETIC RESULTS

Reporting Secondary Findings

In many cases, large-scale exome or genome sequencing will uncover a definitive (or at least plausible) biological explanation for a patient's disorder. It is likely that an additional set of results will also be identified. Known as incidental or **secondary findings**, these include variants that predispose to diseases unrelated to the initial reason for undergoing genomic sequencing. Every genome contains thousands of variants, ranging in frequency from rare to common and carrying functional impacts from inconsequential to harmful. Potentially damaging incidental findings include mutations that lead to adult-onset cancer, those that confer carrier status for recessive disorder, or variants that uncover nonpaternity within a family. The details of this issue are beyond the scope of this chapter, but several groups have recently explored whether researchers and clinicians have a responsibility to actively search for secondary findings and, if so, what specific findings should be assessed (American College of Medical Genetics and Genomics [ACMG], 2012; Clayton et al., 2013; Gliwa & Berkman, 2013; Green et al., 2012). Such discussions would be broached with patients through extensive pretest counseling and informed consent. In 2013, the American College of Medical Genetics and Genomics recommended a minimum set of genes for which variants should always be reported when performing genome- and exome-based sequencing (ACMG, 2013). This list is primarily composed of highly penetrant mutations associated with cancer or cardiac disorders. Based on

---

Box 16-3   Case Study

Sean's clinically relevant genomic variants identified by the testing are returned in a report to Sean's healthcare providers. A follow-up appointment is scheduled for Sean and his family to discuss the results. Testing found that Sean has a rare genetic mutation in the JAG1 gene associated with Alagille syndrome. Upon further reflection, Sean's symptoms are consistent with a diagnosis of Alagille syndrome, although he lacks some of the typical symptoms. These mutations are often not inherited, but arise de novo in the egg or sperm, which explains the lack of family history. Based on this diagnosis, Sean will need to be monitored closely for potential problems with his liver, eyes, growth, and development.

In addition to this diagnosis, exome testing revealed that Sean carries a single nucleotide polymorphism (SNP) that increases the chance he will develop bipolar disease. This result does not impact Sean's current medical care as it is not diagnostic (Sean's risk is somewhat increased, but the SNP is not sufficient to cause the disorder), and there are no currently available interventions to reduce risk or prevent onset of psychiatric conditions such as bipolar disorder.

Lastly, testing revealed that Sean carries a recessive mutation in the CFTR gene associated with cystic fibrosis. This means that Sean is not affected with the condition, but that he (and likely one of his parents) is a carrier for the condition. Sean's parents and Sean's future reproductive partners should be offered cystic fibrosis carrier testing that might help inform reproductive decisions.

Sean's parents are relieved to have an explanation for Sean's medical problems and glad to have an idea of what to expect from Alagille syndrome in the future. However, they are anxious about the increased risk for bipolar disorder and the uncertainty of dealing with this condition in the future. They are not planning to have other children and decline follow-up cystic fibrosis testing but indicate they will discuss the result with Sean when he gets older.

---

currently available data, ACMG estimates secondary variants in these genes would be identified in 1% of all cases.

Genomic Information and Electronic Health Records

Although electronic health records (EHRs) have become a key component of many healthcare systems, very few have historically incorporated genomic information (Hoffman, 2007; Sax & Schmidt, 2005). Most EHR systems do not capture family history or pedigree data in a standardized, queryable form (Scheuner et al., 2009). Similarly, because genomic results are often sent from a testing laboratory to the clinician in narrative, paper-based formats, if these findings are entered into an EHR, they are in free-text, noncoded fields or as scanned images. Details, such as the nucleotide sequence of assessed DNA variants, are often excluded, requiring a clinician to manually search for relevant information (U.S. Department of Health and Human Services [HHS], 2008).

In 2007, NIH established the Electronic Medical Records and Genomics (eMERGE) Network, a consortium of medical institutes dedicated to studying the relationship between genomic information and EHR systems. Along with other organizations, this group is actively identifying how best to incorporate genomic information into the EHR. Simultaneously, groups are exploring interpretive algorithms that incorporate genomic findings to determine individual risk and inform clinical decision support systems (Belmont & McGuire, 2009). Embedded into the EHR, these systems help clinicians interpret actionable findings and guide decisions about care. While the majority of the patient's genomic information will be dormant and never influence health decisions, there will be genetic variants that have event-specific value—shaping drug selection or informing preventative care. This medically relevant genetic information should be highlighted, but only when circumstances call for it.

Aside from the specifics of how it will inform clinical decision making, incorporating genomic information into EHRs faces several practical challenges. What information should be stored in the EHR: the entire genomic sequence, a catalog of all identified variants, or only those identified as clinically relevant? Given that the complete sequence could occupy a gigabyte of storage space or more, will our health systems have sufficient storage capacity? Will the information be searchable and shareable across platforms, or will organizations default to using PDFs or printing the data on paper?

Privacy and Confidentiality of Genomic Information

Before disclosing genetic information or consenting to a genetic test, a patient often asks about risks—"Where will my data be stored?" "Who will have access to the information?" "Will I lose the ability to get insurance?" These are valid questions and concerns about **privacy and confidentiality**. History has taught that it is possible for genetic information to be abused and used to discriminate against and stigmatize a person or population (e.g., the eugenics movement in the early 1900s and sickle cell carrier testing in the 1970s).

There is broad privacy protection for all health information, including genetic information, afforded by the Health Insurance Portability and Accountability Act (HIPAA) and protection against discrimination for individuals with disabilities afforded by the Americans with Disabilities Act (ADA). Whether genetic information requires extra privacy and discriminatory protection, an idea termed *genetic exceptionalism*, continues to be discussed among scientists, lawyers, philosophers, and clinicians (Green & Botkin, 2003). Some argue that genetic information is different from other health information in that it can predict future disease occurrence,

Table 16-2   Definition of Genetic Information
"Genetic Information" as Defined by the Genetic Information Nondiscrimination Act (Hudson, Holohan, & Collins, 2008)
Genetic test results
Family health history
Use of genetic counseling or other genetic services
Participation in genetic research
NOT sex or age
Source: Adapted from www.ginahelp.org

uniquely identify people, and have significant implications for family members. Others argue that these characteristics are not unique to genetic information and therefore genetic information should be treated the same as other personal health information.

The Genetic Information Nondiscrimination Act (GINA) was signed into law May 21, 2008 and offers additional protection on a national level against genetic discrimination in the workplace and in health insurance (Hudson, Holohan, & Collins, 2008). GINA states that employers cannot use an individual's genetic information (defined in **Table 16-2**) to make decisions about hiring, firing, promotion, pay, or privileges or otherwise mistreat an employee. GINA also states that genetic information cannot be used by health insurance companies to make decisions about eligibility, premium, contribution amounts, or coverage terms. Neither employers nor insurance companies can request or require genetic information or tests from individuals.

GINA sets the baseline protection for all Americans, but individual states can pass litigation providing additional protection. While GINA prohibits genetic discrimination in most health insurance and workplace settings, it has several important exclusions (e.g., small business, the military, veterans, and Native Americans) and does not apply to disability or life and long-term care insurance. GINA and many state genetic discrimination laws are relatively new and largely untested in the court systems. Time will tell whether these laws are successful and sufficient in protecting patients from genetic discrimination. More information on GINA and its protections can be found at http://www.ginahelp.org/. A searchable database of state legislations related to genetics and genomics is regularly updated at http://www.genome.gov/PolicyEthics/LegDatabase/pubsearch.cfm.

Nurses and other healthcare professionals need to be aware of national- and state-level legal protections and their limitations, so that they can inform patients of their rights regarding privacy and use of genetic information. Nurses also need to be diligent to abide by these laws and their code of ethics in practice to help safeguard their patients' information (Badzek, Henaghan, Turner, & Monsen, 2013; International Society of Nurses in Genetics [ISONG], 2010).

LOOKING TOWARD THE FUTURE

A number of hurdles still remain before widespread implementation can be considered. Even with the decline in costs, sequencing is still relatively expensive, requires significant computational manipulations, and is uncertain with respect to the clinical significance of many DNA variants. This situation is rapidly evolving and at some future date, it is likely that most single-gene tests will be supplanted by genome-wide approaches.

Much of the current clinical application of whole exome sequencing has been in patients with undiagnosed genetic conditions. This type of analysis has been successful for patients like Sean, the boy in our case study, for whom tests of candidate genes were negative but the constellation of symptoms suggested the presence of some type of genetic disorder. One of the first successes in clinical exome sequencing took place in 2009 for a young boy with an unusual, severe, and unexplained gastrointestinal (GI) disease (Mayer et al., 2011). After exhausting other options, the medical team turned to exome sequencing, which at the time was new and not clinically validated. A rare mutation in the XIAP gene was identified, leading to a stem cell transplant. This has alleviated the boy's GI symptoms and mitigated the risk of additional life-threatening complications associated with XIAP mutations.

The cost of exome sequencing is now comparable to that of most single-gene tests, making it equally or more cost effective to order the broader testing. It is becoming a commonly ordered test in genetics clinics around the country, and laboratories are reporting greater than 25% diagnosis rates (Hayden, 2012; Karow, 2013). It is important to note, however, that even if a definitive diagnosis is obtained, it may not impact patient care. At some point in the future, whole genome sequencing (WGS), will likely replace exome sequencing as the test of preference. Such a move will identify even more disease-related genetic changes, but variants of uncertain significance will become an even greater challenge as laboratories explore regions of the genome that are increasingly less characterized.

The current practice of using clinical sequencing for individuals with rare diseases begins with a relatively narrow question in mind: Can a diagnosis be reached that allows the clinician and patient to understand better the cause and nature of the disease? In contrast, sequencing seemingly healthy individuals for risk prediction, and preventative medicine presents a broad and poorly-defined target that has yet to be validated. In 2010 the genome of Dr. Stephen Quake, a healthy 40-year-old male, was sequenced and analyzed (Ashley et al., 2010). A team of 35 physicians, bioinformaticians, scientists, genetic counselors, and ethicists spent more than 3,000 hours interpreting the genome (N. Lamb, personal communication, September 11, 2010) and determining Quake to be at increased risk for heart disease, type 2 diabetes, and obesity. His increased risk for heart disease was further emphasized by a positive family history. Quake's genome contained three novel mutations in genes associated with the disease hemochromatosis, even though there was no evidence of the disease in Quake or his family members. In addition, 63 clinically relevant pharmacogenomic variants were identified that may be informative for future drug selection and dosing. The interpretation model used with Quake is not scalable in terms of man-hours and personnel. For genome data to be integrated into mainstream health care, the tools that support point-of-care decision making must improve dramatically.

While a person's genome sequence does not significantly change over time, the understanding of the genome and impact of specific genomic variation is fluid. At least in the short term, a patient's genome will need to be periodically re-analyzed. Ideally, EHRs would automatically update with new findings and incorporate the information into a robust decision support system. This would be especially beneficial as the clinical implication of variants of unknown significance becomes clearer. This "sequence once, read often" approach avoids overwhelming physicians with genomic alerts that are not currently relevant, but may be in the future (Manolio et al., 2013). It is important to recognize, however, that recontacting patients with updated information carries with it yet unanswered ethical and legal considerations and may present a significant burden to healthcare providers (Pyeritz, 2011). It is also worth noting that at some point the cost to sequence the genome may become cheaper than the cost to store the genomic information. If that occurs, the approach may change to "sequence often, read often."

AN EDUCATIONAL CHALLENGE

Regardless of work setting or specialty, all nurses and other healthcare professionals need to be armed with the knowledge and skills to incorporate genomic information into practice (Calzone et al., 2010). Unfortunately, the challenge of incorporating genetics and genomics into clinical practice has outpaced the educational training of many healthcare providers. Gaps have emerged relating to genetic and genomic content, including the perception that genetics has little relevance in daily practice, a lack

Table 16-3   Nurses and Genomic Medicine
With respect to genetic and genomic information, nurses should be able to do the following:
1. Understand and be able to explain the role of genetics/genomics in health and disease
2. Use information technology to obtain credible and current information about genetics/genomics
3. Record and interpret a three-generation family health history
4. Incorporate genetic/genomic information into disease risk assessment, taking into account other environmental and medical factors
5. Select and order appropriate genetic/genomic tests
6. Facilitate the informed consent process for genetic/genomic tests
7. Use genetic/genomic information (e.g., test results, family history) to improve patient care
8. Identify patients who would benefit from referral to specialized genetic/genomic services
9. Recruit patients to genetic/genomic research studies
10. Safeguard patients' genetic/genomic privacy and confidentiality
Source: American Nurses Association, 2008; Conley, 2013; NCHPEG, 2007.

of basic genetic knowledge, and an accompanying low personal confidence in discussing genetic concepts (Calzone et al., 2010; McInerney, 2008). As mentioned at the onset of this chapter, genetic and genomics education opportunities for nurses need to be grounded in key skills and competencies. **Table 16-3** lists some **nursing competencies**, which are the expected genomic knowledge, skills, and values needed for clinical practice (American Nurses Association, 2008; Conley et al., 2013; National Coalition for Health Professional Education in Genetics, 2007).

SUMMARY

This chapter has explored the application of genetic and genomic information to health care in the past, present, and future. The size and scope of genomic information presents unique challenges to the healthcare system in terms of gathering, using, and storing patient data. The field of clinical genetics and genomics is continually changing. Healthcare professionals and the public need continued education and resources to maintain a current understanding of the impact of genetics and genomics on health and disease (**Box 16-4**). A list of selected online genetics and genomics resources relevant to nurses is provided in **Table 16-4**. Development of additional educational opportunities and point-of-care resources will be necessary for genomic medicine to reach its full potential.

Box 16-4   A Brief Primer About Genetics

For a deeper understanding of the field, Tonkin, Calzone, Jenkins, Lea, & Prows (2011) have recently reviewed a broad cross-section of genetic education resources of use to nursing students and professionals. A list of selected online resources can be found at the conclusion of this chapter.

DNA

Deoxyribonucleic Acid (DNA) contains the genetic instructions that pass information about the organism from one generation to the next. The DNA is organized into discrete structures known as chromosomes, which consist of long strands of DNA very tightly condensed and wrapped around a protein scaffold (Figure 16-5). In humans, the nucleus contains two (2) sets of chromosomes, one set contributed by each parent. Each set contains 22 autosomes and one sex chromosome for a total of 23 chromosomes per set, or 46 chromosomes per cell. Males have both an "X" and "Y" sex chromosome, while females have two "X" sex chromosomes.

DNA assumes a double helix shape, similar to a twisted ladder. The "rungs" are composed of four chemical building blocks called nucleotides. These nucleotides are Adenine, Thymine, Cytosine and Guanine, abbreviated as A, T, C and G. There are 3.5 billion nucleotides in a complete set of human DNA. The sequence of DNA is the specific order of the nucleotides across a region of DNA.

Genes

A gene is a specific stretch of DNA that provides instructions to the cell. Often, but not always, these instructions tell the cell how to assemble a certain protein. Genes help determine whether we will be male or female, brown or blue-eyed, tall or short. Genes also play major roles in the development of many diseases and disorders. Genes are arranged along the chromosome in a linear fashion, each having a specific location. Only a minority of the human genome is composed of genes (about 1%). The majority of human DNA consists of regulatory and repetitive sequences, fragments of inactive genes and other DNA sequence with yet-unknown functions. Genes generally have a set of sequence-specific characteristics that allow them to be identified. Humans have approximately 21,000 genes (Clamp et al., 2007; International Human Genome Sequencing Consortium, 2004; Lander, 2011).

The genome represents all of the genetic information present in a cell. More precisely, a genome is the specific complement of DNA present on one complete set of chromosomes. Humans therefore have 2 sets of this information (one on the maternal chromosomes and another on the paternal chromosomes). This distinction is often overlooked when individuals speak about the genome of specific organisms.

DNA Changes

A mutation is a permanent change in the DNA sequence. Mutations occur primarily in one of two ways: errors introduced during the process of DNA replication, or failure to repair DNA that has been damaged in some way. DNA damage can be spontaneous or in response to a physical or chemical agent (like ultraviolet light). The vast majority of all DNA mutations are recognized and repaired soon after they occur. A somatic mutation occurs in a subset of cells from a certain tissue—in the lung or breast, for example—and is not passed on to the next generation. In contrast, germline mutations occur in cells that will ultimately develop into eggs or sperm. If a germline mutation occurs in a sperm or an egg that participates in fertilization, all cells in the resulting embryo will contain the mutation, which can then be passed on to future generations. Every individual carries 30-70 of these mutations, introduced in the egg or sperm but not present in the body cells of either parent (Conrad et al., 2011; Roach et al., 2010). Similarly, the mutations we inherit from our parents, which are found in every one of our cells, first originated as a germline mutation in an ancestor from some distant past.

The sequence of DNA in our genome has been estimated to be 99.5% identical between any two humans (Gonzaga-Jauregui, Lupski, & Gibbs, 2012; Levy et al., 2007). Any given individual carries between 4 and 5 million sequence variants. Most of these differences involve one nucleotide of the DNA code (i.e. a C rather than an A) and are known as single nucleotide polymorphisms (SNPs). Other types of variation include insertions or deletions of one or more nucleotides or copy differences around the number of repeated sequences. The alternative forms of a given DNA sequence can also be called alleles.

Within a gene, DNA variation may lead to a protein that functions in a slightly different manner or is present at a different concentration. Many DNA sequence differences have no effect on physical characteristics, whereas other differences are directly responsible for major disease-causing effects. In between these extremes are variations that result in small changes in anatomy, dietary intolerances, organ function, susceptibility to infection, and even some variability in personality, athletic aptitude, and artistic talent. Some alleles function "dominantly", in that a single copy is sufficient to cause a specific trait, regardless of the allele contributed by the other parent. Other alleles act "recessively" and require that both parents contribute similar alleles for the physical characteristic to be manifest.

Note that genetic information is not the sole determinant of these traits—the environment plays a major role as well. In most cases, the trait represents the combined effect of many different genes and environmental factors. For example, it has been estimated that several hundred different genes are involved in human height, with each genetic factor contributing only a few millimeters to the overall total. In the same way, many diseases result from the combined action of environment and genes. The relative genetic role may be very small or very large.

TYPES OF GENETIC DISORDERS

Disorders caused in whole or in part by genetic factors can generally be grouped into single-gene, chromosomal or multifactorial categories, based on their underlying cause.

Single Gene

As their name suggests, single gene defects are caused by mutations in an individual gene. Remember that for most genes, two copies are present (one on the chromosome inherited maternally, the other from the paternal contribution). Single gene disorders, also known as Mendelian disorders, generally have recognizable dominant, recessive or sex-linked inheritance patterns in the family. Most of these defects are rare (usually with a frequency much less than 1 in 1000); however, as a group, single gene disorders are responsible for a significant proportion of disease and death, affecting as many as 2% of the population over an entire life span (Rimoin & Conner, 2002). Some examples of single-gene disorders are cystic fibrosis, Huntington's disease, Tay-Sachs disease, sickle cell anemia, Duchenne muscular dystrophy, and neurofibromatosis.

(continues)

Chromosomal

In chromosomal disorders the defect is not due to a mutation in a single gene, but rather to an excess or deficiency of the genes contained in an entire chromosome or segment of a chromosome. For example, the presence of an entire extra copy of the 21st chromosome leads to a specific defect, trisomy 21 (Down syndrome). There are over 200 genes on chromosome 21, and individuals with trisomy 21 have 3 normal copies of each gene. This increased copy number is believed to disrupt the delicate balance maintained in cells, leading to the specific physical characteristics associated with Down syndrome. As a group, chromosome disorders are quite common, affecting about 1 out of every 150 infants born (American College of Obstetricians and Gynecologists, 2001; Carey, 2003). They are especially common among miscarriages, accounting for about half of all such cases.

Multifactorial

Multifactorial disorders represent a number of both newborn and adult diseases including cleft lip, cardiovascular disease, psychiatric disorders, and cancer. While these diseases have a strong genetic component, they arise from a combination of genetic risk factors that are also influenced by the environment. Few of the contributing genes are believed to make more than a modest contribution to overall risk, perhaps increasing it by 5% or less. It is the specific combination of multiple predisposing alleles and risk-increasing environments that leads to physical symptoms. For this reason, they are often called complex or multifactorial disorders. It is estimated that over 60% of the entire population is impacted by a multifactorial disorder (Wynbrandt & Ludman, 2009).

Table 16-4   Selected Genetics and Genomics Resources

Category	Examples	URL
Background Information	Genetics Home Reference	http://ghr.nlm.nih.gov
	GeneReviews	http://www.ncbi.nlm.nih.gov/sites/GeneTests
	Genetics/Genomics Competency Center for Education	http://www.g-2-c-2.org/index.php
	Public Health Genomics (PHG) Foundation	http://www.phgfoundation.org
	Genetics and Public Policy Center	http://www.dnapolicy.org
	Telling Stories: Understanding Real Life Genetics	http://www.tellingstories.nhs.uk

Table 16-4 *Continued*		
Tools for Your Practice	Genetic Testing Registry	http://www.ncbi.nlm.nih.gov/gtr
	Evaluation of Genomic Applications in Practice and Prevention (EGAPP)	http://www.egappreviews.org
	"My Family Health Portrait"	https://familyhistory.hhs.gov
	National Cancer Institute Breast Cancer Risk Assessment Tool	http://www.cancer.gov/bcrisktool
	National Newborn Screening & Global Resource Center	http://genes-r-us.uthscsa.edu
	National Coalition for Health Professional Education in Genetics	http://www.nchpeg.org
	GINAhelp.org	http://ginahelp.org
Clinical Genetics Professional Organizations	International Society of Nurses in Genetics	http://www.isong.org
	National Society of Genetic Counselors	http://www.nsgc.org
	American College of Medical Genetics and Genomics	http://www.acmg.net
	American Society of Human Genetics	http://ashg.org
Patient Support and Advocacy Organizations	Genetic Alliance	http://www.geneticalliance.org
	National Organization for Rare Disorders	http://www.rarediseases.org
Nursing CEU Opportunities	Genetics Education Program for Nurses	http://www.cincinnatichildrens.org/education/clinical/nursing/genetics/default/

For a full suite of assignments and additional learning activities, use the access code located in the front of your book and visit www.jblearning.com. If you do not have an access code, you can obtain one at the site.

REFERENCES

Acheson, L. S., Wiesner, G. L., Zyzanski, S. J., Goodwin, M. A., & Stange, K. C. (2000). Family history-taking in community family practice: Implications for genetic screening. *Genetics in Medicine, 2*(3), 180–185.

Allegra, C. J., Jessup, J. M., Somerfield, M. R., Hamilton, S. R., Hammond, E. H., Hayes, D. F., . . . Schilsky, R. L. (2009). American Society of Clinical Oncology Provisional clinical opinion: Testing for KRAS gene mutations in patients with metastatic colorectal carcinoma to predict response to anti-epidermal growth factor receptor monoclonal antibody therapy. *Journal of Clinical Oncology, 27*(12), 2091–2096. doi:10.1200/JCO.2009.21.9170

American College of Medical Genetics and Genomics. (2013). ACMG Recommendations for reporting of incidental findings in clinical exome and genome sequencing. *Genetics in Medicine, 15*, 565–574.

American College of Medical Genetics and Genomics Board of Directors. (2012). Points to consider in the clinical application of genomic sequencing. *Genetics in Medicine, 14*, 759–761.

American Nurses Association. (2008). *Essentials of genetic and genomic nursing competencies, curricula guidelines, and outcome indicators* (2nd ed.). Bethesda, MD: Author.

Amir, E., Evans, D. G., Shenton, A., Lalloo, F., Moran, A., Boggis, C., . . . Howell, A. (2003). Evaluation of breast cancer risk assessment packages in the family history evaluation and screening programme. *Journal of Medical Genetics, 40*(11), 807–814. doi:10.1136/jmg.40.11.807

Ashley, E. A., Butte, A. J., Wheeler, M. T., Chen, R., Klein, T. E., Dewey, F. E., . . . Altman, R. B. (2010). Clinical assessment incorporating a personal genome. *Lancet, 375*, 1525–1535. doi:10.1016/S0140- 6736(10)60599-5

Badzek, L., Henaghan, M., Turner, M., & Monsen, R. (2013). Ethical, legal, and social issues in the translation of genomics into health care. *Journal of Nursing Scholarship, 45*(1), 15–24. doi:10.1111/jnu.12000

Bainbridge, M. N., Wiszniewski, W., Murdock, D. R., Friedman, J., Gonzaga-Jauregui, C., Newsham, I., . . . Gibbs, R. A. (2011). Whole-genome sequencing for optimized patient management. *Science Translational Medicine, 3*(87), 87re3. doi:10.1126/scitranslmed.3002243

Baldwin, E. L., Lee, J. Y., Blake, D. M., Bunke, B. P., Alexander, C. R., Kogan, A. L., . . . Martin, C. L. (2008). Enhanced detection of clinically relevant genomic imbalances using a targeted plus whole genome oligonucleotide microarray. *Genetics in Medicine, 10*(6), 415–429. doi:10.1097/GIM.0b013e318177015c

Belmont, J., & McGuire, A. L. (2009). The futility of genomic counseling: Essential role of electronic health records. *Genome Medicine, 1*(5), 48. doi:10.1186/gm48

Brock, J. A., Allen, V. M., Keiser, K., & Langlois, S. (2010). Family history screening: Use of the three generation pedigree in clinical practice. *Journal of Obstetrics and Gynaecology Canada, 32*(7), 663–672.

Calzone, K. A., Cashion, A., Feetham, S., Jenkins, J., Prows, C. A., Williams, J. K., & Wung, S-F. (2010). Nurses transforming health care using genetics and genomics. *Nursing Outlook, 58*(1), 26–35. doi:10.1016j.outlook.2009.05.001

Cavallari, L. H., & Limdi, N. A. (2009). Warfarin pharmacogenomics. *Current Opinion in Molecular Therapeutics, 11*(3), 243–251.

Chitty, L. S., Hill, M., White, H., Wright, D., & Morris, S. (2012). Noninvasive prenatal testing for aneuploidy-ready for prime time? *American Journal of Obstetrics & Gynecology, 206*(4), 269–275. doi:10.1016/j.ajog.2012.02.021

Chiu, R. W. K., Akolekar, R., Zheng, Y. W. L., Leung, T. Y., Sun H., Allen Chan, K. C., . . . Dennis Lo, Y. M. (2011). Non-invasive prenatal assessment of trisomy 21 by multiplexed maternal plasma DNA sequencing: Large scale validity study. *British Medical Journal, 342*, 1–9. doi:10.1136/bmj.c7401

Claassen, L., Henneman, L., Janssens, A. C. J. W., Wijdenes-Piji, M., Qureshi, N., Walter, F. M., . . . Timmermans, D. R. M. (2010). Using family history information to promote healthy lifestyles and prevent diseases; a discussion of the evidence. *BMC Public Health, 10*(1), 248. doi:10.1186/1471-2458-10-248

Clayton, E. W., Haga, S., Kuszler, P., Bane, E., Shutske, K., & Burke, W. (2013). Managing incidental genomic findings: Legal obligations of clinicians. *Genetics in Medicine, 15*(8), 624–629. doi: 10.1038/gim.2013.7

Conley, V. P., Biesecker, L. G., Gonsalves, S., Merkle, C. J., Kirk, M., & Aouizerat, B. E. (2013). Current and emerging technology approaches in genomics. *Journal of Nursing Scholarship, 45*(1), 5–14. doi:10.1111/jnu.12001

Consensus Panel on Genetic/Genomic Nursing Competencies. (2009). *Essentials of genetic and genomic nursing: Competencies, curricula guidelines, and outcome indicators* (2nd ed.). Silver Spring, MD: American Nurses Association.

Doerr, M., & Teng, K. (2012). Family history: Still relevant in the genomics era. *Cleveland Clinic Journal of Medicine, 79*(5), 331–336. doi:10.3949/ccjm.79a.11065

Domcheck, S. M., Eissen, A., Calzone, K., Stopfer, J., Blackwood, A., & Weber, B. L. (2003). Application of breast cancer risk prediction models in clinical practice. *Journal of Clinical Oncology, 21*(4), 593–601. doi:10.1200/JCO.2003.07.007

Eiland, E. H., Beyda, N., Han, J., Lindgren, W., Ward, R., English, T. M., . . . Hathcock, K. (2010). The utility of rapid microbiological and molecular techniques in optimizing antimicrobial therapy. *Scholarly Research Exchange Pharmacology, 2010*, 1–7. doi:10.3814/2010/395215

Feero, W. G., Guttmacher, A. E., & Collins, F. S. (2010). Genomic medicine—An updated primer. *New England Journal of Medicine, 362*(21), 2001–2011. doi:10.1056/NEJMra0907175

Giovanni, M. A., & Murray, M. F. (2010). The application of computer-based tools in obtaining the genetic family history. *Current Protocols in Human Genetics, 9*(21), 1–9. doi:10.1002/0471142905. hg0921s66

Gliwa, C., & Berkman, B. E. (2013). Do researchers have an obligation to actively look for genetic incidental findings? *American Journal of Bioethics, 13*(2), 32–42.

Green, M. J., & Botkin, J. R. (2003). "Genetic exceptionalism" in medicine: Clarifying the differences between genetic and nongenetic tests. *Annals of Internal Medicine, 138*(7), 571–575.

Green, R. C., Berg, J. S., Berry, G. T., Biesecker, L. G., Dimmock, D. P., Evans, J. P., . . . Jacob, H. J. (2012). Exploring concordance and discordance for return of incidental findings from clinical sequencing. *Genetics in Medicine, 14*(4), 405–410. doi:10.1038/gim.2012.21

Guttmacher, A. E., Collins, F. S., & Drazen, J. M. (2004). *Genomic medicine*. Baltimore, MD: Johns Hopkins University Press.

Hayden, E. C. (2012). Sequencing set to alter clinical landscape. *Nature, 482*(7385), 288.

Hoffman, M. A. (2007). The genome-enabled electronic medical record. *Journal of Biomedical Informatics, 40*(1), 44–46. doi:10.1016/j.jbi.2006.02.010

Hudson, K. L., Holohan, M. K., & Collins, F. S. (2008). Keeping pace with the times—The genetic information nondiscrimination act of 2008. *New England Journal of Medicine, 358*(25), 2661–2663. doi:10.1056/NEJMp0803964

International Society of Nurses in Genetics. (2010). *Position statement: Privacy and confidentiality of genetic information: The role of the nurse*. Retrieved from http://www.isong.org/pdfs2013/PS_Privacy_Confidentiality.pdf

Karow, J. (2013). Q&A: Sharon Plon on Baylor College of Medicine's first year of clinical exome sequencing. *News Archives*. Texas Children's Cancer and Hematology Centers. Retrieved from http://txch.org/qa-sharon-plon-on-baylor-college-of-medicines-first-year-of-clinical-exome-sequencing/

Kirk, M., McDonald, K., Longley, M., & Anstey, S. (2003). *Fit for practice in the genetics era: Defining what nurse, midwives and health visitors should know and be able to do in relationship to genetics*. Glamorgan, UK: University of Glamorgan.

Larach, M. G., Gronert, G. A., Allen, G. C., Brandom, B. W., & Lehman, E. B. (2010). Clinical presentation, treatment, and complications of malignant hyperthermia in North America from 1987 to 2006. *Anesthesia & Analgesia, 110*(2), 498–507. doi:10.1213/ANE.0b013e3181c6b9b2

Lux, M. P., Fasching, P. A., & Beckmann, M. W. (2006). Hereditary breast and ovarian cancer: Review and future perspectives. *Journal of Molecular Medicine, 84*(1), 16–28. doi:10.1007/s00109-005-0696-7

Manning, M., & Hudgins, L. (2010). Array-based technology and recommendations for utilization in medical genetics practice for detection of chromosomal abnormalities. *Genetics in Medicine, 12*(11), 742–745. doi:10.1097/GIM.0b013e3181f8baad

Manolio, T. A., Chisholm, R. L., Ozenberger, B., Roden, D., Williams, M. S., Wilson, R., . . . Ginsburg, G. S. (2013). Implementing genomic medicine in the clinic: The future is here. *Genetics in Medicine, 15*(4), 258–267. doi: 10.1038/gim.2012.157

Mardis, E. (2011). A decade's perspective on DNA sequencing technology. *Nature, 470*(7333), 198–203. doi:10.1038/nature09796

Mayer, A. N., Dimmock, D. P., Arca, M. J., Bick, D. P., Verbsky, J. W., Worthey, E. A., . . . Margolis, D. A. (2011). A timely arrival for genomic medicine. *Genetics in Medicine, 13*(3), 195–196. doi:10.1097/GIM.0b013e3182095089

McInerney, J. D. (2008). Genetics education for health professionals: A context. *Journal of Genetic Counseling, 17*(2), 145–151. doi:10.1007/s10897–007–9126-z

Moorthie, S., Hall, A., & Wright, C. F. (2013). Informatics and clinical genome sequencing: Opening the black box. *Genetics in Medicine, 15*(3), 165–171. doi:10.1038/gim.2012.116

National Coalition for Health Professional Education in Genetics. (2007). *Core competencies in genetics for health professionals* (3rd ed.). Retrieved from http://www.nchpeg.org/index.php?option=com_content&view=article&id=237&Itemid=84

Pletcher, B. A., Toriello, H. V., Noblin, S. J., Seaver, L. H., Driscoll, D. A., Bennett, R. L., & Gross, S. J. (2007). Indications for genetic referral: A guide for healthcare providers. *Genetics in Medicine, 9*(6), 385.

Pyeritz, R. E. (2011). The coming explosion in genetic testing—Is there a duty to recontact? *New England Journal of Medicine, 365*(15), 1367–1368.

Sax, U., & Schmidt, S. (2005). Opportunities and dilemmas. *Methods of Information in Medicine, 44*, 546–550.

Scheuner, M. T., de Vries, H., Kim, B., Meili, R. C., Olmstead, S. H., & Teleki, S. (2009). Are electronic health records ready for genomic medicine? *Genetics in Medicine, 11*(7), 510–517. doi:10.1097/GIM.0b013e3181a53331

Scheuner, M. T., Wang, S., Raffel, L. J., Larabell, S. K., & Rotter, J. I. (1997). Family history: A comprehensive genetic risk assessment method for the chronic conditions of adulthood. *American Journal of Medical Genetics, 71*(3), 315–324. doi:10.1002/(SICI)1096-8628(19970822)71:3<315::AID-AJMG12>3.0.CO;2-N

Shaffer, L. G., Ledbetter, D. H., & Lupski, J. R. (2006). Molecular cytogenetics of contiguous gene syndromes: Mechanisms and consequences of contiguous gene dosage imbalance. In D. Valle (Ed.), *Scriver's online metabolic and molecular basis of inherited disease.* Retrieved from http://www.ommbid.com/

Speicher, M. R., & Carter, N. P. (2005). The new cytogenetics: Blurring the boundaries with molecular biology. *Nature Reviews Genetics, 6*(10), 782–792. doi:10.1038/nrg1692

U.S. Department of Health and Human Services. (2008). *Personalized healthcare detailed use case.* Rockville, MD: Author.

Wetterstrand, K. A. (2013). DNA sequencing costs: Data from the NHGRI Genome Sequencing Program (GSP). Retrieved from http://www.genome.gov/sequencingcosts

RESOURCE

American College of Obstetricians and Gynecologists. (2001). Prenatal diagnosis of fetal chromosomal abnormalities. *ACOG Practice Bulletin, 27.*

CHAPTER 17

Digital Patient Engagement and Empowerment

Xiaohua Sarah Wu, MSN, RN, FNP-BC
Ellise D. Adams, PhD, RN, CNM

CHAPTER LEARNING OBJECTIVES

1. Understand patient engagement and empowerment and the role of the Internet.
2. Explore current perspectives on digital patient engagement and empowerment.
3. Discuss the challenges and issues related to the use of the Internet in patient engagement and empowerment.
4. Describe the revolutionary digital changes in healthcare delivery systems.
5. Recognize future trends in patient engagement and empowerment in the digital era.

KEY TERMS

Digital divide
Health literacy
Internet
Patient empowerment
Patient engagement

Personal health record (PHR)
Shared decision making
Social media
Telehealth

CHAPTER OVERVIEW

This chapter reviews the healthcare information technology revolution and the innovations that impact interactions between healthcare providers (HCPs) and patients. Its specific focus is on the ways in which patients engage and are empowered by use of the Internet, social media, and personal health records. While advancements in technology promise an endless number of possibilities for accessing healthcare information, there are challenges that should not be overlooked. Recognizing and addressing challenges can make these technologies more useful in providing patient-centered health care and improving patient engagement and empowerment.

INTRODUCTION

Traditional methods of patient engagement in health care include printed educational materials and face-to-face encounters between HCPs and patients. The onset of the information age has led to revolutionary changes in the delivery of health care. The capacities of the information age and the needs of patients have led HCPs to alter old methods and develop new methods of engaging patients and promoting patient engagement and empowerment. As public health promotion becomes an increasingly significant priority, methods that lead to improved collaboration between patients and HCPs will continue to be an important trend in the evolution of health care.

ENGAGEMENT AND EMPOWERMENT

Patient engagement is a set of reciprocal tasks performed by patients and HCPs in a collaborative effort to promote and support active patient involvement in their own health care (Coulter, 2011). When more than one viable treatment or screening option exists, patient engagement can raise the patient's awareness and understanding of treatment options and possible outcomes. **Patient empowerment** is the practice of maximizing the number of opportunities made available to patients to endow them with a better sense of control over their own health care, which can only lead to well-informed decisions and an improved collaborative dynamic with HCPs (Coulter, Safran, & Wasson, 2012). Empowerment encourages patients to share their preferences and values with HCPs to form plans of care that are based on the best available evidence and that also reflect patients' best interests. For example, the anterior cruciate ligament (ACL) is a commonly injured ligament of the knee. With the same severity of injury, the treatment plans for ACL injury can vary from altered activity level with conservative management to surgical intervention to repair or even replace the injured ligament. The different approaches for treatment are dependent on a patient's goal of activity level. An 18-year-old football player who wants to play ball in college may choose to have his torn ACL reconstructed surgically, but a 30-year-old working mother may opt for an alteration of her level of activity rather than having surgery. Allowing patients to make these types of decisions about their care is one of the primary means of empowering patients with regard to their own health care.

The integration of the Internet into day-to-day life and the tremendous access to healthcare information the Internet provides have transformed patients into more active healthcare consumers, particularly in terms of how they accept medical advice. As the Internet has started to bridge the information gap, patients have begun to transition from being passive recipients of the healthcare plans or decisions made by their HCP to being more actively engaged in the decisions surrounding their own health care (White & Herzlinger, 2004). The patients of today acquire access to their personal health data and then join appropriate groups, using avenues such as social media, to share experiences and coping mechanisms. It is common to see patients arrive for a visit with a stack of printouts from online resources already in hand, as well as a list of questions on which they wish to consult with their HCPs.

When the visit with the HCP becomes more collaborative, it is the perfect time to encourage patients to engage in decisions about their health. **Shared decision making** is most effective whenever patients are fully aware of the risks, benefits, and their own preferences (or values). HCPs can use clinical informatics tools to integrate patients' values with scientific evidence in an effort to provide treatment alternatives that are amenable with the patients' goals. However, HCPs must always be sure to impress upon patients the objective risks and benefits of each alternative (Eysenbach, 2000). When patients make more responsible choices, they will in turn experience positive results, which help to further reinforce those healthy choices (Juengst, Flatt, & Settersten, 2012). Shared decision making is becoming more and more valuable in management of chronic diseases, such as diabetes. A patient's increased involvement in decision making about his or her own health management, which may include lifestyle changes, diet modification, medication regimens, and regularly scheduled appointments with the HCP, may maximize the likelihood of the patient's compliance with the plan of care (Muhlbacher, Stoll, Mahlich, & Nubling, 2013). Furthermore, contemporary health care tries to focus on the value or efficacy of decisions from the perspective of the patients, another way to encourage patient engagement and self-care. Patients are truly empowered by efforts that help them engage in the planning of their care, as well as by tools that help improve their ability to understand, cope, and manage health in their lives (Mittler, Martsolf, Telenko, & Scanlon, 2013).

Often, patients who are geographically challenged, such as those living in rural areas, find it difficult to receive timely and consistent treatment and to provide feedback to their providers. This is especially problematic in management of chronic diseases, such as diabetes, cancer, heart disease, and acute diseases that require frequent and intense follow ups, reminders, and support for patients. Consumer-centered health care and shared decision making work in tandem to create options that promote patient engagement and empowerment, and contemporary methods of communication can help bridge this gap between isolated patients and HCPs.

In order to have patient engagement, empowerment, and shared decision making, patients must be able to understand information about their own health. The term **health literacy** is used to describe "the degree to which individuals can obtain, process, and understand the basic health information and services they need to make appropriate health decisions" (Institute of Medicine [IOM], 2004, p. 1). Just as one's level of education plays a role in health literacy, many other skills, such as communicating, having adequate background information, and advocating for one's self, are also critical components of health literacy. In the United States, 36% of adults have low levels of health literacy, meaning they have difficulty in locating, comprehending, and applying health information (Sheridan et al., 2011).

In the digital era, patients with low levels of health literacy may be at a serious disadvantage. Without the ability to interpret health-related information, the increased use of information technology in health care means little to these patients. A patient who is without health literacy skills can make few or no well-informed decisions, which directly impairs patient empowerment. In 2010, the U.S. Department of Health and Human Services (HHS) released a national action plan to improve health literacy, in which they hope to bridge the chasm of knowledge between what professionals know and what patients know. The plan includes: (1) simplifying and standardizing the health information available to patients; (2) providing clinicians with formal training in communicating with lower level literacy patients; (3) expanding community services in terms of providing culturally and linguistically appropriate health information; and (4) increasing the use of evidence-based health literacy research, practices, and interventions (HHS, 2010). These efforts to improve communication between HCPs and low health literacy patients can greatly foster patient engagement and empowerment.

HEALTHCARE INFORMATION REVOLUTION

There is little doubt that the Internet has taken over the global communication landscape. The revolutionary impact of the Internet, sometimes called the "third industrial revolution," has changed the way HCPs share data and communicate (Rifkin, 2011). The use of personal computers, laptops, and mobile Internet devices such as smartphones and tablets has dramatically changed the means by which patients seek access to healthcare information. Widespread use of the Internet has led developers of healthcare information systems to shift their focus toward developing products for patients (Eysenbach, 2000). In the late 1990s, Eysenbach (2000) foresaw an "information age healthcare system" in which patients would use technology to gain access to information and assume more responsibility for their own health care (p. 1715). It is believed that patient empowerment will result in more efficient use of healthcare resources, with an emphasis on preventive care

(Eysenbach, 2000). Legislation designed to promote the implementation of patient-centered healthcare information technologies, such as the Health Information Technology for Economic and Clinical Health (HITECH) Act of 2009, ensures that healthcare delivery systems will continue to address patients' needs, values, and preferences (Eysenbach, 2000).

Internet

The **Internet** has "world-wide broadcasting capability, a mechanism for information dissemination, and a medium for collaboration and interaction between individuals and their computers without regard for geographic location" (Leiner et al., 1997). The Internet is proving to be a major source of health information for patients (Moretti, deOliveira, & Koga da Silva, 2012). In 2010, a survey showed that three-quarters of adults in the United States use the Internet, and 59% of all adults have looked online for healthcare information, such as specific disease information or treatment options (Fox, 2011). The range of available healthcare information has expanded through the use of Internet-based tools such as email, websites, search tools, discussion forums, blogs, and videos, with websites being the tool that people choose to browse most frequently (Pew Internet & American Life Project, 2013).

There are two general categories of healthcare-related websites: government-sponsored and nongovernmental, which can be either commercial or nonprofit. HCPs should understand the need for a thorough evaluation of healthcare information that is present on the Internet. In general, websites sponsored by schools of medicine, nursing, or allied health professions, medical centers, or the U.S. government are more likely to provide accurate and thorough information. **Table 17-1** provides a short list of trustworthy websites for consumer health information.

Websites that seek to provide healthcare information should also be evaluated in terms of effectiveness from the perspective of the patient. Research suggests that the effectiveness can be assessed in four dimensions: accessibility, content, marketing, and technology (Ford, Huerta, Schilhavy, & Menachemi, 2012). Definitions of these dimensions and their contributory elements are provided in **Table 17-2**.

Today, websites often represent the initial point of contact that patients establish with healthcare organizations such as hospitals, government agencies, and insurance companies (Ford et al., 2012). Websites that are designed to engage and empower patients send a clear message that patients' interests and needs are now the focus of the healthcare system.

Table 17-1 Trustworthy Websites for Consumer Health Information	
Title of Agency or Organization	**Website**
American Association of Retired Persons	http://www.aarp.org/health/
Agency for Healthcare Research and Quality	http://www.ahrq.gov/patients-consumers/
Centers for Medicare & Medicaid Services	http://www.cms.gov
Leapfrog Group	http://www.leapfroggroup.org
Mayo Clinic	http://www.mayoclinic.com
Medical Library Association	http://www.mlanet.org/resources/consumr_index.html
PubMed	http://www.ncbi.nlm.nih.gov/pubmed
U.S. Centers for Medicare & Medicaid Services	https://www.healthcare.gov/
U.S. Department of Health and Human Services	http://www.hhs.gov/ocr/privacy/hipaa/understanding/consumers/
U.S. Department of Labor	http://www.dol.gov/ebsa/consumer_info_health.html

Quality Control of Information Available to Patients

The rapid growth of health-related information available on the Internet could be overwhelming to patients. Research suggests that less than one-third of Internet users who follow medical advice or seek health information online describe the data as helpful (Fox, 2011). Approximately 3% of adults say they or others they know have been harmed in some way by online healthcare-related information (Fox, 2011). Finding useful and valid information on the Internet can be challenging and time-consuming for patients, because it is difficult to filter out applicable and credible information from other less trustworthy information (Jadad, 1999).

One strategy to help patients judge the quality of a website's information is website certification (Moretti et al., 2012). Five "C's" can be used to assess the quality of information on any website containing health-related information—credibility, currency, content, construction, and clarity (Roberts, 2010). The 5C Evaluation tool, as described by Roberts, contains numerous questions in the five categories to guide an extensive assessment of any website.

Table 17-2 Website Effectiveness Assessment

Website Assessment Dimension	Definition	Utilization	Contributory Elements
Accessibility	A website's ease of use for healthcare patients with lower computer literacy levels	To reach as many users (patients) as possible	1. Spiderability: To ensure interoperability with search engines. This enables patients to easily find the healthcare information they need without navigating a complex site hierarchy. 2. Flash reliance: To avoid features relying on Flash that systematically limit some users' access levels, especially for Apple mobile products users. 3. Use of link states: To help patients move across the site with effective visual cues, such as use of color, to identify potential new links. 4. Use of alternative text: To convert images to text-only healthcare information that enables sight-impaired patients to navigate web pages through screen readers.
Content	A website's overall content quality without taking into consideration the technical limitations of the site	Promote and maintain effective consumer engagement	1. Quality: Well-chosen titles and descriptions can encourage consumer engagement. Ensure grammatically correct text and the right number of words on the web page. 2. Freshness: Up-to-date content is a positive indicator to patients that the organization is engaged in state-of-the-art activities. 3. Readability and visual interests: Healthcare web pages should use words and grammar consistent with 8th–11th grade reading levels. Striving to increase the interest of websites leads to consumer engagement.
Marketing	How readily and reliably information is accessed using search engines	Become more accessible to search engines to increase a website's popularity	1. The amount of content: Content within a page becomes more accessible to search engines, which results in more consumer visits. 2. Popularity: More site traffic indicates higher popularity.
Technology	How well a website is designed, built, and maintained	Provide user-friendly website	1. Website download speed: The ideal loading time for a webpage is 0.5 second or less. 2. Site structure and code quality: To build and maintain a well-performing website. 3. Content organization: Adding healthcare education video and graphics as web page content is a trend in healthcare consumer empowerment.

Source: Ford, Huerta, Schilhavy, & Menachem, 2012, January–February. Effective US health system websites: Establishing benchmarks and standards for effective consumer engagement. *Journal of Healthcare Management 57*(1), 47–64.

When patients come to HCPs with health-related information obtained from online sources, they should be advised that while the Internet provides tools to promote healthcare information exchange, the quality of the information is not standardized. Patients should be directed only to websites that have been thoroughly evaluated and deemed trustworthy by HCPs. Still, direct instructions from a patient's HCP remain the most reliable information in forming a healthcare plan.

As wireless technologies grow and electronic medical information expands, mobile medical and health applications (apps) continue to impact the cyber infrastructure of health care (Abernethy, Wheeler, & Bull, 2011). As of May 2012, there were 10,000 apps available in the "medical section" of Apple's "App store" and more than 3,000 on the Google Play store (Buijink, Visser, & Marshall, 2013). Although there is a promising future in apps for public health, challenges remain. Wireless medical device and software regulations to ensure the quality of health apps are set by different governmental agencies such as the Federal Communications Commission (FCC) and the U.S. Food and Drug Administration (FDA).

Social Media

Social media is increasingly becoming the mechanism that patients use to seek and share healthcare information (Pho, 2013). **Social media** is defined as "the use of web-based and mobile technologies to turn communication into interactive dialogues" (Bradley, 2011). In an online environment, social media creates a powerful platform for the mass collaboration of people, who may or may not have had preexisting connections, to exchange user-generated content (Kaplan & Haenlein, 2010). While social media is similar to television, radio, and newspaper in that it is a format that delivers a message, it is unique in its capability to create a platform for two-way communication, a dynamic known as "social networking" (French, 2010).

Use of Social Networks by Patients

When social networking enables conversation with patients, rather than lecture, it becomes an act of engagement. Facebook and Twitter, well-known social networking media, have become venues of information exchange for patients. According to the Pew Research Center, a nonpartisan source of data analysis, 72% of adult Internet users report use of a social network for procuring health-related information about drugs or other treatments and for following healthcare organizations for information updates or procedure videos (Pew Internet & American Life Project, 2013). The percentage of adult Internet users who use a social network for health-related information has increased elevenfold when compared to Pew Research Center's report in 2011 (Fox, 2011).

As a teaching tool that increases patient awareness, information from social networking was found to be useful in facilitating self-care in terms of supporting diagnoses, managing conditions, and monitoring treatments and preventing disease (Griffiths et al., 2012). Latino and African American men who voluntarily used Facebook to post and discuss human immunodeficiency virus (HIV)-related topics were more likely to request an HIV testing kit (Young & Jaganath, 2013). Facebook was found to have a positive impact on allowing patients to shift from being mere passengers to responsible drivers of their health for a wide variety of issues, including maternal and infant care, depression, general wellness, and weight management (Prasad, 2013).

More than simply educating patients with medical knowledge, social media can provide an online environment for patients to discuss their health in virtual support groups. Some patients share their personal stories, including side effects of treatments and the psychological aspects of their illness. Patients with chronic illness, cancer, and rare diseases have found social media useful as a means for sharing stories, learning from others, and instilling hope to other members of the virtual group (Fox & Purcell, 2010).

Use of Social Networks by Nurses

Social media can be a tool for professional connections among nurses and can enrich nurses' knowledge when it is used mindfully and in accordance with professional standards. However, nurses must understand that posting information on social media outlets can be widely and rapidly disseminated to individuals other than those for whom the post was intended. In the social media environment, privacy is typically only an illusion. In October 2011, the American Nurses Association (ANA) released two guiding documents on social networking for nurses: *Social Networking Principles for Nurses* and *Fact Sheet—Navigating the World of Social Media* that can be found on the ANA website. Strategies that nurses can use to avoid breaches of patient privacy and confidentiality with social media have also been identified by the National Council of State Boards of Nursing (NCSBN). These strategies address the maintenance of professional boundaries and employer policies, professional behavior in the online environment, and specifically recommend that nurses refrain from posting patient-related images or information that could lead to the identification of a patient (NCSBN, 2011). In addition, the NCSBN also recommends that nurses avoid posting disparaging remarks about patients, employers, or coworkers.

Use of Social Networks by Healthcare Organizations

The increasingly popular practice of patients using social networking for health-related information has resulted in the widespread adoption of social networking by healthcare organizations. A recent survey conducted by the Mayo Clinic found that 1,264 hospitals actively used and maintained officially sponsored accounts on Facebook, while 976 hospitals mentioned the exchange of healthcare information with their patients on Twitter (Bennett, 2013).

Many organizations have adopted Facebook to increase awareness and promote the healthcare system. The United Network for Organ Sharing (UNOS), which manages the U.S. organ transplant and organ procurement system, advocates for organ donation awareness on Facebook. They see Facebook as a key opportunity for broadening public awareness of the organ shortage and promoting the decision to become an organ donor. As of May 2012, Facebook users can share their organ share status by accessing "Life event," selecting "Health and Wellness," and adding "choose Organ Donor" to be a registered donor. On the first day of the change, about 13,000 people in the United States registered to become organ donors. That is 20 times more than the average number of daily registrations (Stobbe, 2012).

Concerns and Future of Social Media

Although social networking is becoming more accepted as a vehicle for exchanging healthcare information, there are concerns associated with the use of large social networks as platforms for healthcare delivery. Confidentiality has been cited as the most troubling factor (Tang, Ash, Bates, Overhage, & Sands, 2006). Because the networks are social in nature, certain groups, such as patient support groups and fundraising groups, may prompt users to "surrender" their confidentiality by exchanging names, locations, symptoms, or lab results (Farmer, Burckner Holt, Cook, & Hearing, 2009). In light of this concern, patients and their caregivers must be made aware of the security risks involved in the disclosure of personal details on public networking sites.

Just as there are obvious benefits to patients who now have access to others with similar medical conditions, the practice of comparing treatment plans, procedure processes, and practice protocols may also create anxiety. Much of the information found on social networks, even the so-called "scientific" content, is often unauthorized, leaving many to question its accuracy and applicability (Farmer et al., 2009). With these concerns in mind, healthcare-focused networking, which is akin to Facebook but exclusive to HCPs and patients, seems to be an ideal solution. In 2013, Dabo Health, partnering with the Mayo Clinic, launched a full version of a healthcare-focused networking site (https://www.dabohealth.com/welcome) that is limited to use by HCPs. Though the site remains in development, Dabo Health is striving to reach the goal of providing relevant and accurate healthcare-related content to users. Another healthcare-focused networking site is called Sharecare, which is found at http://www.sharecare.com. At Sharecare, experts in particular healthcare topics answer questions posed by consumers. Nurses who are members of Sigma Theta Tau International Honor Society of Nursing can apply to become experts for Sharecare.

Personal Health Records

In 2005, President George W. Bush and Secretary Mike Leavitt set a specific goal for health care. By 2014, the U.S. Government would implement a program to "create a personal health record that patients, doctors, and other health care providers could securely access through the Internet no matter where a patient is seeking medical care" (HHS, 2006). Since then, there has been remarkable adoption of **personal health records (PHR)** at all levels of government and health care.

Despite the increased attention, there is no uniform definition of PHR. One of the most often cited definitions comes from the Markle Foundation (2003), a private foundation that promotes the use of information technology in health and national security. Its definition of PHR is "An electronic application through which individuals can access, manage and share their health information, and that of others for whom they are authorized, in a private, secure, and confidential environment" (p. 3). The American Health Information Management Association (AHIMA e-HIM Personal Health Record Work Group, 2005) adds the following:

> The personal health record is an electronic, universally available, lifelong resource of health information needed by individuals to make health decisions. Individuals own and manage the information in the PHR, which comes from health care providers and the individual. The PHR is maintained in a secure and private environment, with the individual determining rights of access. The PHR is separate from and does not replace the legal record of any provider. (p. 64)

Data Entry and Management

A PHR is an individualized, web-based, decision-support tool that patients can access from home computers or other mobile devices. A PHR is different from an electronic health record (EHR), which is often used by HCPs for entering healthcare documentation and data on patients. Unlike with an EHR, the patient plays a pivotal role in the collaborative process of PHR data entry and retrieval. Although HCPs may import healthcare data to PHR, patients should be the only individuals who have the access to maintain information, manage, and make decisions based on their own health information. A PHR provides patients with healthcare information that is truly customized and accurate, such as patients' allergies, lab results, pathology reports, prescribed medication lists, diagnoses, health insurance, and scheduled appointments.

Advantages of Adapting PHRs

The unique PHR data-entry method shared online by patients and providers has direct benefits such as automated services, up-to-date consumer information, and improved consumer satisfaction (Klein-Fedyshin, 2002). Patients can request routine appointments, outpatient procedures, medicine refills, and referrals to specialists through PHR automated services. Automated services can provide efficient medical attention to patients and ease HCPs' workload by shortening communication time between patients and providers.

PHRs have the capacity to facilitate record-keeping processes between patients and HCPs. Traditionally, patient demographics and insurance information are often not current in medical records, which can result in miscommunication and patient dissatisfaction. Patients who have access to PHRs tend to check and update the data regularly (Ash, Berg, & Coiera, 2004). Effective communication and efficient medical services can improve overall consumer satisfaction.

The ultimate goal of PHRs is for patients to leverage their own health information and have ongoing communication with their providers in order to engage in health-promoting behaviors and to develop continuity among HCPs (Tang et al., 2006). Although PHRs benefit patients the most, they are certainly advantageous to individuals involved in the process at all levels. **Table 17-3** summarizes potential benefits for patients, HCPs, payers, employers, and public health (HHS, 2006).

Challenges and Concerns

Although the PHR offers great potential in empowering patients, those who need it most may find it challenging to enter and maintain their data. Groups who have experienced disparities in health care, such as the poor, uneducated, elderly, unemployed, and disabled, often lack access to information resources on the Internet (O'Grady et al., 2012). The **digital divide** includes a technical divide based on the availability of infrastructure and a social divide resulting from the skills required to manipulate and utilize healthcare resources. These skills are often referred to as health information literacy.

Table 17-3   Key Potential Benefits of PHRs and PHR Systems

Roles	Benefits
Patients and their Caregivers	• Support wellness activities • Improve understanding of health issues • Increase sense of control over health • Increase control over access to personal health information • Support timely, appropriate preventive services • Support healthcare decisions and responsibility for care • Strengthen communication with providers • Verify accuracy of information in provider records • Support home monitoring for chronic diseases • Support understanding and appropriate use of medications • Support continuity of care across time and providers • Manage insurance benefits and claims • Avoid duplicate tests • Reduce adverse drug interactions and allergic reactions • Reduce hassle through online appointment scheduling and prescription refills • Increase access to providers via e-visits • Improve documentation of communication with patients
Healthcare Providers	• Improve access to data from other providers and the patients themselves • Increase knowledge of potential drug interactions and allergies • Avoid duplicate tests • Improve medication compliance • Provide information to patients for healthcare and patient services purposes • Provide patients with convenient access to specific information or services (e.g., lab results, Rx refills, e-visits) • Improve documentation of communication with patients
Payers	• Improve customer service (transactions and information) • Promote portability of patient information across plan • Support wellness and preventive care • Provide information and education to beneficiaries
Employers	• Support wellness and preventive care • Provide convenient service • Improve workforce productivity • Promote empowered healthcare patients • Use aggregate data to manage employee health
Public Health Benefits	• Strengthen health promotion and disease prevention • Improve the health of populations • Expand health education opportunities

Source: U.S. Department of Health and Human Services, 2006; http://www.ncvhs.hhs.gov/0602nhiirpt.pdf

Bridging the digital divide and lessening disparity will require action from various government (federal, state, and local) agencies and stakeholders. In 2000, President Bill Clinton argued, "We must close the digital divide between those who've got the tools and those who don't." Hence, he proposed $2.25 billion of initiatives to bridge the digital divide (U.S. White House, 2000). In 2009, the stimulus package allocated $4.7 billion to the Broadband Technology Opportunities Program, of which a sum of no less than $2 billion was made available for competitive grants in an effort to expand public computer center capacity (U.S. Department of Commerce, 2009). These efforts clearly indicate that the development of a national information infrastructure has and continues to be a key priority for the federal government. As time progresses, the government should be able to utilize that infrastructure to reduce the costs of health care.

THE FUTURE OF E-HEALTH APPLICATIONS

Inherently, a healthcare system is labor intensive, and HCPs play important roles in the provision of effective and high-quality health care. Imbalances in the geographic distribution of skilled HCPs have a huge impact on the provision of high-quality health care for all patients (Nouhi, Fayaz-Bakhsh, Mohamadi, & Shafii, 2012). Today, healthcare technology is used widely to improve patient access to HCPs and promote patient empowerment. Along with technology innovation, more and more virtual healthcare teams are used to bridge the gaps in time, distance, and quality of health care. Virtual health care provides Internet-based, advanced care that monitors and manages patient care remotely. Trauma surgeons at the University of Arizona have developed a Voice-over-Internet-Protocol (VoIP) to provide real-time guidance in remote airway intubation by using video-laryngoscope and Skype over 3G wireless networks (Mosier, Joseph, & Sakles, 2013). Remote operators perform (or facilitate the performance of) procedures that can help ensure patient safety and improve outcomes (see **Figures 17-1, 17-2,** and **17-3**).

Based on the virtual healthcare concept, the virtual intensive care unit (vICU) is a model of future care that uses state-of-the-art technology to leverage the expertise and knowledge of experienced ICU HCPs to perform virtual rounds and critically ill patient management. The vICU was the idea of two intensivists from Johns Hopkins Hospital, Brian Rosenfeld, MD, and Michael Breslow, MD (Breslow et al., 2004; Nowlin, 2004). Imagine an extremely ill patient is connected to tubes and monitors that calculate every change in vital signs. In the meantime, ICU physicians and nurses who may be hundreds of miles away from the patients monitor these changes. Live

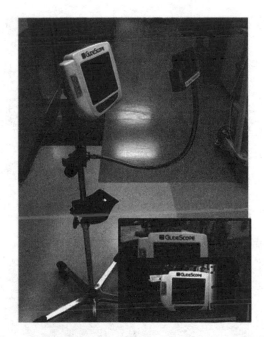

FIGURE 17-1   GlideScope telebation unit.

Source: Mosier, Joseph, & Sakles, (2013). Telebation: Next-generation telemedicine in remote airway management using current wireless technologies. *Telemedicine and e-Health, 19*(2), 95–98. doi:10.1089/tmj.2012.0093

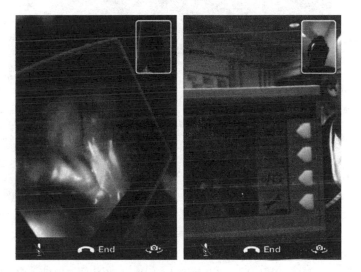

FIGURE 17-2   iPhone view of telebation. Right picture is KingVision and left picture is C-MAC videolaryngoscopes.

Source: Mosier, Joseph, & Sakles, (2013). Telebation: Next-generation telemedicine in remote airway management using current wireless technologies. *Telemedicine and e-Health, 19*(2), 95–98. doi:10.1089/tmj.2012.0093

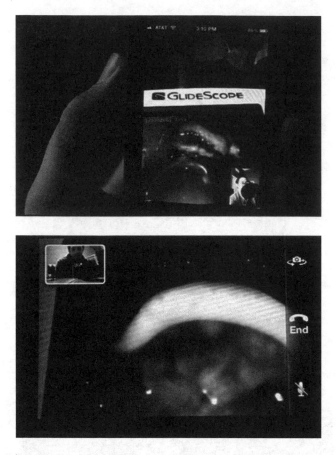

FIGURE 17-3   iPhone view of GlideScope from remote hospital. Top picture view using skype via Wi-Fi. Bottom picture view using view via FaceTime.

Source: Mosier, Joseph, & Sakles, (2013). Telebation: Next-generation telemedicine in remote airway management using current wireless technologies. *Telemedicine and e-Health, 19*(2), 95-98. doi:10.1089/tmj.2012.0093

audio and video are used to assess a patient. When something triggers an alarm, the vICU nurse can direct a camera in the patient's room to zoom in and visually examine the patient. The vICU nurse can then alert and coach the actual bedside nurse to provide appropriate nursing intervention. vICUs will not only bring the resources and expert care of experienced specialists to rural facilities but also provide an extra layer of safety to patient care.

Remote monitoring and management can be used for those who need chronic disease and/or post-acute care management at home. Patients or caregivers can use devices to upload blood pressure, heart rate, body temperature, weight, blood glucose levels, post-surgery drain output, and other relevant, measurable data. When multiple

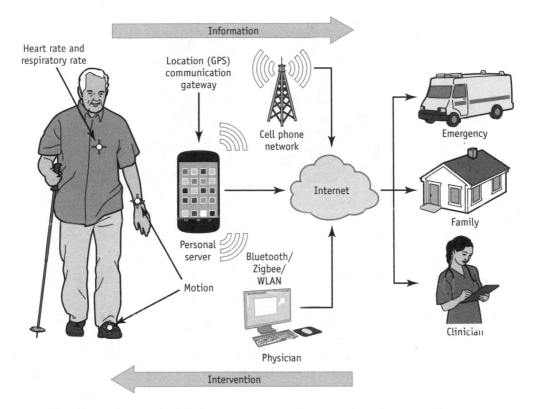

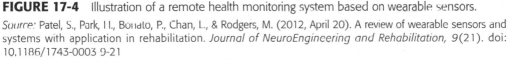

FIGURE 17-4   Illustration of a remote health monitoring system based on wearable sensors.

Source: Patel, S., Park, H., Bonato, P., Chan, L., & Rodgers, M. (2012, April 20). A review of wearable sensors and systems with application in rehabilitation. *Journal of NeuroEngineering and Rehabilitation, 9*(21). doi: 10.1186/1743-0003 9-21

comorbidities compound the challenges in self-reporting and patient data collection, invasive or noninvasive devices that automatically record data and detect changes are utilized to ensure patient safety (Bui & Fonarow, 2012). Noninvasive, wearable sensors have been widely used to collect and forward patient information to one or multiple recipients who can then provide appropriate feedback and/or responses (see **Figure 17-4**).

European pain management groups have put forth major efforts to develop wearable motion sensors within interactive garments to provide an engaging way to perform home-based therapeutic exercises in back pain management. The system allows patients to increase the amount of motor exercise they perform independently with real-time feedback based on data collected via wearable sensors embedded in the garment across the upper limb and trunk. A patient's activity-associated data are

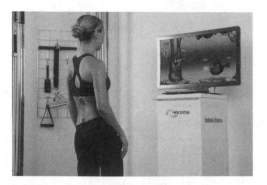

FIGURE 17-5 Low back pain therapy system with wireless wearable motion sensors and interactive games to perform therapeutic exercises.
Source: Courtesy of Hocoma AG.

then stored in a central location where clinicians can access and review statistics (Patel, Park, Bonate, Chan, & Rodgers, 2012; **Figure 17-5**).

One such noninvasive, wearable garment system was implemented for remote fetal monitoring during a pregnancy to allow pregnant women to remain at home as much as possible. A group of experts received the recorded signals and then provided prompt feedback about the fetal condition. The system allowed a reduction in the costs inherent in fetal monitoring, improved the assessment of fetal conditions, and, most importantly, guaranteed a continuous and deep screening of the fetal health state whenever a particular pregnant woman was at home (Fanelli et al., 2010).

Patients with heart failure can benefit from implanting a hemodynamic monitoring device via right heart catheterization, which monitors intracardiac and pulmonary artery pressure when patients are at home. This monitoring device provides an early warning of potential decompensation and facilitates the day-to-day management by titrating medications on the basis of reliable physiological data (Bui & Fonarow, 2012; see **Figure 17-6**). Digital technology improvements, such as 4G network and wireless devices, have made prompt clinician feedback possible for those patients who choose to manage their health at home.

SUMMARY

Health information technology is changing the ways in which patients access and manage their own health care. Technologies such as the Internet, PHRs, and social media, promote patient engagement and empowerment. **Telehealth** technologies

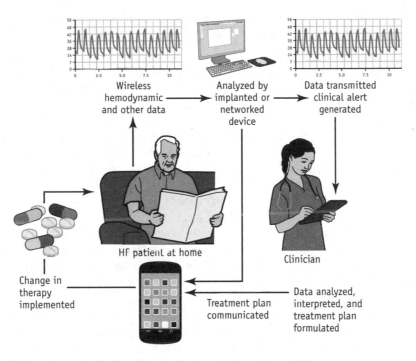

FIGURE 17-6 Home hemodynamic monitoring of chronic heart failure.

Source: Reprinted from *Journal of the American College of Cardiology, 59*(2), Bui AL & Fonarow, GC, Home monitoring for heart failure management, pp. 97–104, Copyright 2012, with permission from Elsevier.

make it possible to deliver healthcare services to patients in a remote fashion, thereby equipping patients with tools to take control of their health. Healthcare information technology offers many opportunities for patients and HCPs, but issues of privacy and security of protected health information need to be addressed. In addition, people with low health literacy or lack of access to technology can be left out of the movement toward patient engagement and empowerment.

For a full suite of assignments and additional learning activities, use the access code located in the front of your book and visit www.jblearning.com. If you do not have an access code, you can obtain one at the site.

Box 17-1   Case Study

Charlotte is a certified nurse-midwife (CNM) who is opening a freestanding birth center within 5 miles of a major community hospital. The birth center is accredited by the American Association of Birth Centers and has a collaborative agreement, including a transfer agreement with the community hospital and an obstetric practice consisting of three physicians and a women's health nurse practitioner.

In order to promote patient engagement and to provide a PHR, Charlotte installs iPad stations in her waiting rooms and antepartum assessment rooms. Using these electronic stations, pregnant women provide their health history and update their health status throughout pregnancy. The PHR is also accessible online and can be viewed by patients and HCPs at the birth center, obstetrician's office, and the hospital. This allows for a seamless, continuity of care should risks develop and the patient need to transfer to an obstetrician's care.

Although intrapartum transfers from birth center to hospital comprised less than 12% of the population of women using a birth center, it is important for Charlotte to develop policies in conjunction with the obstetric practice and hospital to promote maternal and newborn safety. One reason for emergent transfer in the immediate postpartum period is postpartum hemorrhage (PPH). By using the protocols outlined in the *Obstetric Hemorrhage Toolkit* (California Maternal Quality Care Collaborative, 2007), Charlotte is able to provide the women and families the best care (see http://www.cmqcc.org/). This clinical information document provides antepartum, admission, and ongoing risk assessment procedures to identify patients at highest risk for PPH, parameters to diagnosis PPH, and a protocol for management. For example, patients are screened for antepartum risks including severe anemia, history of labor uterine fibroids, body mass index greater than 35, estimated fetal weight greater than 4 kg, more than 4 previous vaginal births, history of bleeding disorders, and a lack of consent to receive blood products in an emergency. The protocols for management of PPH include active management of the third stage of labor by the CNM. Active management procedures are administration of 10 units Pitocin intramuscularly and vigorous fundal massage following delivery of the placenta. Also, all birth center staff are educated in accurately estimating blood loss and implementing appropriate transfer protocols. Not only does this toolkit promote standardized, quality care between the healthcare professionals but, when shared with the birth center patients, it promotes shared decision making and patient empowerment.

REFERENCES

Abernethy, A. P., Wheeler, J. L., & Bull, J. (2011). Development of a health information technology-based data system in community-based hospice and palliative care. *American Journal of Preventive Medicine, 40*(5S2), S162–S172.

AHIMA e-HIM Personal Health Record Work Group. (2005). The role of the personal health record in the EHR. *Journal of AHIMA, 76*(7), 64A–64D.

American Nurses Association [ANA]. (2011). *Social networking principles for nurses.* Retrieved from http://www.nursingworld.org/FunctionalMenuCategories/AboutANA/Social-Media/Social-Networking-Principles-Toolkit

American Nurses Association. (2011). *Fact sheet: Navigating the world of social media.* Retrieved from http://www.nursingworld.org/FunctionalMenuCategories/AboutANA/Social-Media/Social-Networking-Principles-Toolkit/Fact-Sheet-Navigating-the-World-of-Social-Media.pdf

Ash, J. S., Berg, M., & Coiera, E. (2004). Some unintended consequences of information technology in health care: The nature of patient care information system-related errors. *Journal of the American Medical Informatics Association, 11*(2), 104–112.

Bennett, E. (2013). *Health care social media list.* Retrieved from http://network.socialmedia.mayoclinic.org/hcsml-grid/

Bradley, A. (2011, March 8). Defining social media: Mass collaboration is its unique value. *Gartner Blog Network.* Retrieved from http://blogs.gartner.com/anthony_bradley/2011/03/08/defining-social-media-mass-collaboration-is-its-unique-value/

Breslow, M. J., Rosenfeld, B. A., Doerfler, M., Burke, G., Yates, G., Stone, D. J., . . . Plocher, D. W. (2004). Effect of a multiple-site intensive care unit telemedicine program on clinical and economic outcomes: An alternative paradigm for intensivist staffing. *Critical Care Medicine, 32*(7), 1632.

Bui, A. L., & Fonarow, G. C. (2012). Home monitoring for heart failure management. *Journal of the American College of Cardiology, 59*(2), 97–104. doi: 10.1016/j.jacc.2011.09.044

Buijink, A. W., Visser, B. J., & Marshall, L. (2013). Medical apps for smartphones: Lack of evidence undermines quality and safety. *Evidence-Based Medicine, 18*(3), 90–92. doi: 10.1136/eb-2012-100885

California Maternal Quality Care Collaborative. (2007). *Obstetric hemorrhage toolkit.* Retrieved from https://www.cmqcc.org/ob_hemorrhage

Coulter, A. (2011). *Engaging patients in healthcare.* Maidenhead, England: Open University Press.

Coulter, A., Safran, D., & Wasson, J. H. (2012). On the language and content of patient engagement. *Journal of Ambulatory Care Management, 35*(2), 78–79. doi: 10.1097/JAC.0b013e31824a5676

Eysenbach, G. (2000). Consumer health informatics. *British Medical Journal, 320*(7251), 1713–1716.

Fanelli, A., Ferrario, M., Piccini, L., Andreoni, G., Matrone, G., Magenes, G., & Signorini, M. G. (2010). Prototype of a wearable system for remote fetal monitoring during pregnancy. *Conference Proceeding IEEE Engineering Medicine and Biology, 2010,* 5815–5818. doi: 10.1109/IEMBS.2010.5627470

Farmer, A. D., Bruckner Holt, C. E. M., Cook, M. J., & Hearing, S. D. (2009). Social networking sites: A novel portal for communication. *Postgraduate Medical Journal, 85*(1007), 455–459.

Ford, E. W., Huerta, T. R., Schilhavy, R. A., & Menachemi, N. (2012). Effective US health system websites: Establishing benchmarks and standards for effective consumer engagement. *Journal of Healthcare Management, 57*(1), 47–64.

Fox, S. (2011). *The social life of health information, 2011.* Washington, DC: Pew Research Center's Internet & American Life Project. Retrieved from http://pewinternet.org/Reports/2011/Social-Life-of-Health-info.aspx

Fox, S., & Purcell, K. (2010). Chronic disease and the Internet. Pew Internet and American Life Project. Retrieved from http://pewinternet.org/~/media/Files/Reports/2010/PIP_Chronic_Disease_with_topline.pdf

French, D. (2010). The social media mindset: A narrative view of public relations and marketing in the Web 2.0 environment. *Media Psychology Review, 3*(1).

Griffiths, F., Cave, J., Boardman, F., Ren, J., Pawlikowska, T., Ball, R., . . . Cohen, A. (2012). Social networks—the future for health care delivery. *Social Science & Medicine, 75*(12), 2233–2241.

Institute of Medicine. (2004). *Health literacy: A prescription to end confusion.* Retrieved from http://www.iom.edu/~/media/Files/Report%20Files/2004/Health-Literacy-A-Prescription-to-End-Confusion/healthliteracyfinal.pdf

Jadad, A. R. (1999). Promoting partnership: Challenges for the Internet age. *British Medical Journal, 319,* 761–764.

Juengst, E. T., Flatt, M. A., & Settersten, R. A. (2012). Personalized genomic medicine and the rhetoric of empowerment. *The Hastings Center Report, 42*(5), 34–40.

Kaplan, A., & Haenlein, M. (2010). Users of the world, unite! The challenges and opportunities of social media. *Business Horizons, 53*(1), 61.

Klein-Fedyshin, M. S. (2002). Consumer health informatics: Integrating patients, providers and professionals online. *Medical References Services Quarterly, 21*(3), 35–50.

Leiner, B. M., Cerf, V. G., Clark, D. D., Kahn, R. E., Kleinrock, L., Lynch, D. C., . . . Wolff, S. (1997). A brief history of the Internet. *e-OTI: OnTheInternet. An International Electronic Publication of the Internet Society.* Retrieved from www.isoc.org/oti/printversions/0797prleiner.html

Markle Foundation. (2003). *Final report, Personal Health Working Group.* Retrieved from www.markle.org/downloadable_assets/final_phwg_report1.pdf

Mittler, J. N., Martsolf, G. R., Telenko, S. J., & Scanlon, D. P. (2013). Making sense of "consumer engagement" initiatives to improve health and health care: A conceptual framework to guide policy and practice. *Milbank Memorial Fund, 91*(1), 37–77. doi: 10.1111/milq.12002

Moretti, F. A., de Oliveira, V. E., & Koga da Silva, E. M. (2012). Access to health information on the Internet: A public health issue? *Journal of the Brazilian Medical Association, 58*(6), 650–658.

Mosier, J., Joseph, B., & Sakles, J. C. (2013). Telebation: Next-generation telemedicine in remote airway management using current wireless technologies. *Telemedicine and e-Health, 19*(2), 95–98. doi:10.1089/tmj.2012.0093

Muhlbacher, A. C., Stoll, M., Mahlich, J., & Nubling, M. (2013). Patient preference for HIV/AIDS therapy—a discrete choice experiment. *Health Economics Review, 3*(1), 14. doi: 10.1186/2191-1991-3-14

National Council of State Boards of Nursing. (2011). *White paper: A nurse's guide to the use of social media.* Retrieved from https://www.ncsbn.org/Social_Media.pdf

Nouhi, M., Fayaz-Bakhsh, A., Mohamadi, E., & Shafii, M. (2012). Telemedicine and its potential impacts on reducing inequalities in access to health manpower. *Telemedicine and e-Health, 18*(8), 648–653. doi:10.1089/tmj.2011.0242

Nowlin, A. (2004). Get ready for the virtual ICU. *Registered Nurse, 67,* 52.

O'Grady, L., Wathen, C. N., Charnaw-Burger, J., Betel, L., Shachak, A., Luke, R., . . . Jadad, A. R. (2012, January). The use of tags and tag clouds to discern credible content in online health message forums. *International Journal of Medical Informatics, 81*(1), 36–44.

Patel, S., Park, H., Bonato, P., Chan, L., & Rodgers, M. (2012). A review of wearable sensors and systems with application in rehabilitation. *Journal of NeuroEngineering and Rehabilitation, 9*(21). doi: 10.1186/1743-0003-9-21

Pew Internet & American Life Project. (2013). *Pew Internet: Health.* Retrieved from http://www.pewinternet.org/Commentary/2011/November/Pew-Internet-Health.aspx

Pho, K. (2013, February 3). *3 reasons why patients should use social media*. Retrieved from http://www.kevinmd.com/blog/

Prasad, B. (2013). Social media, health care, and social networking. *Gastrointestinal Endoscopy*, 77(3), 492–495.

Rifkin, J. (2011). *The Third Industrial Revolution: How lateral power is transforming energy, the economy, and the world*. New York, NY: Palgrave Macmillan.

Roberts, L. (2010). Health information and the Internet: The 5 Cs website evaluation tool. *British Journal of Nursing*, 19(5), 322–325.

Sheridan, S. L., Halpern, D. J., Viera, A. J., Berkman, N. D., Donahue, K. E., & Crotty, K. (2011). Interventions for individuals with low health literacy: A systematic review. *Journal of Health Communication*, 16(3), 30–54.

Stobbe, M. (2012). 100,000 Facebook users use new organ donor option. *USA Today News*. Retrieved from http://usatoday30.usatoday.com/news/health/story/2012-05-02/facebook-organ-donation-option/54690366/1

Tang, P. C., Ash, J. S., Bates, D. W., Overhage, J. M., & Sands, D. Z. (2006). Personal health records: Definitions, benefits, and strategies for overcoming barriers to adoption. *Journal of the American Medical Informatics Association*, 13, 121–126.

U.S. Department of Commerce, National Telecommunications & Information Administration. (2009). American Recovery and Reinvestment Act of 2009. Retrieved from http://www.ntia.doc.gov/page/2011/american-recovery-and-reinvestment-act-2009

U.S. Department of Health and Human Services, National Committee on Vital and Health Statistics. (2006). *Report recommendation: Personal health records and personal health record systems*. Retrieved from http://www.ncvhs.hhs.gov/0602nhiirpt.pdf

U.S. Department of Health and Human Services. (2010). *National action plan to improve health literacy*. Retrieved from http://www.health.gov/communication/hlactionplan/pdf/Health_Literacy_Action_Plan.pdf

U.S. White House. (2000). *The Clinton-Gore administration: From digital divide to digital opportunity*. Retrieved from http://clinton4.nara.gov/WH/New/digitaldivide/digital1.html

White, T., & Herzlinger, R. E. (2004). *Consumer-driven health care: Implications for providers, payers, and policymakers*. San Francisco, CA: Jossey-Bass.

Young, S. D., & Jaganath, D. (2013). Online social networking for HIV education and prevention: A mix-methods analysis. *Sexually Transmitted Diseases*, 40(2), 162–167. doi: 10.1097/OLQ.0b013e318278bd12

access control tools Safety measures to protect information built into EHR systems, such as user-specific passwords and personal identification numbers.

Agency for Healthcare Research and Quality (AHRQ) U.S. government agency within the U.S. Department of Health and Human Services whose mission is to improve the quality, safety, efficiency, and effectiveness of health care for all Americans.

alert fatigue When false alerts occur frequently, staff members experience a lack of responsiveness to them, or a "cry wolf" bias.

algorithms A set of mathematical steps used for calculation, data processing, and automated reasoning.

analytic validity Refers to how well a test predicts the presence or absence of a particular gene or genetic change.

anthropometry Workplace design principle that plays an important role in the design of the workplace in that it allows the worker to assume a comfortable working posture and promotes safety and efficiency as tasks are carried out.

artificial intelligence The ability of a computer to perform human-like behavior and/or analysis.

artificial neural network An information-processing system that is based on biological neural networks such as are present in the human nervous system.

association rules Rules designed to capture information about items that are frequently associated with each other; often used in business applications such as market-basket analysis to find relationships present among attributes in large datasets.

Bayesian modeling Based on Bayes' theorem, it is used to estimate the conditional probability of a given data point belonging to a particular class using a probabilistic approach for data classification and is based on the assumption that attributes in the training examples are governed by probability distributions.

bioinformatics The storage, organization, and retrieval of large sets of genetic data and the computing power and programming needed to analyze genetic data.

biometric identifiers Unique biological identification measures such as fingerprints and voice prints.

Boolean operators "And," "or," "not"; used to combine words or phrases in key word searches.

breach A failure or disruption of a system.

business associate A person or organization that uses protected health information to perform activities on behalf of a covered entity but is not part of the covered entity's workforce.

business intelligence Using data to understand why buyers make purchasing decisions and developing well-defined techniques that increase a business's ability to understand what makes a business successful.

Census Data Mapper An application that allows users to create custom maps containing county-level demographic data.

Centers for Disease Control and Prevention (CDC) The national public health institute of the United States, whose main goal is to protect public health and safety through the control and prevention of disease, injury, and disability.

cite while you write References are cited in the narrative and added to a reference list in the word-processing document in real time using software.

clinical decision rules Rules that inform clinical decision-support systems based on best practices.

clinical decision-support systems (CDSS)   Computer systems designed to impact clinical decision making about individual patients at the moment those decisions are made.

clinical informatics   A broad term that encompasses all medical and health specialties, including nursing, and addresses the ways information systems are used in the day-to-day operations of patient care.

clinical microsystem   A small group of people who work to provide care to a particular group of patients.

clinical validity   Refers to how well the genetic variant being analyzed is related to the presence, absence, or risk of a specific disease.

clinical vocabulary   A common terminology that can be used globally in all computerized health information systems.

Cochrane Library   A library built by healthcare professionals who author Cochrane Reviews, which are the gold standard for pre-appraised research evidence.

commission   An error caused by doing something wrong.

community   Groups of people may be designated a community based on their own unique characteristics and dynamics. Those who reside in the community have similarities because they share a common greater environment and experience similar social interactions. Community residents may have shared histories, values, and concerns.

computerized provider order entry   Refers to any system in which clinicians directly enter medication orders (and, increasingly, tests and procedures) into a computer system, which then transmits the order directly to the pharmacy.

continuing education   To stay current in practice, meet state-mandated continuing education units, and fulfill requirements for certification/recertification in specialty practice.

covered entity   (1) providers (ranging from an individual provider to a large organization), (2) health plans that provide or pay for health care, and (3) healthcare clearinghouses.

Cumulative Index to Nursing and Allied Health Literature (CINAHL)   Database that indexes a comprehensive body of healthcare literature.

data   Data are values or measurements, bits of information that can be collected and transformed, allowing one to answer a question or to create an end product, such as an image.

data display   Data presented in an understandable manner, such as in flowcharts, Pareto charts, Gantt charts, run charts, control charts, scatterplots, force field analysis, and fishbone charts.

data mining   An important component within the process of analytics, in which a particular mining algorithm is used to extract patterns from the dataset.

data quality and validity   The state of completeness, validity, consistency, timeliness, and accuracy that makes data appropriate for a specific use; can be enhanced by using specific terminology and tools such as drop-down menus.

data warehouse   A collection of databases designed and optimized with specific applications in mind, consisting of several components including various external sources. Decision support systems are used in the warehouse to provide specific analyses, reports, mining, and other processing that users seek from the data. In a data warehouse, queries are optimized to provide efficient access to data for analysis, reporting, and mining. For example, a data warehouse of a healthcare system may keep aggregated data values of all of its patient records.

database   A collection of related data.

database management system   Software that enables users to create and maintain a database.

decision tree   Often used for patient protocols as an aid to decision making, and in analytical research; often represented as a tree-shaped diagram, with each branch used to represent a possible decision or occurrence. The structure of the branches can illustrate how one decision may lead to another.

decryption   Translation or access to encrypted information.

defects   Errors.

descriptive algorithm   Generally used to explore data and identify patterns or relationships within them; examples of descriptive algorithms include clustering, summarization, and association rules.

dialogue   Interaction between display of information and operation.

dialogue principles   Suitability for the task, self-descriptiveness, controllability, conformity with user expectations, error tolerance, suitability for individualization, suitability for learning.

digital divide   A technical divide based on the availability of infrastructure, and a social divide resulting from the skills required to manipulate and utilize health IT resources.

digital era   Late 1980s; integrated computerized information that could transmit voice and video data at high speeds.

Directory of Open Access Journals (DOAJ)   Database of journals that are open access.

DNA (deoxyribonucleic acid)   A nucleic acid that creates the genetic instructions for the processes that support the life of all organisms, and many viruses.

effectiveness   Accuracy and completeness with which users achieve specified goals.

efficiency   Resources expended in relation to the accuracy and completeness with which users achieve goals.

electronic health record (EHR)   A longitudinal electronic record of patient health information generated by one or more encounters in any care-delivery setting. Included in this information are patient demographics, progress notes, problems, medications, vital signs, past medical history, immunizations, laboratory data, and radiology reports. The EHR automates and streamlines the clinician's workflow.

embedded relational database   Packaged as part of other software or hardware applications; for example, local databases used by a mobile application to store phone numbers can be considered an embedded relational database.

encryption   Stored information frequently undergoes encryption, meaning that it cannot be interpreted by anyone unless it is translated by an authorized person who has a specialized key for decryption of the information.

epidemiology   A field of science that studies health and disease in defined populations or communities.

ergonomics   The scientific discipline concerned with the understanding of the interactions among humans and other elements of a system, and the profession that applies theoretical principles, data, and methods to design in order to optimize human wellbeing and overall system performance.

errors   Risks that pass through gaps in protective barriers that normally defend patients from harm.

ethics   A branch of philosophy that is concerned with the values of human behavior; can be subjective; it incorporates moral values and requires examination of the issues involved.

evidence-based practice (EBP)   A core skill necessary to improve nursing care and enhance the safety of patients; the components of EBP include a systematic and critical evaluation of the current literature, the nurse's clinical expertise and available resources, and patients' values and preferences. This information is used to make deliberate clinical decisions based on theory and relevant research to guide patient care.

exome   The approximately 1% of the genome that primarily encodes proteins.

flat database model   Only one table is used, and the attributes are defined as separate columns of the table.

flowchart   Graphical display tool used to show documents, tasks, decisions, and interactions associated with care delivery and/or to show work across time and roles; helpful for illustrating the relationship of tasks among providers.

forms   The traditional interface to databases that offer a simple visual mechanism for users to insert new data into relational databases.

fragmentation   Disconnected healthcare delivery; multiple healthcare providers may make decisions for a single patient resulting in fragmentation of care, which ultimately places patients at greater risk for poor outcomes, particularly if those patients have multiple or chronic conditions (e.g., patients with chronic diseases such as type 2 diabetes mellitus are at risk for multiple complications that often necessitate management by subspecialists, such as ophthalmologists, nephrologists, podiatrists, and cardiologists, making referrals and follow-ups for such patients an arduous task).

gap analysis   The inefficiencies represent a gap between the current, inefficient workflow and the future, desired workflow with health IT; a formal report of this gap is the gap analysis.

genetic/risk assessment   Analysis of genes/genomes to provide insight into a patient's future risk of disease.

genetics   The study of individual genes.

genomic variation   Variation in alleles of genes, occurs both within and among populations.

genomics   The study of all the genes in the human genome, including the interactions between genes and with the environment, and the influence of cultural and psychosocial factors.

genomic medicine   The application of genetics in clinical care of patients.

Google Scholar   A web-based search engine for scholarly literature across a broad range of disciplines, including literature from free and paid repositories, professional societies, academic publishers, and other sources across the web.

graphical user interface (GUI)   A complex platform that allows users to interact with the computer through electronic devices or the computer mouse; interaction is facilitated by visual elements such as icons (symbols, pictograms).

hardware ergonomics   Supplies the technical framework and sets the conditions for optimal human–computer interactions.

health information technology (health IT)   The comprehensive management of health information across computerized systems and its secure exchange between consumers, providers, government and quality entities, and insurers.

Health Information Technology for Economic and Clinical Health (HITECH) Act   A section of the American Recovery and Reinvestment Act of 2009 that: (1) modifies HIPAA regulations to make business associates directly liable for compliance with HIPAA regulations, to limit the use of protected health information (PHI) for marketing and fundraising purposes, and to allow individuals to receive electronic copies of PHI; (2) establishes increased, tiered civil money penalties; (3) establishes an objective breach standard; and (4) prohibits health plans from using or disclosing genetic information for underwriting purposes.

Health Insurance Portability and Accountability Act of 1996 (HIPAA)   Federal law regarding ethical and regulatory guidelines for confidentiality; also includes sections promoting continuity of health insurance coverage for employed people, reducing Medicare fraud and abuse, simplifying health insurance administration, and protecting the privacy and security of health information.

health literacy The degree to which individuals can obtain, process, and understand the basic health information and services they need to make appropriate health decisions.

health maintenance A systematic program or procedure planned to prevent illness, maintain maximum function, and promote health; it is central to health care, especially nursing care.

healthcare providers (HCPs) Those who deliver health care, including doctors and nurses.

human–computer interaction (HCI) A natural way for users to interact with the system through information input, information processing, decision making, and information storage. The starting point is the perception of stimuli from the environment via visual, acoustic, and tactile stimuli.

index patient The first known case of a disease.

inefficiency The lack of ability to do something or produce something without wasting materials, time, or energy.

information Structured data that are understandable and meaningful.

information gain A measure of how well a given attribute separates a subset of the whole dataset (also known as training sample data) to achieve the target classification.

information literacy The ability to identify information needed for a specific purpose, locate pertinent information, evaluate the information, and apply it correctly.

information management The process of collecting data, processing, and presenting and communicating the data as information or knowledge.

information processing Perceived information is subconsciously compared with an inner, dynamic perspective and used to initiate motor processes.

information systems The software and hardware systems that support data-intensive applications.

instance-based learning classifiers As a new sample is presented to these classifiers, it is matched against a set of similar stored instances in order to assign a classification label.

integrity rules Rules that protect the validity of the data used in relational databases (e.g., if entity integrity is enforced, then every record will have its own specific identity and there will be no duplicate records).

interactivity A key component of computer applications depending on user input or given parameters.

interface Point at which separate systems meet and communicate.

interlibrary loan A service whereby a user of one library can borrow books or receive photocopies of documents that are owned by another library.

International Organization for Standardization (ISO) International standards are issued by the ISO and are based on firmly established scientific principles and are determined on an international level and adopted by majority decision.

Internet World-wide broadcasting system, a mechanism for information dissemination, and a medium for collaboration and interaction between individuals and their computers without regard for geographic location.

Internet era 1990s–present; has enabled telehealth services such as video-conferencing, remote access to patient data and information, and rapid communication between patients and providers.

interoperability The ability of different information technology systems and software applications to communicate, exchange data, and use the information that has been exchanged.

iterative Each step informs the next, resulting in health IT that is suited to the needs of healthcare providers.

K-means   A partitional clustering algorithm where the desired number of clusters to partition the data is specified.

knowledge   Information that has been synthesized so that relationships are identified and formalized.

knowledge base   Essential elements to most clinical decision-support systems derived from research literature that are considered best evidence.

knowledge-based error   Errors that occur when an individual does not possess the information needed to determine the appropriate action.

knowledge creation   Structuring raw data into understandable, meaningful information.

law   An objective rule.

literature search   A systematic approach to reviewing healthcare literature to improve practice.

Medical Subject Headings (MeSH)   A controlled vocabulary thesaurus used in PubMed in place of key words.

mHealth   An emerging practice of medicine and public health and wellness enabled and supported by mobile communication devices such as smartphones and tablets.

mobile apps   Software applications used on mobile devices such as smartphones.

mobile health monitoring   Monitoring of particular health parameters from any location.

modeling   A set of mathematical terms used to create a computer application capable of anticipating a response to a situation.

My National Center for Biotechnology Information (My NCBI)   A cloud-based folder provided by PubMed that stores search histories.

National Guideline Clearinghouse   A database of systematic reviews and current practice guidelines.

National Library of Medicine (NLM)   A service of PubMed that is an extensive index of published medical literature with more than 22 million citations.

natural language processing   A method of taking free text from progress notes, nursing documentation, discharge summaries, or radiology reports, for example, and analyzing them for patterns and added meaning to create added rules and generate more individualized patient-specific alerts.

natural user interfaces   User interfaces that avail themselves of the natural finger and hand movements of the user on a touch screen, allowing for intuitive use of interactive devices.

need to know   Law requires that access to PHI be given only to those with a need to know, and that only the minimum amount of information needed to accomplish the purpose be released. (For example, a nurse would have a greater need for access to PHI than would a billing clerk; a nurse not involved in an individual's care would *not* have any need to know.)

Notice of Privacy Practices   First, the law requires that a Notice of Privacy Practices be given to a patient upon the first contact with a covered entity and at other times upon request; the notice must be written in language that is easy for patients to understand and explain how the covered entity will use the patient's protected health information.

nursing competencies   The expected genetic/genomic knowledge, skills, and values needed for clinical practice.

nursing informatics   The science and practice that integrates nursing, its information, and knowledge with management of information and communication technologies to promote the health of people, families, and communities worldwide.

nursing intelligence data warehouse   A collection of nursing-relevant data elements that can be mined to answer clinical questions, examine results of practice changes, and compare the effectiveness of different nursing interventions on patient outcomes.

omission   Error caused by failing to do the right thing.

open access   Freely available articles provided by publishers.

open source relational database   Open source databases, such as MySQL (http://www.mySQL.com) and PostGIS (http://postgis.net), freely available for use.

out-of-range alarms   Triggered when a patient's value is above or below a set parameter; these high and low limits can be set manually by the nursing staff or to a default determined by the institution.

patient empowerment   The practice of maximizing the number of opportunities made available to patients to endow them with a better sense of control over their own health care, which can only lead to well-informed decisions and an improved collaborative dynamic with HCPs.

patient engagement   A set of reciprocal tasks performed by patients and HCPs in a collaborative effort to promote and support active patient involvement in their own health care.

patient safety   Freedom from unacceptable risk of harm.

Patient Safety and Quality Improvement Act of 2005 (PSQIA)   The PSQIA created a voluntary system for reporting medical errors without fear of liability. The patient safety information is considered a "patient safety work product" and can be shared by HCPs and organizations within a protected legal environment, with a common goal of improving patient safety and quality of care.

patient safety organization (PSO)   A PSO can be public or private, for profit or not for profit. Insurance companies are not eligible to be designated as PSOs.

penetration testing   A method that has been used in other areas of electronic information management to assess the security of systems.

personal health record (PHR)   An electronic, universally available, lifelong resource of health information needed by individuals to make health decisions. Individuals own and manage the information in the PHR, which comes from healthcare providers and the individual. The PHR is maintained in a secure and private environment, with the individual determining rights of access. The PHR is separate from and does not replace the legal record of any provider.

Plan-Do-Study-Act (PDSA)   A cyclical process that is made up of alternating phases of enacting changes and then assessing the effects of those changes.

point of care   The time of care when healthcare providers deliver healthcare products and services to patients.

point-of-care data entry   Allows the nurse to capture the activities of care as they occur, including the administration of medications, assessment of vital signs, physical exam, updating of medical histories, or other nursing duties.

population   Those living in a specific geographic area or those in a particular group who experience a disproportionate burden of poor health outcomes.

predictive algorithm   An algorithm that makes predictions about values of data using a set of known results.

privacy   A patient's right to protection and confidentiality of health information.

privacy and confidentiality   There is broad privacy protection for all health information, including genetic information, afforded by the Health Insurance Portability and Accountability Act (HIPAA) and protection against discrimination for individuals with disabilities afforded by the Americans with Disabilities Act (ADA).

process mapping   Map of workflow.

productivity   The rate at which work is completed.

proprietary relational database   Licensed by vendors, proprietary relational databases provide a robust set of management tools that includes creation of a data warehouse.

protected health information (PHI)   To be considered PHI three criteria must be met: (1) information that could reasonably identify the person such as name, address, date of birth, and social security number; (2) past, current, or future information about the patient's physical or mental conditions, information about the provision of care, and information about payment for care; and (3) it must be held or transmitted electronically by the covered entity or business associates.

public health informatics   The use of nursing informatics within the field of public health.

PubMed   Database that indexes a comprehensive body of healthcare literature.

PubMed Advanced Search Builder   An advanced search engine within PubMed with drop-down menus that can be set to MeSH terms and uses Boolean operators.

PubMed Clinical Queries   Displays citations filtered to a specific clinical study category and scope.

PubMed LinkOut   A service that allows the user to link directly from PubMed and other NCBI databases to a wide range of information and services beyond the NCBI systems. LinkOut aims to facilitate access to relevant online resources in order to extend, clarify, and supplement information found in NCBI database.

PubMed sidebar filters   Filters that can be added to limit the search to a number that is more manageable, including categorizing by article type (clinical trials, systematic reviews, practice guidelines, etc.), text availability (abstract available, free full text available, or full text available), and publication date.

qualitative method   Use of interviews, focus groups, text, video, or audio to uncover why usability problems exist and sometimes how to fix them. Qualitative data can be converted to quantitative data by counting, for example, instances of users having difficulty finding information on a website.

quantitative method   Produce numbers such as counts, frequencies, and ratios and might include assessments of tasks, surveys, usage logs, and error logs.

query   An operation that is used to directly retrieve and update data from a database table.

real time applications   Take place when the capture and transfer of information occur simultaneously.

reasoning engine   Essential elements to most clinical decision-support systems that function as a series of logic schemes for eventual output.

recovery capabilities   Mechanisms to retrieve necessary data during downtime to carry on normal operating procedures and to prevent the loss of data when downtime occurs suddenly.

reference maps   Designed to show geographic locations and features such as rivers but do not contain demographic data.

relational database model   A collection of tables linked together by relationship between attributes within the separate tables and/or operations within the tables.

remote access   Users use their own computers to remotely access EHR systems from their homes or offices.

Rich Site Summary (RSS feeds)   Simplified, aggregated summaries of the information provided on whole websites.

risk assessment   Following a breach, a risk assessment must be conducted, which includes an assessment of the PHI involved, the person who used or to whom the PHI was disclosed, whether the PHI was actually viewed, and the extent of the risk.

rule-based error   When a good rule is applied in the wrong situation.

satisfaction   Freedom from discomfort; positive attitudes of the user of the product.

secondary findings   Also known as incidental findings, these include variants that predispose to diseases unrelated to the initial reason for undergoing genomic sequencing.

security   Measures implemented to prevent unauthorized access.

security risk analysis   Compares present security measures in the EHR to those that are legally required to safeguard patient information, and the analysis can help in identifying high-priority threats and vulnerabilities; it is the initial step in creating an effective action plan for addressing threats and vulnerabilities of a system.

selective attention   Ability to concentrate on relevant stimuli and ignore irrelevant information.

sequencing   This technology identifies single nucleotide changes, plus small insertions and deletions that can impact the function of the encoded protein. The gene of interest, or a panel of candidate genes, is divided into small overlapping fragments and analyzed using a method called capillary-based Sanger sequencing.

shared decision making   A patient's increased involvement in decision making about his or her own health management, which may include lifestyle changes, diet modification, medication regimens, and regularly scheduled appointments with the HCP.

simulation   A model that uses mathematical terms to create a computer application capable of anticipating a response to a situation in order to imitate reality for purposes such as training or entertainment.

slip   A type of error in which a person knows the correct actions, yet at the time

care is delivered, an incorrect action is taken.

smartphones   A mobile phone built on a mobile operating system, with more advanced computing capability and connectivity than a feature phone.

social media   Web-based and mobile technologies that turn communication into interactive dialogues among many users.

software ergonomics   Deals with the analysis, evaluation, and optimization of user interfaces by applying various strategies to meet the needs of the user and enhance the display of information and the interaction between information and subsequent operations. *See also* **human–computer interaction (HCI)**.

standardized/controlled data   Accepted laboratory values, vital signs, and pre-accepted items (typically made available via a drop-down menu).

store and forward applications   Capture data and store it for review at a later date.

structured query language (SQL)   A common database language that standardizes the ways to perform operations in various implementations of relational databases.

support vector machine modeling   Informs the program to learn from the data; can be used in analyses of healthcare coverage in large populations of people.

system development life cycle   Employs user-centered design to meet the needs, desires, and limitations of users in order to create the optimal system design.

system downtime   Downtime can occur for reasons as simple as short-term power outages, or can be prolonged if natural disasters, such as floods, affect healthcare facilities.

system fault alarms   Triggered when there is an ineffective reading, potentially caused by displaced leads or other system malfunction(s).

task analysis   A qualitative and quantitative method for understanding the activities associated with a particular goal of patient care.

task design for individuality   Requires user-centered tasks, versatility, completeness of job, significance, degree of autonomy, feedback, and opportunities for development.

telecommunications   Communication over a distance by cable, telegraph, telephone, or other broadcasting mechanism; an essential component of telehealth.

telecommunications era   1970s–1980s; characterized by television and broadcast technologies.

teleconsult   Remote consultation with a specialist by a healthcare provider.

telehealth   The process of using technological communication systems in the assessment and management of patients.

telemonitoring   Patient data such as blood pressure, weight, and pulse are delivered to HCPs so that they can keep track of condition of a patient remotely.

telerehabilitation   The use of telecommunications and information technology to deliver rehabilitation services remotely.

teletrauma   The remote treatment of trauma situations.

televisit   An encounter involving a patient and a healthcare provider that is enabled by telecommunications technologies.

testing technologies   Technologies (e.g., sequencing) that allow the genetic diagnosis of vulnerabilities to inherited diseases and can produce massive amounts of data quickly and relatively inexpensively.

thematic maps   Display of the socioeconomic, demographic, or business-related data about an area that may build on reference maps.

usability testing   A technique used to evaluate a product or information system by testing it with representative users.

user-centered design (UCD)   A method for assessing usability throughout the system development life cycle; UCD means that the needs, desires, and limitations of users are the driving factors for design, not the technology capabilities. UCD requires developers to understand human–computer interaction and to design a natural way for users to interact with the system that satisfies, rather than frustrates, them.

user experience (UX)   A person's behaviors, attitudes, and emotions about using a particular product, system, or service.

user interface   Input devices (e.g., keyboard or mouse) and output devices (e.g., screen, loudspeaker, or printer) that constitute the operational platform of a computer system in combination with software.

Variant   A possible change that can be detected, such as in a gene.

Vendor   Developers of electronic health record systems that in turn market them to health care settings, such as hospitals.

virtual private network (VPN)   Enables the remote user to access the EHR network remotely through a tightly configured firewall.

visual display terminal (VDT)   The computer display; based on ergonomic guidelines, the dimensions of the workstation and the arrangement of the individual elements (e.g., table, chair, and computer) should reduce the demands on the musculoskeletal system and the eyes.

vital statistics   Data points such as births, deaths, marriages, divorces, and fetal death.

voice user interfaces   Human–machine interactions made possible through a voice or synthesized speech platform; input requires a speech recognition system, commonly called voice recognition (VR) software.

wearable sensors   Sensors that transmit data by wireless technology to a patient's smartphone or other mobile communication device.

wisdom The proper use of knowledge to solve real-world problems and aid continuous improvement.

workarounds Nurses and other healthcare providers who experience workflow problems after implementation of health IT will often develop workarounds, which are unauthorized ways to use health IT.

Workflow Clinical processes; the flow of people, equipment (including machines and tools), information, and physical and mental tasks, in different places, at different levels, at different timescales continuously and discontinuously, that are used or required to support the goals of the clinical work domain. Workflow also includes communication, coordination, searching for information, interacting with information, problem solving, and planning.

workflow analysis A method to avoid the consequences of poorly designed health IT and its impact on workflow.

workflow redesign The process of mapping out current workflows and analyzing how an organization gets work done (the current state) and planning for the future by mapping out how EHRs will create new workflow patterns to improve the organization's efficiency and healthcare quality (the future state).

workload Includes all external influences acting on humans; the workload of nurses is measured by counting the number of patients per nurse for inpatient care and the number of patient visits per day in ambulatory settings

work systems Humans and computers form a complex sociotechnical work system.

Zotero A software program that can be added to a web browser and word-processing program to assist in citing while writing.

INDEX

Note: Page numbers followed by *b*, *f*, or *t* indicate material in boxes, figures, or tables, respectively.